Orthopedics: Physical Assessment and Rehabilitation

Orthopedics: Physical Assessment and Rehabilitation

Editor: Nicholas Roche

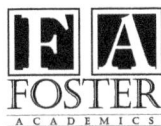

FA
FOSTER
ACADEMICS

www.fosteracademics.com

www.fosteracademics.com

FA
FOSTER
ACADEMICS

Cataloging-in-Publication Data

Orthopedics : physical assessment and rehabilitation / edited by Nicholas Roche.
    p. cm.
Includes bibliographical references and index.
ISBN 978-1-63242-561-4
1. Orthopedics. 2. Physical orthopedic tests. 3. People with disabilities--Rehabilitation.
I. Roche, Nicholas.
RD731 .O78 2018
617--dc23

Foster Academics,
118-35 Queens Blvd., Suite 400,
Forest Hills, NY 11375, USA

ISBN 978-1-63242-561-4 (Hardback)

TABLE OF CONTENTS

Permissions

List of Contributors

Index

Preface

Over the recent decade, advancements and applications have progressed exponentially. This has led to the increased interest in this field and projects are being conducted to enhance knowledge. The main objective of this book is to present some of the critical challenges and provide insights into possible solutions. This book will answer the varied questions that arise in the field and also provide an increased scope for furthering studies.

This book discusses the fundamental as well as modern approaches of orthopedics. Orthopedics as a field of medical science deals with the prevention and treatment of diseases occurring in our musculoskeletal system. It is mainly concerned with the diseases like neoplasm, spinal herniation, spina bifida, inflammatory bowel disease, Parkinson's disease, osteoporosis, osteoarthritis, etc. This book includes some of the vital pieces of work being conducted across the world, on various topics related to orthopedics. It aims to shed light on some of the unexplored aspects of the field and the recent researches in this area. It will provide comprehensive knowledge to the readers.

I hope that this book, with its visionary approach, will be a valuable addition and will promote interest among readers. Each of the authors has provided their extraordinary competence in their specific fields by providing different perspectives as they come from diverse nations and regions. I thank them for their contributions.

Editor

A Case of Successful Foraminotomy for Severe Bilateral C5 Palsy following Posterior Decompression and Fusion Surgery for Cervical Ossification of Posterior Longitudinal Ligament

Yoshifumi Kudo,[1] Tomoaki Toyone,[1] Toshiyuki Shirahata,[1] Tomoyuki Ozawa,[1] Akira Matsuoka,[1] Yoichi Jin,[2] and Katsunori Inagaki[1]

[1]*Department of Orthopaedic Surgery, Showa University School of Medicine, 1-5-8 Hatanodai, Shinagawa-ku, Tokyo 142-8666, Japan*
[2]*Department of Orthopaedic Surgery, Ebara Hospital, 4-5-10 Higashiyukigaya, Ota-ku, Tokyo 145-0065, Japan*

Correspondence should be addressed to Yoshifumi Kudo; kudo_4423@yahoo.co.jp

Academic Editor: Taketoshi Yasuda

We report a very rare (5~7%) case of bilateral C5 palsy after cervical surgery. A 71-year-old male patient with cervical ossification of posterior longitudinal ligament (OPLL) with foraminal stenosis at bilateral C4/5 underwent posterior decompression and fusion surgery. After surgery, muscle weakness in his both deltoid and biceps was detected and gradually deteriorated to complete paralysis. Postoperative MRI showed sufficient decompression of the spinal cord and posterior shifting. Subsequently, an additional bilateral foraminotomy at C4/5 was performed, with a suspicion that bilateral foraminal stenosis at C4/5 may have been the cause of the paresis. After foraminotomy, muscular contraction was seen in both deltoid and biceps. Finally, complete motor recovery was achieved in a year. Although the gold standard procedure for the prevention and treatment of postoperative C5 palsy has not yet been established, an additional foraminotomy may be recommended for severe C5 palsy in cases of foraminal stenosis even after the occurrence of palsy.

1. Introduction

C5 palsy is well known as one of the most common complications of cervical spine surgery [1, 2], and its incidence has been reported as 4.6% (0~30%) [3, 4]. Most of the paresis (93~95%) occur unilaterally, but the remaining (5~7%) have developed bilaterally [5, 6]. Bilateral cases are very rare and only few reports have been described in detail before [7, 8]. Although there are many reports describing C5 palsy, its pathomechanisms are still controversial [4, 9–12] and prevention of C5 palsy has not yet been established. We encountered a patient with progressing bilateral severe C5 palsy following posterior decompression and fusion for cervical ossification of posterior longitudinal ligament (OPLL). In this male patient complete strength recovery as measured by manual muscle testing (MMT) was achieved almost a year after an additional foraminotomy of C4/5. In this report, this rare case of severe bilateral C5 palsy with complete recovery in MMT is presented and its assumed pathomechanisms are discussed.

2. Case Presentation

A 71-year-old man complained of unstable gait and numbness in his left upper extremity. On physical examination, numbness was detected in his left upper extremity including C5/6 areas. No muscle weakness was detected including bilateral deltoid and biceps, and deep tendon reflexes were accentuated. Mixed type-OPLL was seen at C4/5/6/7 on the lateral view of the cervical spine X-ray (Figure 1(a)) and sagittal CT (Figure 1(b)). Alignment of the cervical spine was lordotic and ossification did not exceed the "K-Line" [13]. Foraminal stenosis was seen at bilateral C4/5 (1.5 mm on the left side and 2.5 mm on the right side) on CT and

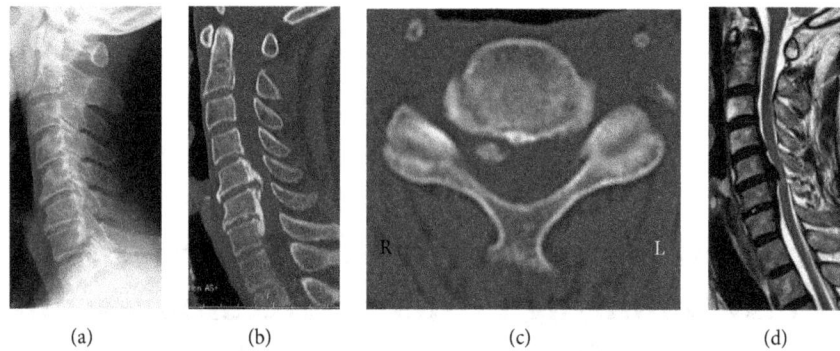

FIGURE 1: Preoperative radiological findings. (a) and (b): mixed type ossification of the posterior longitudinal ligament was observed on the lateral view of the cervical spine radiograph and sagittal view on computed tomography (CT). Alignment was lordotic and ossification did not exceed the "K-line." (c): Foraminal stenosis was detected at bilateral C4/5 (1.5 mm on the left side and 2.5 mm on the right side) on axial view CT. (d): high-intensity areas in the spinal cord were not evident on magnetic resonance imaging.

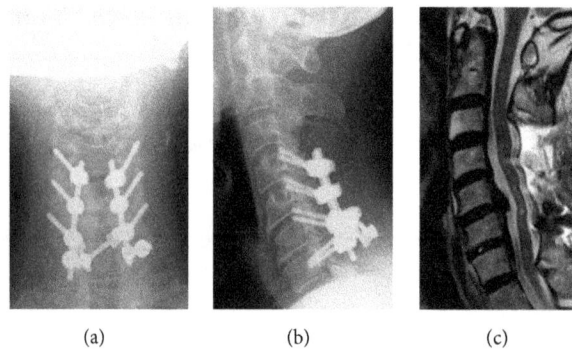

FIGURE 2: Postoperative X-ray and magnetic resonance imaging. (a) and (b): anteroposterior and lateral view X-ray of the cervical spine. (c): magnetic resonance imaging showed sufficient decompression of the spinal cord and posterior shifting, without high-intensity areas at C3/4.

high-intensity areas in the spinal cord were not evident on MRI (Figure 1(c)). Posterior decompression (laminectomy) at C3–7 and in situ fusion at C4–7 were performed using instrumentation (Figure 2(a)). On the next day of surgery, this patient started to walk and his unstable gait got better with no muscle weakness on deltoid and biceps. But, on the second day, he started to complain of severe pain in his left scapula, and muscle weakness was detected in his left deltoid and biceps. Postoperative MRI showed sufficient decompression of the spinal cord and posterior shifting (3.8 mm), without high-intensity areas at C3/4 (Figure 2(b)). There were no changes in anteroposterior diameters of the bilateral C4/5 foramen and no malposition of the screws on postoperative CT. Although we performed posterior fusion in situ, lordotic angle at the operated segment (C4–7) increased by 5 degrees compared to the preoperative angle (Figures 3(a), 3(b), and 3(c)). Five days after surgery, he recognized severe pain in his right scapula and muscle weakness in his right deltoid and biceps. Paresis in bilateral deltoids and biceps gradually deteriorated and MMT finally became of grade 0~1 ten days after surgery. Subsequently, we decided to perform an additional bilateral foraminotomy at C4/5 (Figure 3(d)), with a suspicion that foraminal stenosis may have been the cause of the paresis. However, no remarkable change was seen immediately after foraminotomy. One week after the additional operation, electromyographic (EMG) studies were performed. Acute denervation patterns in bilateral C5 > C6 muscle groups were detected with muscular activities remaining in the deltoid and biceps. The patient underwent physical therapies of muscle strengthening exercise and range of motion exercise of the shoulder and elbow joints. Two weeks after foraminotomy, muscular contraction was seen in both deltoid and biceps, followed by grade 2 recovery in these muscles at four weeks. Muscle strength in bilateral biceps and right deltoid recovered completely 3 month after foraminotomy, but grade 3 muscle weakness remained in the left deltoid. Finally, complete motor recovery was achieved in a year. The changes of muscle strength in bilateral biceps and deltoid were shown in a timeline based graph (Figure 4).

3. Discussion

Postoperative C5 palsy is a well-recognized complication of cervical decompression surgery. The incidence of C5 palsy is around 4.6% (0~30%) in patients who receive laminoplasty, and bilateral cases are very rare (5%). Although many authors have suggested the mechanisms of C5 palsy, major mechanisms are as follows: (1) nerve root traction as "tethering phenomenon" [2, 4, 9, 14, 15] and (2) disorders occurring at the spinal cord [10–12], but controversies still remain.

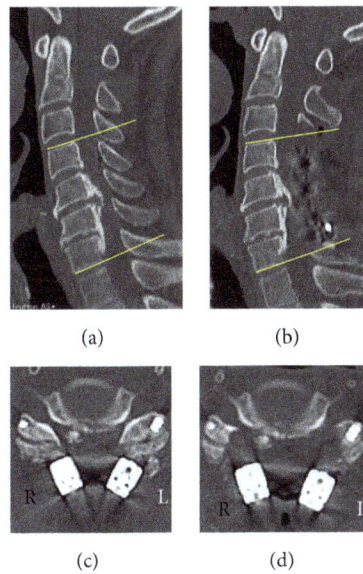

FIGURE 3: Pre- (a) and postoperative ((b) and (c)) and postadditional foraminotomy (d) computed tomography (CT). (a) and (b): lordosis angle at the operated segment (C4–7) increased by 5 degrees compared to the preoperative angle. (c): there were no changes in anteroposterior diameters of the bilateral C4/5 foramen and no malposition of the screws on postoperative CT. (d): Additional bilateral foraminotomy at C4/5 was performed.

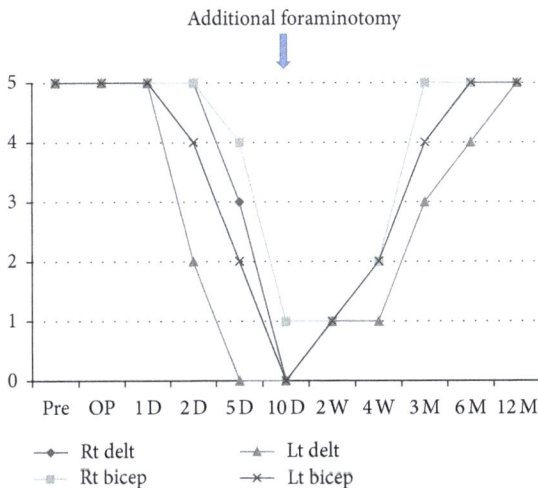

FIGURE 4: A timeline based graph for the changes of muscle strength (MMT) in bilateral deltoid and biceps. The palsy started on the left side in which foraminal stenosis is more severe on the second day after laminectomy and fusion and then extended on to the right side on the fifth day. Paresis gradually deteriorated and manual muscle testing finally became of grade 0-1 at 10 days after surgery, on which day we performed additional foraminotomy. Muscular contraction was seen at 2 weeks after foraminotomy and gradually improved. The weakness of left deltoid remained. Finally, complete recovery was achieved in a year after additional foraminotomy.

"Tethering phenomenon" is the hypothesis that tethering of the nerve root might cause C5 palsy as a result of posterior shift of the spinal cord in association with anchoring of the nerve root at the edge of the superior facet. Some authors have proposed that OPLL and foraminal stenosis at C4/5 could be the risk factors of C5 palsy in radiographic analysis [6, 16–18] and prophylactic foraminotomy could prevent postoperative C5 palsy [4, 12, 17, 19].

Matsunaga et al. [17] have reported that there was a significant difference in anteroposterior diameters of the C4/5 foramen between the palsy side (2.3 mm) and the side without palsy (3.3 mm) and have recommended foraminotomy for cases when the diameter is less than 2.5 mm. Nakashima et al. [20] have described that the cut-off values of the pre- and postoperative widths of the C5 intervertebral foramen for C5 palsy were 2.2 and 2.3 mm, respectively. Furthermore, iatrogenic foraminal stenosis could be a cause of C5 palsy after rearrangement of cervical alignment with instrumentation. Takemitsu et al. [21] reported that the risk of developing C5 palsy with instrumentation was 11.6-fold greater than that without instrumentation. In this case, foraminal stenosis was seen at bilateral C4/5 (1.5 mm on the left side and 2.5 mm on the right side) on preoperative CT, while iatrogenic foraminal stenosis was not detected on postoperative CT. Imagama et al. [6] reported that the mean postoperative posterior shift of the spinal cord at C4/5 was 3.9 mm in C5 palsy cases and 3.0 mm in control and have stated that this results in traction and impingement of C5 nerve root as a "tethering phenomenon." We performed posterior fusion in situ. But, actually, the lordotic angle increased by 5 degrees at C4–7 compared from that of preoperation. This could be a cause of greater posterior shift of the spinal cord (3.8 mm), resulting in the C5 palsy in this case (Figures 5(a) and 5(b)). Some authors have suggested the disorder of the spinal cord, detected by the high frequency of high-intensity area at C3/4 on postoperative MRI, to be the mechanism of C5 palsy [10, 11]. Chiba et al. proposed an etiology that postoperative upper extremity paresis might be associated with deterioration of gray matter such as focal reperfusion injury after acute decompression

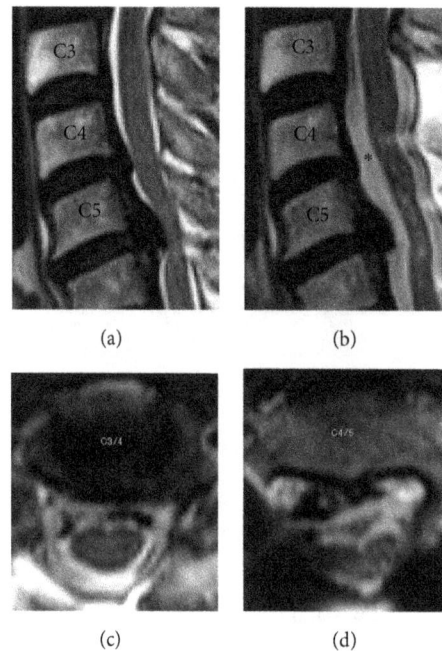

FIGURE 5: Pre- and postoperative magnetic resonance imaging. (a) and (b): posterior shift of the spinal cord at C4/5 (∗) was 3.8 mm. (c) and (d): sufficient decompression of the spinal cord was achieved and high-intensity areas in the spinal cord at C3/4 were not detected.

procedure against ischemic condition of the spinal cord [10]. In our case, no high-intensity area was observed at C3/4 on postoperative MRI, and it is hard to explain that the cause of the C5 palsy originated from the spinal cord even if the paralysis had occurred bilaterally (Figures 5(c) and 5(d)).

We believe that the palsy of this patient might have been caused by multifactorial etiology. Therefore, bilateral foraminal stenosis at C4/5 and posterior shift of the spinal cord which were thought to have been caused by laminectomy and unintentionally gained lordosis might have resulted in the kinking of bilateral C5 nerve roots. Then, the palsy may have started on the left side in which foraminal stenosis is more severe extending on to the right side.

To our knowledge, no report has described severe (grade 0~1) bilateral C5 palsy with full recovery to date. Only two case reports on bilateral grade 2~3/5 C5 palsy have been reported. One is the case report of bilateral C5 palsy following anterior cervical surgery by David and Rao [7], and the other is of anteroposterior decompression and fusion surgery by Jeon and Kim [8]. Spontaneous motor recoveries were achieved with conservative treatment in these cases. In many cases, conservative treatment resulted in complete recovery from postoperative C5 palsy. On the other hand, Imagama et al. reported that 33% of the patients of C5 palsy exhibited residual paralysis, and significantly worse recovery occurred if the patient was severely paralysed at the onset. They also suggested that an additional foraminotomy at an early stage may be useful to treat patients with a severe C5 palsy (MMT = 0 or 1) even after laminoplasty and it may shorten the recovery period [6].

The gold standard procedure for the prevention and treatments of postoperative C5 palsy has not yet been established. Furthermore, the suitable timing of the additional surgery

like foraminotomy is debatable. Katsumi et al. presented a prospective study to investigate the effectiveness of prophylactic bilateral C4/5 foraminotomy to prevent postoperative C5 palsy. They reported that prophylactic foraminotomy significantly decreased the incidence of C5 palsy to 1.4% compared with 6.4% in patients without foraminotomy [19]. Practically, prophylactic foraminotomy should be performed when the foraminal stenosis is obvious in preoperative CT. However, if prophylactic foraminotomy prevents postoperative C5 palsy, additional foraminotomy could be effective for recovery even after the occurrence of severe paresis. It might be preferable that surgeons consider the additional foraminotomy in case of progressing severe (MMT0~1) C5 palsy at early stage. Future research is needed to establish the guideline for prevention and treatments for postoperative C5 palsy.

4. Conclusion

We experienced a very rare case of severe bilateral C5 palsy following posterior decompression and fusion for cervical OPLL. Multifactorial etiology including foraminal stenosis and posterior shift of the spinal cord due to laminectomy and unintentionally gained lordosis with posterior fusion may be responsible causes for the palsy. An additional foraminotomy at early stage may be recommended for severe C5 palsy in cases of foraminal stenosis even after the occurrence of severe palsy.

Abbreviations

OPLL: Ossification of the posterior longitudinal ligament
MMT: Manual muscle testing

MRI: Magnetic resonance imaging
CT: Computed tomography.

Consent

The patient gave consent for submitting his data for publication.

Competing Interests

The authors declare that they have no competing interests.

References

[1] W. B. Scoville, "Cervical spondylosis treated by bilateral facetectomy and laminectomy," *Journal of Neurosurgery*, vol. 18, pp. 423–428, 1961.

[2] K. Yonenobu, N. Hosono, M. Iwasaki, M. Asano, and K. Ono, "Neurologic complications of surgery for cervical compression myelopathy," *Spine*, vol. 16, no. 11, pp. 1277–1282, 1991.

[3] H. Sakaura, N. Hosono, Y. Mukai, T. Ishii, and H. Yoshikawa, "C5 palsy after decompression surgery for cervical myelopathy: review of the literature," *Spine*, vol. 28, no. 21, pp. 2447–2451, 2003.

[4] K. Sasai, T. Saito, S. Akagi, I. Kato, H. Ohnari, and H. Iida, "Preventing C5 palsy after laminoplasty," *Spine*, vol. 28, no. 17, pp. 1972–1977, 2003.

[5] A. Nassr, J. C. Eck, R. K. Ponnappan, R. R. Zanoun, W. F. Donaldson III, and J. D. Kang, "The incidence of C5 palsy after multilevel cervical decompression procedures: a review of 750 consecutive cases," *Spine*, vol. 37, no. 3, pp. 174–178, 2012.

[6] S. Imagama, Y. Matsuyama, Y. Yukawa et al., "C5 palsy after cervical laminoplasty: a multicentre study," *The Journal of Bone & Joint Surgery—British Volume*, vol. 92, no. 3, pp. 393–400, 2010.

[7] K. S. David and R. D. Rao, "Bilateral C5 motor paralysis following anterior cervical surgery—a case report," *Clinical Neurology and Neurosurgery*, vol. 108, no. 7, pp. 675–681, 2006.

[8] H. S. Jeon and K. N. Kim, "Delayed bilateral C5 palsy following circumferential decompression and fusion in patient with cervical spondylotic myelopathy," *Korean Journal of Spine*, vol. 12, no. 3, pp. 200–203, 2015.

[9] N. Tsuzuki, R. Abe, K. Saiki, and L. Zhongshi, "Extradural tethering effect as one mechanism of radiculopathy complicating posterior decompression of the cervical spinal cord," *Spine*, vol. 21, no. 2, pp. 203–211, 1996.

[10] K. Chiba, Y. Toyama, M. Matsumoto, H. Maruiwa, M. Watanabe, and K. Hirabayashi, "Segmental motor paralysis after expansive open-door laminoplasty," *Spine*, vol. 27, no. 19, pp. 2108–2115, 2002.

[11] T. Shimizu, H. Shimada, and H. Edakuni, "Post-laminoplasty palsy of upper extremities, with special reference to the spinal cord factors," *Bessatsu Seikeigeka*, vol. 29, pp. 188–194, 1996 (Japanese).

[12] M. Komagata, M. Nishiyama, K. Endoh, H. Ikegami, S. Tanaka, and A. Imakiire, "Clinical study of the postoperative C5 palsy after cervical expansive laminoplasty; efficacy of bilateral partial foraminotomy for the prevention the C5 palsy," *Journal of Japanese Spine Research Society*, vol. 131, p. 237, 2002 (Japanese).

[13] T. Fujiyoshi, M. Yamazaki, J. Kawabe et al., "A new concept for making decisions regarding the surgical approach for cervical ossification of the posterior longitudinal ligament: the K-line," *Spine*, vol. 33, no. 26, pp. E990–E993, 2008.

[14] Y. Uematsu, Y. Tokuhashi, and H. Matsuzaki, "Radiculopathy after laminoplasty of the cervical spine," *Spine*, vol. 23, no. 19, pp. 2057–2062, 1998.

[15] T. Sodeyama, S. Goto, M. Mochizuki, J. Takahashi, and H. Moriya, "Effect of decompression enlargement laminoplasty for posterior shifting of the spinal cord," *Spine*, vol. 24, no. 15, pp. 1527–1531, 1999.

[16] S. Kaneyama, M. Sumi, T. Yano et al., "Prospective study and multivariate analysis of the incidence of C5 palsy after cervical laminoplasty," *Spine*, vol. 35, no. 26, pp. E1553–E1558, 2010.

[17] H. Matsunaga, M. Inada, M. Takeuchi, Y. Matsumoto, and N. Suzuki, "Pathogenesis and prevention of C5 palsy after cervical laminoplasty," *The Japanese Orthopaedic Association*, vol. 68, pp. 134–147, 1994 (Japanese).

[18] K. Katsumi, A. Yamazaki, K. Watanabe, M. Ohashi, and H. Shoji, "Analysis of C5 palsy after cervical open-door laminoplasty: relationship between C5 palsy and foraminal stenosis," *Journal of Spinal Disorders and Techniques*, vol. 26, no. 4, pp. 177–182, 2013.

[19] K. Katsumi, A. Yamazaki, K. Watanabe, M. Ohashi, and H. Shoji, "Can prophylactic bilateral C4/C5 foraminotomy prevent postoperative C5 palsy after open-door laminoplasty?: a prospective study," *Spine*, vol. 37, no. 9, pp. 748–754, 2012.

[20] H. Nakashima, S. Imagama, Y. Yukawa et al., "Multivariate analysis of C-5 palsy incidence after cervical posterior fusion with instrumentation: clinical article," *Journal of Neurosurgery: Spine*, vol. 17, no. 2, pp. 103–110, 2012.

[21] M. Takemitsu, K. M. C. Cheung, Y. W. Wong, W.-Y. Cheung, and K. D. K. Luk, "C5 nerve root palsy after cervical laminoplasty and posterior fusion with instrumentation," *Journal of Spinal Disorders and Techniques*, vol. 21, no. 4, pp. 267–272, 2008.

2

Sword-Like Trauma to the Shoulder with Open Head-Splitting Fracture of the Head

Andreas Panagopoulos, Konstantinos Pantazis, Ilias Iliopoulos, Ioannis Seferlis, and Zinon Kokkalis

Department of Shoulder & Elbow Surgery, Patras University Hospital, Papanikolaou 1, 26504 Patras, Greece

Correspondence should be addressed to Andreas Panagopoulos; andpan21@gmail.com

Academic Editor: Byron Chalidis

Head-splitting fractures occur as a result of violent compression of the head against the glenoid; the head splits and the tuberosities may remain attached to the fragments or split and separate. Isolated humeral head-splitting fractures are rare injuries. Favorable results with osteosynthesis can be difficult to achieve because of the very proximal location of the head fracture and associated poor vascularity. We present a case of a 67-year-old man who sustained a severe, sword-like trauma to his left shoulder after a road traffic accident with associated isolated open Gustilo-Anderson IIIA humeral head-splitting fracture. Bony union was achieved with minimal internal fixation but the clinical outcome deteriorated due to accompanying axillary nerve apraxia. To our knowledge, this type of sword-like injury with associated humeral head-split fracture has not previously been reported.

1. Introduction

Head-splitting fractures are extremely rare and indicate a severe trauma to the shoulder joint. The head is violently compressed against the glenoid and split with or without associated dislocation. We present a case of an isolated open Gustilo-Anderson IIIA humeral head-splitting fracture after a road traffic accident treated with minimal internal fixation. To our knowledge, this type of sword-like injury has not previously been reported.

2. Case Presentation

A 67-year-old man was admitted to our department following a high-speed road traffic accident. He was sited at the back of a car when a lateral-frontal collision happened crushing the back door to his left shoulder. He sustained an open, Gustilo-Anderson IIIA fracture of the proximal humerus with a large overlying sword-like contaminated wound and significant skin loss (Figure 1(a)). There was no neurovascular deficit to the distal forearm and hand. He sustained also fractures of the 1st, 2nd, and 6th rib without any intrathoracic injury. Plain radiographs and CT scan indicated an anteroposterior directed head-splitting fracture of the humeral head involving ~30% of the lateral articular surface with a sagittal extension pattern of the greater tuberosity and without any evidence of humeral head dislocation (Figures 1(b) and 1(c)). He was transferred immediately to the operating theatre as there was uncontrolled bleeding from the wound and hemoglobin level had been dropped by 4 degrees during resuscitation.

At surgery, thorough debridement was carried out and foreign bodies (glass particles) were removed where possible. There was a large circumferential wound to the deltoid involving its anterior, middle, and part of its posterior fibers. The platysma muscle was also ruptured exposing the medial and lateral end of the clavicle. The fractured head was palpable under the deltoid being totally uncovered from rotator cuff muscles. Severe bleeding was detected from the posterior circumflex artery and vein; both vessels were ligated. The axillary artery and the brachial plexus were recognized unmarked. We were not able to identify the axillary nerve at that time. The fractured humeral head was reduced with pointed clamps and fixed with two 4 mm AO cancellous screws (Figure 1(e)). The torn RC was repaired primarily with transosseous nonabsorbable sutures. Deep soft tissue closure was achieved by loosely approximated absorbable

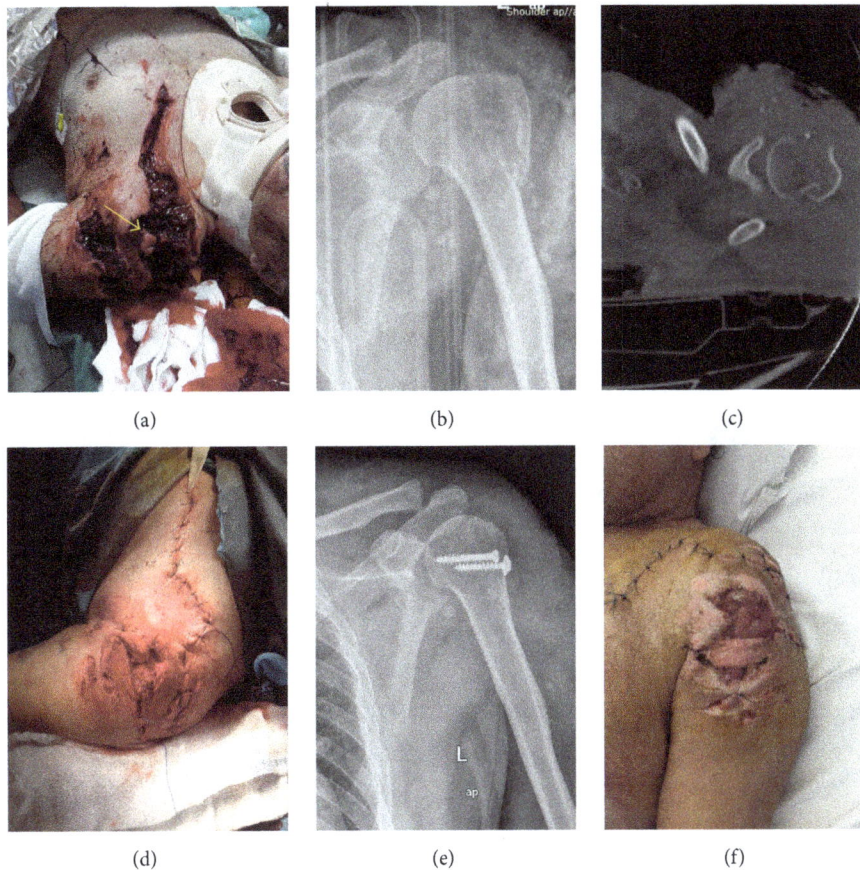

FIGURE 1: (a) Photography of the trauma during patient resuscitation indicated severe, sword-like injury to the left shoulder, with open fracture of the humeral head (arrow). (b) Preoperative anteroposterior X-ray of the left shoulder showing head-splitting fracture of the proximal humerus and presence of multiple foreign bodies (glass). (c) CT scan of the left shoulder indicating involvement of ~30% of the articular surface and the greater tuberosity. (d) Intraoperative picture after muscle and skin closure. (e) Postoperative X-ray of the left shoulder showing adequate reduction of the fragment. (f) Condition of the skin at the 10th postoperative day just before a split skin graft was about to apply.

sutures (Figure 1(d)). Skin has been closed partially and a Penrose drain was applied. From the wound was cultivated *E. coli* and *Staphylococcus warneri*. The patient was treated with intravenous antibiotics for 3 weeks and oral administration for another 3 weeks after his discharge. At the 10th postoperative day, the wound showed signs of reepithelialization and a split-thickness skin graft was applied for terminal closure (Figure 1(f)).

The arm was placed in a sling for 4 weeks. Shoulder physiotherapy and passive assisted mobilization were commenced as soon as the wound was closed, at the second postoperative week. Soft tissue and bony healing occurred without further surgical intervention. The humeral head fracture united with no evidence of avascular necrosis, confirmed radiologically within 12 months (Figures 2(a)–2(c)). The patient unfortunately did not recover shoulder abduction and forward elevation as an ENG assessed a complete neurapraxia of the axillary nerve (Figures 2(d)–2(f)). He had a Constant score of 47 at the latest clinical follow-up 17 months postoperatively. A nerve transfer has been offered to him but he denied any further surgical intervention.

3. Discussion

Head-splitting fractures indicate a severe trauma to the shoulder joint. The head is violently compressed against the glenoid and split. A segment of the humeral head is fractured and is subluxated or dislocated, while the articular surface of the unfractured part of the head remains attached to the shaft. Neer II [1] defined splitting fractures as those in which the fractured fragments measure more than 20% of the articular surface. Classic radiographic "trauma series" of the shoulder and computed tomography are valuable for delineating the configuration of the fracture and helping to plan surgical reconstruction [2, 3]. Robinson et al. [4] proposed two patterns of injury in complex humeral head fractures with dislocation (or splitting) depending on a prospective assessment of the pattern of soft tissue and bony injury and the degree of devascularisation of the humeral head. In type I injuries, the head retains capsular attachments and arterial back-bleeding whereas in type II injuries the head is devoid of significant soft tissue attachments with no active arterial bleeding. ORIF is recommended in type I injuries

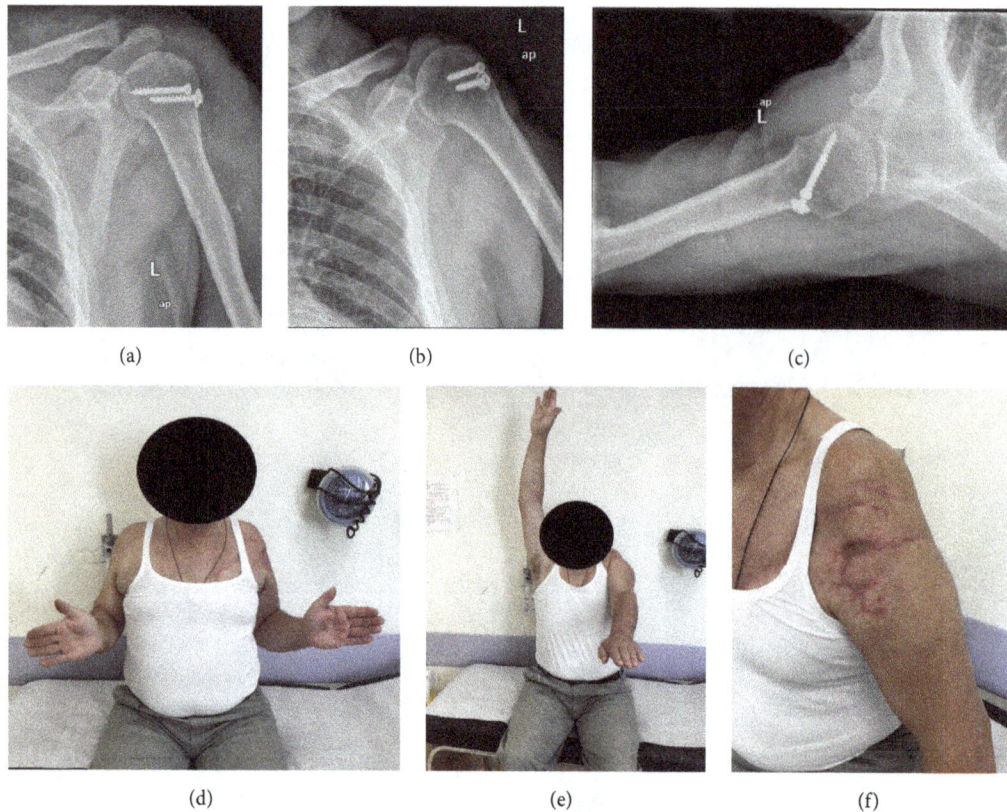

FIGURE 2: ((a)–(c)) Radiological examination at 12 months with anteroposterior views in external (a) and internal (b) rotation as well as axillary view of the shoulder (c) indicated solid union of the fracture. ((d)-(e)) Poor clinical outcome especially in forward elevation due to axillary nerve neurapraxia. (f) Clinical picture of the wound at 17 months after surgery.

as only two of 23 patients with type I injuries developed radiological evidence of osteonecrosis of the humeral head, compared with four of seven patients with type II injuries. The mechanism of injury in our case was more unique as the split in the humeral head was probably caused by direct extrinsic trauma to the shoulder by the distorted metallic parts of the back door during the crush. This explains the severe damage to deltoid and rotator cuff muscles as well as the neurologic damage to the axillary nerve.

The outcome of head-split fractures, regardless of management, is thought to be worse than other types of humeral head fractures because of a perceived higher energy of injury and disruption of the terminal blood supply to the articular fragments [5]. Lee and Hansen [6] reported on 19 patients with displaced 4-part fracture or fracture dislocation treated with ORIF and having no signs of AVN after a mean follow-up period of 23.6 months. They hypothesized a mechanism of revascularization with capillary ingrowth sequence and new bone formation during the healing process (e.g., creeping substitution). As the humeral head is surrounded by rich vascular tissue and has wide fractured surfaces relative to the thickness of the head, a reduced mechanical stress is expected as the healing is progressed, thus reducing the incidence of AVN. The available evidence on optimal treatment of head-splitting fractures is scarce: apart from some case reports [7–9], only two case series have been published on minimal [10]

or locking plate osteosynthesis [11], one case series has been published on hemiarthroplasty [12], and two recent studies have been published on reverse shoulder arthroplasty [13, 14] of isolated head-splitting fractures.

Collopy and Skirving [7] reported on a 20-year-old patient who sustained a "transchondral fracture dislocation" involving 60% of the articular surface and fixed with two 4.0 mm cancellous screws; at 7-year follow-up, the patient had full range of motion and no evidence of AVN or arthritis. Gokkus et al. [8] reported a complex head-splitting fracture with anterior dislocation of the fractured part on a 40-year-old patient. Surgery was performed within 6 hours and the osteochondral fragment, carrying approximately 65% of the articular surface, was found firmly entrapped between the anterior glenoid rim and the subscapularis. Anatomical reduction was achieved with two k-wires and three 4 mm AO cancellous screws. After the 15-month follow-up, the patient had 130° of forward elevation, no shoulder pain, and a Constant score of 76 points. Bailie and McAlinden [9] reported a case of a 17-year-old man with a compound comminuted fracture of the proximal third of the humeral shaft with complete head-splitting extension and a large overlying contaminated wound with skin loss (Gustilo-Anderson grade IIIB). This is the only case in the literature describing an open head-splitting fracture. The mechanism of injury was high-speed road traffic accident. At surgery, fixation with a bridging plate was impossible as the proximal third of the humeral shaft was found to be highly comminuted with marked degloving and soft tissue stripping of multiple fragments in this segment. Fixation of the head part was achieved with two fully threaded AO cancellous screws. The humeral shaft fracture united fully both clinically and radiologically within 3 months without the need for further surgery or bone grafting. At the final follow-up, 8 months after surgery, the patient recovered shoulder abduction and flexion >130°.

Chesser et al. [10] reported on 8 patients with head-splitting fractures; five were diagnosed at presentation and treated with minimal fixation (3 cases), primary hemiarthroplasty (1 case), and closed reduction (1 case). In three cases, the injury was initially unrecognized; two developed a painless bony ankyloses and one was scheduled for hemiarthroplasty. At the latest follow-up (minimum of two years), all ORIF patients had no signs of AVN of the humeral head. Gavaskar and Tummala [11] reported the largest study so far including 15 patients <55 years old treated with locking plate fixation. Five fractures were classified as simple (isolated head-splitting fractures) and 11 as complex (associated tuberosity fractures). None of the patients with simple fracture developed AVN; a nonunion rate of 20% and AVN rate of 40% in complex fractures indicated the inherent severity of these injuries. The mean Constant (66.5) and DASH score (21) showed significantly better outcomes in simple fractures. Greiwe et al. [12] reported the outcome of primary hemiarthroplasty in 8 head-splitting fractures in contrast to 22 patients with complex 3- and 4-part fractures. Head-split fractures demonstrated improved range of motion (mean 138°), complication rate (12.5%), and revision rate (0) compared with standard fractures at an average of 3.6 years postoperatively. Finally, primary reverse shoulder arthroplasty for isolated head-splitting fractures or split fractures with long segment diaphyseal extension is another treatment option in older patients (>65 years old) as indicated by two recent reports describing mixed population of complex fractures of the proximal humerus [13, 14].

4. Conclusion

In our case, the mechanism of injury was direct open trauma not previously reported. A head preserving treatment was considered within few hours of the injury. The humeral head was reduced and fixed with minimal internal fixation and soft tissue handling paying attention to avoiding excessive soft tissue stripping. Clinical and radiological healing was uncomplicated. Final outcome was poor due to axillary nerve apraxia but the patient refused any further intervention. There is little advice about the optimal treatment of splitting fractures of the humeral head in the literature. Internal fixation is mandatory for younger patients but the results are worse in more complex fracture patterns, including fractures of tuberosities. Hemiarthroplasty or reverse arthroplasty can be used in older, low demanded patients.

Consent

Written informed consent was obtained from the patient for publication of this case report and any accompanying images.

Disclosure

Konstantinos Pantazis, Ilias Iliopoulos, Ioannis Seferlis, and Zinon Kokkalis are coauthors.

Competing Interests

The authors declare that they have no competing interests.

References

[1] C. S. Neer II, "Four-segment classification of proximal humeral fractures: purpose and reliable use," *Journal of Shoulder and Elbow Surgery*, vol. 11, no. 4, pp. 389–400, 2002.

[2] C. A. Rockwood Jr. and M. A. Wirth, "Subluxations and dislocations about the glenohumeral joint," in *Rockwood and Green's Fractures in Adults*, C. A. Rockwood, R. W. Bucholz, D. P. Green, and J. D. Heckman, Eds., pp. 1221–1227, Lippincott-Raven, Philadelphia, Pa, USA, 4th edition, 1996.

[3] A. J. Ramappa, V. Patel, K. Goswami et al., "Using computed tomography to assess proximal humerus fractures," *The American Journal of Orthopedics*, vol. 43, no. 3, pp. E43–E47, 2014.

[4] C. M. Robinson, L. A. K. Khan, and M. A. Akhtar, "Treatment of anterior fracture-dislocations of the proximal humerus by open reduction and internal fixation," *Journal of Bone and Joint Surgery—Series B*, vol. 88, no. 4, pp. 502–508, 2006.

[5] R. Hertel, A. Hempfing, M. Stiehler, and M. Leunig, "Predictors of humeral head ischemia after intracapsular fracture of the proximal humerus," *Journal of Shoulder and Elbow Surgery*, vol. 13, no. 4, pp. 427–433, 2004.

[6] C. K. Lee and H. R. Hansen, "Post-traumatic avascular necrosis of the humeral head in displaced proximal humeral fractures," *The Journal of Trauma*, vol. 21, no. 9, pp. 788–791, 1981.

[7] D. Collopy and A. Skirving, "Transchondral fracture dislocation of the shoulder," *The Journal of Bone & Joint Surgery—British Volume*, vol. 77, no. 6, pp. 975–976, 1995.

[8] K. Gokkus, E. Agar, E. Sagtas, and A. T. Aydin, "Proximal humerus head-splitting fracture associated with single-part anterior dislocation," *BMJ Case Reports*, 2014.

[9] A. G. Bailie and M. G. McAlinden, "Complex head-splitting fracture-dislocation of the proximal humerus successfully treated with minimal internal fixation: a case report and discussion," *Injury Extra*, vol. 37, no. 2, pp. 82–85, 2006.

[10] T. J. S. Chesser, I. J. Langdon, C. Ogilvie, P. P. Sarangi, and A. M. Clarke, "Fractures involving splitting of the humeral head," *Journal of Bone and Joint Surgery B*, vol. 83, no. 3, pp. 423–426, 2001.

[11] A. S. Gavaskar and N. C. Tummala, "Locked plate osteosynthesis of humeral head-splitting fractures in young adults," *Journal of Shoulder and Elbow Surgery*, vol. 24, no. 6, pp. 908–914, 2015.

[12] R. M. Greiwe, R. Vargas-Ariza, L. U. Bigliani, W. N. Levine, and C. S. Ahmad, "Hemiarthroplasty for head-split fractures of the proximal humerus," *Orthopedics*, vol. 36, no. 7, pp. e905–e911, 2013.

[13] R. Garofalo, B. Flanagin, A. Castagna, E. Y. Lo, and S. G. Krish-
     nan, "Long stem reverse shoulder arthroplasty and cerclage for
     treatment of complex long segment proximal humeral fractures
     with diaphyseal extension in patients more than 65 years old,"
     Injury, vol. 46, no. 12, pp. 2379–2383, 2015.

[14] F. Grubhofer, K. Wieser, D. C. Meyer et al., "Reverse total
     shoulder arthroplasty for acute head-splitting, 3- and 4-part
     fractures of the proximal humerus in the elderly," *Journal of
     Shoulder and Elbow Surgery*, 2016.

3

Stenosing Tenosynovitis of the Flexor Hallucis Longus Tendon Associated with the Plantar Capsular Accessory Ossicle at the Interphalangeal Joint of the Great Toe

Song Ho Chang, Takumi Matsumoto, Masashi Naito, and Sakae Tanaka

Department of Orthopaedic Surgery, Faculty of Medicine, The University of Tokyo, 7-3-1 Hongo, Bunkyo-ku, Tokyo 113-8655, Japan

Correspondence should be addressed to Takumi Matsumoto; matumot-tky@umin.ac.jp

Academic Editor: Stamatios A. Papadakis

This report presents a case of stenosing tenosynovitis of the flexor hallucis longus tendon associated with the plantar capsular accessory ossicle at the interphalangeal joint of the great toe, which was confirmed by intraoperative observation and was successfully treated with surgical resection of the ossicle. As the plantar capsular accessory ossicle was not visible radiographically due to the lack of ossification, ultrasonography was helpful for diagnosing this disorder.

1. Introduction

Portions of the general population have a plantar capsular accessory ossicle at the interphalangeal joint (IPJ) of the great toe [1–5]. Although usually asymptomatic, this accessory ossicle sometimes becomes troublesome, causing painful plantar callosities [6, 7], inflammation of the ossicle [8], inflammation of the flexor hallucis longus (FHL) tendon [9], or irreducible interphalangeal joint dislocation due to its interposition [10, 11]. In cases that do not respond to conservative treatment, surgery may be the best treatment option. To the best of our knowledge, this is the first documented case of stenosing tenosynovitis of the FHL among literatures written in English, associated with an IPJ plantar capsular accessory ossicle, leading to pain at the IPJ and significantly reduced IPJ flexion, which was successfully resolved through surgical removal of the ossicle.

2. Case Report

A previously healthy, 28-year-old male complained of persistent pain at the IPJ and inability to flex the IPJ of the great toe for the past month. One week prior to noticing the loss of IPJ flexion, he had discomfort at the IPJ after exercise, although he had had no apparent episode of trauma. His doctor ordered an MRI, but no definite diagnosis was established at that time. His doctor recommended conservative treatment—including protected weight-bearing and use of anti-inflammatory medication—but this failed to relieve the patient's symptoms. He presented to our hospital two months after the onset of symptoms. On examination, the patient had difficult IPJ active flexion, acute tenderness at the plantar aspect of the IPJ, and pain with passive flexion of the IPJ. Plain radiography and computed tomography (CT) showed no significant abnormality (Figure 1). Magnetic resonance imaging (MRI) showed a single elliptical nodule in the plantar capsule at the IPJ of the great toe, distinct from the FHL tendon, and showed fluid accumulation in the IPJ and the tendon sheath of the FHL indicative of tenosynovitis (Figure 2). Dynamic observation via ultrasonography showed continuity of the FHL tendon from the toe to the ankle, ruling out FHL tendon rupture as a cause of inability to flex the IPJ. Ultrasonography of the plantar aspect of the IPJ revealed fluid retention around the nodule and FHL tendon on the affected side, but not the healthy side (Figure 3). From these observations we suspected that the stenosing tenosynovitis of the FHL was associated with the IPJ plantar capsular accessory ossicle. Local infiltration with 0.5 mL of 1%

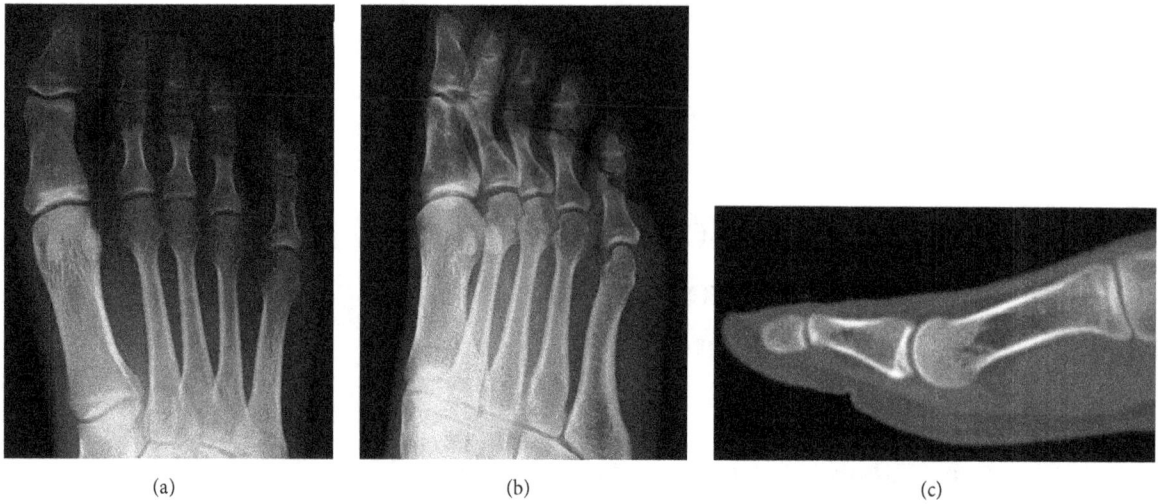

FIGURE 1: Plain radiographs and computed tomography showed no significant abnormality. (a) Anteroposterior radiograph of the foot. (b) Oblique radiograph of the foot. (c) Sagittal plane of the great toe in computed tomography.

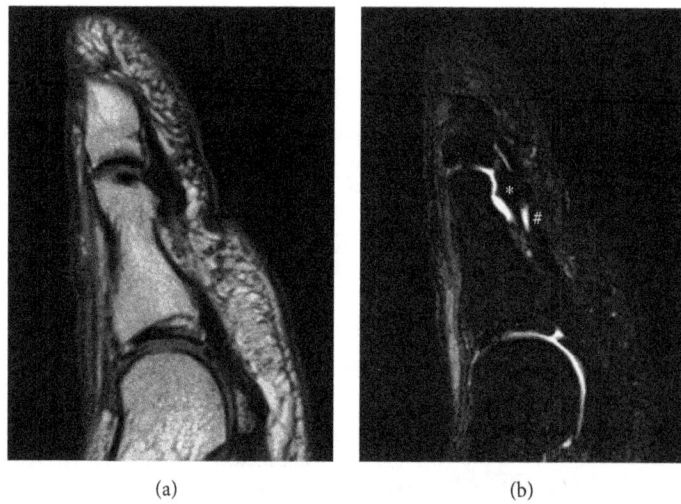

FIGURE 2: Sagittal T1 and T2 weighted magnetic resonance (MR) images showed a nodule in the plantar capsule at the interphalangeal joint of the great toe and fluid retention around it and the flexor hallucis longus tendon. (a) T1 weighted MR image. (b) T2 weighted MR image. *Plantar capsule nodule. #Flexor hallucis longus.

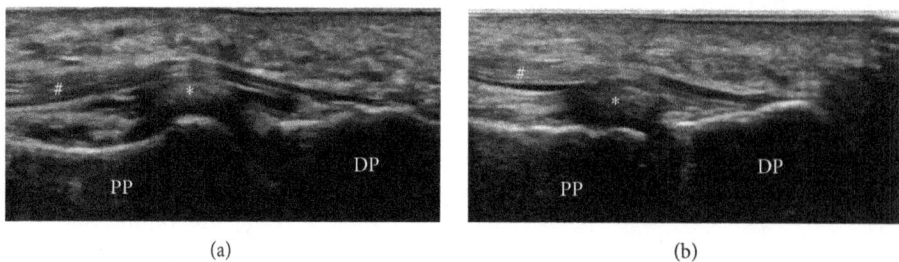

FIGURE 3: Ultrasonography image of the interphalangeal joint (IPJ) showed fluid retention around the plantar capsule nodule and flexor hallucis longus tendon on the affected side, but not on the healthy side, of the great toe. (a) Affected side. (b) Healthy side. DP: distal phalanx and PP: proximal phalanx. *Plantar capsule nodule. #Flexor hallucis longus.

(a)

(b)

(c)

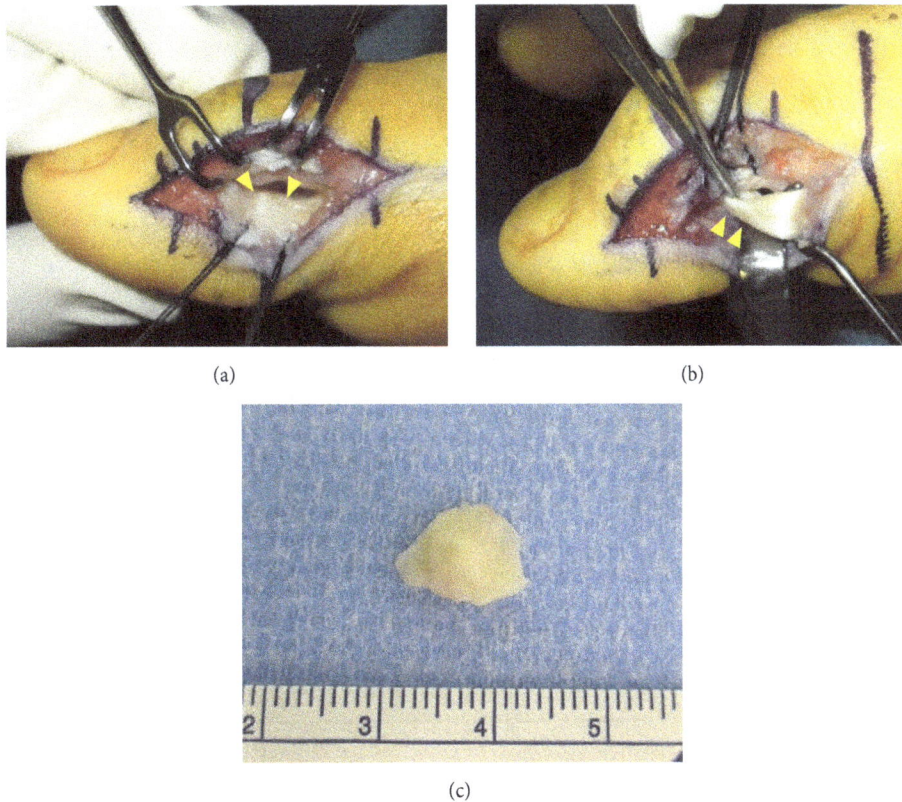

FIGURE 4: Surgical resection of the plantar capsular accessory ossicle at the interphalangeal joint (IPJ) via medial approach. (a) The IPJ plantar capsular ossicle (arrow heads). (b) The constricted flexor hallucis longus tendon at the level of the IPJ plantar capsular ossicle (arrow heads). (c) Removed IPJ plantar capsular accessory ossicle.

lidocaine mixed with 10 mg of triamcinolone acetonide had limited effect, only partially relieving the pain for a week. We proposed surgical treatment and the patient agreed.

The procedure was performed via a longitudinal 2 cm skin incision over the medial side of the IPJ of the great toe. The digital nerve was identified and retracted below the surgical field. The capsule was opened and a firm round nodule approximately 1 cm by 1 cm was seen to be embedded in the plantar capsule. The nodule had the cartilaginous appearance at its intra-articular aspect (Figure 4). The FHL ran through the tendon sheath as part of the plantar capsule of the IPJ. The FHL tendon was constricted beneath the tendon sheath so tightly that we had difficulty passing the tip of a small bone elevator between the tendon and tendon sheath. We opened a 3 mm length of the tendon sheath from its proximal end and visualized the FHL tendon at the level of the nodule (Figure 4). The nodule was detached from the capsule using surgical scissors. The procedure did not damage the plantar capsule in any way. The FHL tendon could slide easily once the nodule was removed. No postoperative external fixation was used. Postoperative recovery was uneventful. Follow-up six months later found the patient had returned to normal activity without any pain or functional impairment.

3. Discussion

The reported incidence of the ossicle at the plantar aspect of the hallucial IPJ varies widely, from 2% to 96% [1–5]. A possible explanation for this extreme difference in reported rates is the difference in observational methods between plain radiography and studies of cadavers. Racial and geographical variation may also cause discrepancies in observed rates. The accessory ossicle was found in 96% of Japanese cadavers [3], but in only 73% of British Caucasian cadavers [12]. Radiographic observation found the ossicle in 91% of Japanese subjects [3], 86% of Thai subjects [13], 13% of North American subjects [14], and only 2% of Turkish subjects [5].

This condition can result in several different clinical presentations including painful plantar callosities [6, 7], inflammation of the ossicle and/or FHL tendon [8, 15], and irreducible IPJ dislocation due to the interposition of the ossicle [10, 11]. However, to our knowledge, stenosing tenosynovitis of the FHL by the plantar capsular accessory ossicle presenting with limited IPJ flexion has not been previously reported.

A sesamoid is a bone, embedded within a tendon, which serves to modify pressure and alter the direction of muscle forces [2]. In earlier literature the term sesamoid was used to describe the ossicle at the plantar aspect of the IPJ, because it was assumed that the ossicle lies within the fibers of the FHL [16]. Later, better defined dissection studies proved that, in fact, the ossicle lies within the plantar capsule and therefore the term accessory ossicle or intra-articular ossicle was proposed [12, 13]. The theory that this ossicle is derived from a rudiment of the lost middle phalanx of the great toe is generally accepted [17].

Diagnosing IPJ plantar capsular ossicle disorder is often difficult. The ossicles are easily overlooked on radiography, especially in cases with incomplete ossification. Because they are small, oval, rough, and convex in shape, their contours on radiographs often are obscured by the opacity of the phalanges [12, 13, 15]. Ultrasonography and MRI are both useful tools for detecting small cartilaginous nodules that cannot be detected with radiography [8, 15]. However, ultrasound is superior to MRI in that it can provide dynamic anatomical information of both the ossicle and FHL tendon.

Conservative treatment of a symptomatic IPJ plantar capsular accessory ossicle of the great toe includes rest, use of a pad for decompression, shaving of hyperkeratotic lesions, and local corticosteroid injection [2, 15]. In cases where conservative treatment is ineffective, surgical removal should be considered [9]. In our case intractable pain and persistent IPJ flexion disorder was unresponsive to conservative treatment but the removal of the IPJ plantar capsular ossicle relieved both symptoms completely. This result demonstrated that the symptoms were caused by irritation of the FHL tendon related to pathology of the IPJ plantar capsular ossicle.

A number of procedures for surgical removal of the accessory ossicle are in use [16–19]; they are generally divided into medial, plantar, and dorsal approaches. Each has distinct advantages and disadvantages over the others. The plantar approach provides the most direct approach to the ossicle and offers the possibility of concomitant resection of plantar hyperkeratotic lesion; however, this approach is frequently complicated by residual hypertrophic scar tissue formation. The dorsal approach is often used in cases of ossicle interposition associated with IPJ dislocation [11]; however, extensive invasions—including tenotomy, capsulotomy, and collateral ligament release—are required to achieve complete exposure of the ossicle in nondislocated cases [16]. The medial approach creates an incision extending from just distal to the first metatarsophalangeal joint to the base of the distal phalanx of the great toe. With a plantarflex position of the IPJ, the FHL is relaxed and allows direct visualization of the plantar ossicle. This approach provides the least surgical exposure, avoids neurovascular bundles, and does not cross lines of flexion and extension of the great toe [6, 17]. These are significant advantages since they prevent painful hypertrophic scar tissue formation in a weight-bearing area. For these reasons, we chose the medial approach, and we had no postoperative complications.

4. Conclusion

We conclude that stenosing tenosynovitis of the FHL tendon associated with the IPJ plantar capsular accessory ossicle

should be taken into consideration in the differential diagnosis of IPJ flexion disorder. Further, cases unresponsive to conservative treatments may benefit from surgical removal of the ossicle.

Competing Interests

The authors declare that there is no conflict of interests regarding the publication of this paper.

References

[1] A. H. Bizarro, "On sesamoid and supernumerary bones of the limbs," *Journal of Anatomy*, vol. 55, part 4, pp. 256–268, 1921.

[2] M. H. Jahss, "The sesamoids of the hallux," *Clinical Orthopaedics and Related Research*, vol. 157, pp. 88–97, 1981.

[3] T. Masaki, "An anatomical study of the interphalangeal sesamoid bone of the hallux," *Nihon Seikeigeka Gakkai Zasshi*, vol. 58, no. 4, pp. 419–427, 1984 (Japanese).

[4] A. S. Dharap, H. Al-Hashimi, S. Kassab, and M. F. Abu-Hijleh, "Incidence and ossification of sesamoid bones in the hands and feet: a radiographic study in an Arab population," *Clinical Anatomy*, vol. 20, no. 4, pp. 416–423, 2007.

[5] N. Coskun, M. Yuksel, M. Cevener et al., "Incidence of accessory ossicles and sesamoid bones in the feet: a radiographic study of the Turkish subjects," *Surgical and Radiologic Anatomy*, vol. 31, no. 1, pp. 19–24, 2009.

[6] S. M. Sharon, "Interphalangeal joint hallux ossicle," *Journal of Foot Surgery*, vol. 16, no. 2, pp. 69–72, 1977.

[7] K. J. Dennis and S. McKinney, "Sesamoids and accessory bones of the foot," *Clinics in Podiatric Medicine and Surgery*, vol. 7, no. 4, pp. 717–723, 1990.

[8] S. Kumar, R. Kadavigere, R. Puppala, A. Ayachit, and R. Singh, "Subhallucal interphalangeal sesamoiditis: a rare cause of chronic great toe pain," *Journal of Clinical and Diagnostic Research*, vol. 9, no. 5, pp. TD01–TD02, 2015.

[9] G. Del Rossi, "Great toe pain in a competitive tennis athlete," *Journal of Sports Science and Medicine*, vol. 2, no. 4, pp. 180–183, 2003.

[10] T. Miki, T. Yamamuro, and T. Kitai, "An irreducible dislocation of the great toe. Report of two cases and review of the literature," *Clinical Orthopaedics and Related Research*, no. 230, pp. 200–206, 1988.

[11] M. Hatori, M. Goto, K. Tanaka, R. A. Smith, and S. Kokubun, "Neglected irreducible dislocation of the interphalangeal joint of the great toe: a case report," *Journal of Foot and Ankle Surgery*, vol. 45, no. 4, pp. 271–274, 2006.

[12] M. B. Davies and S. Dalal, "Gross anatomy of the interphalangeal joint of the great toe: implications for excision of plantar capsular accessory ossicles," *Clinical Anatomy*, vol. 18, no. 4, pp. 239–244, 2005.

[13] P. Suwannahoy, T. Srisuwan, N. Pattamapaspong, and P. Mahakkanukrauh, "Intra-articular ossicle in interphalangeal joint of the great toe and clinical implication," *Surgical and Radiologic Anatomy*, vol. 34, no. 1, pp. 39–42, 2012.

[14] M. S. Burman and P. W. Lapidus, "The functional disturbances caused by the inconstant bones and sesamoids of the foot," *Archives of Surgery*, vol. 22, no. 6, pp. 936–975, 1931.

[15] H. Y. Shin, S. Y. Park, H. Y. Kim, Y. S. Jung, S. An, and D. H. Kang, "Symptomatic hallucal interphalangeal sesamoid bones

successfully treated with ultrasound-guided injection," *Korean Journal of Pain*, vol. 26, no. 2, pp. 173–176, 2013.

[16] T. S. Roukis and J. S. Hurless, "The hallucal interphalangeal sesamoid," *Journal of Foot and Ankle Surgery*, vol. 35, no. 4, pp. 303–308, 1996.

[17] D. J. McCarthy, T. Reed, and N. Abell, "The hallucal interphalangeal sesamoid," *Journal of the American Podiatric Medical Association*, vol. 76, no. 6, pp. 311–319, 1986.

[18] W. A. Miller and B. P. Love, "Cartilaginous sesamoid or nodule of the interphalangeal joint of the big toe," *Foot and Ankle*, vol. 2, no. 5, pp. 291–293, 1982.

[19] J. J. Genakos, "Clinical sign consistent with the hallucal interphalangeal sesamoid," *Journal of the American Podiatric Medical Association*, vol. 83, no. 12, pp. 696–697, 1993.

4

Spinous Process Osteochondroma as a Rare Cause of Lumbar Pain

Bárbara Rosa,[1] **Pedro Campos,**[1] **André Barros,**[1] **Samir Karmali,**[1] **Esperança Ussene,**[2] **Carlos Durão,**[1] **João Alves da Silva,**[1] **and Nuno Coutinho**[1]

[1]*Trauma and Orthopaedics Department, Hospital Vila Franca de Xira, 2600 009 Lisbon, Portugal*
[2]*Department of Pathology, Hospital Vila Franca de Xira, 2600 009 Lisbon, Portugal*

Correspondence should be addressed to Carlos Durão; drcarlosdurao@hotmail.com

Academic Editor: Koichi Sairyo

We present a case of a 5th Lumbar Vertebra (L5) spinous process osteochondroma as a rare cause of lumbar pain in an old patient. A 70-year-old male presented with progressive and disabling lower lumbar pain. Tenderness over the central and left paraspinal area of the lower lumbar region and a palpable mass were evident. CT scan showed a mass arising from the spinous process of L5. Marginal resection of the tumor was performed through a posterior approach. The histological study revealed an osteochondroma. After surgery, pain was completely relieved. After one year there was no evidence of local recurrence or symptoms. Osteochondromas rarely involve the spine, but when they do symptoms like pain, radiculopathy/myelopathy, or cosmetic deformity may occur. The imagiologic exam of election for diagnosis is CT scan. When symptomatic the treatment of choice is surgical resection. The most concerning complication of osteochondromas is malignant transformation, a rare event.

1. Introduction

Osteochondroma is a benign outgrowth of bone and cartilage and is one of the most common bone tumors that usually occurs in long bones but rarely involves the spine [1], affecting mainly the cervical and upper dorsal segments [2]. They are more common in males and have an average age at presentation of approximately 32 ± 4.6 years [3]. Lumbar osteochondromas can be asymptomatic or cause symptoms like pain, radiculopathy/myelopathy, or cosmetic deformity [3–10]. The imagiologic exam of election for diagnosis is CT scan [4, 11]. When symptomatic the treatment of choice is surgical resection. The most concerning complication of osteochondromas is malignant transformation, a rare event [2, 12].

We have found in the literature one case of a symptomatic lumbar osteochondroma presenting in the 6th decade of life [5]. We report a case of a lumbar osteochondroma presenting in the 8th decade of life causing lumbar back pain. Despite being rare, we must consider osteochondroma as a cause of lumbar back pain, even in older patients.

2. Case Report

A 70-year-old male, with history of hypertension, dislipidemia, and hyperuricemia, presented to our institution with a one-year long history of progressive and intense lower lumbar pain causing great limitation of daily activities. Physiotherapy or medication was ineffective. The patient reported a palpable mass on this region for years but with neither symptoms nor size progression. He had no constitutional or neurologic symptoms. On examination, there were tenderness over the central and left paraspinal area and a fixed palpable mass of size approximately 7×5 cm, hard in consistency, and no pulse. The pain aggravated with flexion, extension, and rotational trunk movements. Neurologic examination was normal. Radiographs showed a bony mass protruding posteriorly, apparently from the L5 vertebra. CT scan showed a 7 cm long well-limited mass with an apparent cartilage cap arising from the spinous process of L5. It was lateralized to the left with adjacent paraspinal muscle compression (Figure 1). Under general anesthesia, the tumor was marginally resected along with the L5 spinous process through a posterior

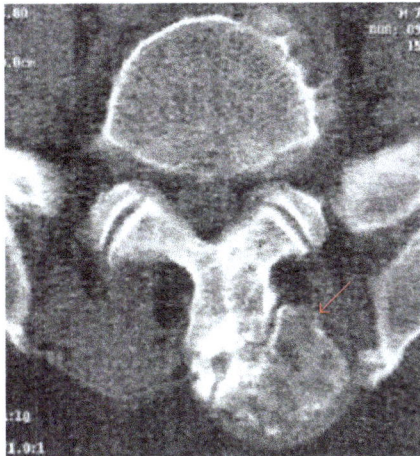

FIGURE 1: CT scan. Axial view showing a well-limited mass with a cartilage cap arising from the spinous process of L5 lateralized to the left (arrow).

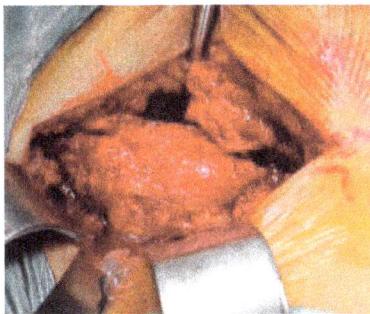

(a)

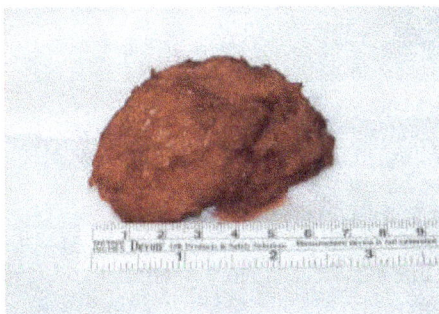

(b)

FIGURE 2: (a) Intraoperative picture showing a lumbar spine midline approach, exposing the tumor *in situ* in contiguous to the spinous process of L5 causing adjacent left paraspinal muscular compression. (b) Intraoperative picture of the resected tumor with an approximately 7 cm axis-length.

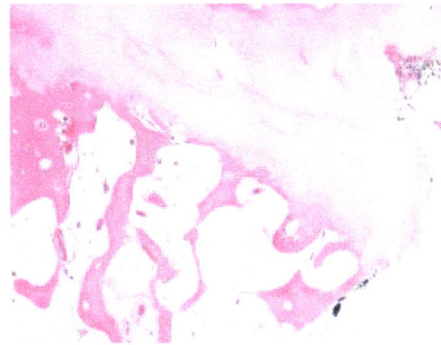

(a)

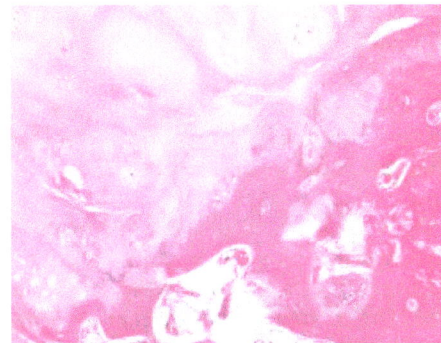

(b)

FIGURE 3: (a) Hematoxylin-eosin stain, original magnification ×2.5, and (b) Hematoxylin-eosin stain, original magnification ×10. Junction of cartilage cap and underlying bone without atypia and resemblance to an epiphyseal plate with enchondral ossification.

3. Discussion

Osteochondroma is a benign outgrowth of bone and cartilage and is one of the most common bone tumors that usually occurs in long bones but rarely involves the spine [1]. Only 1,3% to 4,1% of solitary osteochondromas arise in spine and occur in approximately 9% of patients who are affected by hereditary multiple exostosis [4, 11]. They are more common in males and according to Gaetani et al. [3] the average age at presentation is approximately 32 ± 4.6 years. Only five cases of lumbar osteochondroma out of 17 occurred in the L5 level. We have found in the literature one case of a symptomatic lumbar osteochondroma presenting in the 6th decade of life [5]. Until now, the oldest case of spinal osteochondroma reported in the literature occurred in a 73-year-old female in the cervical spine [2]. We report a case of a lumbar osteochondroma presenting in the 8th decade of life.

The tumors are thought to arise through a process of progressive endochondral ossification of aberrant cartilage of a growth plate following surgery or fracture or as a consequence of a congenital perichondral deficiency and are the most common radiation-induced benign tumors [1, 4, 6]. Choi et al. [5] reported a case in which the osteochondroma arose from a spondylolytic lamina and speculate that the fibrous cartilage of spondylolysis served as the origin of aberrant cartilaginous tissue.

approach (Figure 2). Histologic examination has shown a specimen composed of trabecular bone with focus on bone marrow covered by lobules of cartilaginous tissue, without cellular atypia, consistent with osteochondroma (Figure 3). After surgery pain was completely relieved, and neurologic function was normal. At one-year follow-up there was no evidence of local recurrence or symptoms.

The tumor affects mainly the cervical and dorsal spine, probably related to different durations of the ossification processes that occur in the secondary centers of ossification. It can be speculated that the more rapidly the ossification process of these centers develops, the greater the probability that aberrant cartilage will form is. In adolescence, secondary ossification centers, which lie in the spinous process, transverse process, articular process, and the endplate of vertebral body, complete the growth of the vertebral column. These secondary ossification centers appear in children between the ages of 11 and 18 years. They develop into complete ossification in the cervical spine during adolescence and in the thoracic and the lumbar spine during the end of the second decade of life [4, 13].

In most reported cases we have found in the current literature, involving the lumbar spine, the tumor is included in posterior arch elements, more commonly the lamina [3–10, 14]. We have found only two reported cases like this one with involvement of the spinous process [7, 14].

The tumor can be asymptomatic or symptomatic, either causing pain by pressure on adjacent soft tissue structures when it grows posteriorly, or, more rarely, causing radicular or spinal compression symptoms, when it grows into the spinal canal [3, 4, 6–9]. The tumor can also cause cosmetic deformity, as occurred in a case of an 8-year-old girl presenting with an atypical spinal curvature caused by a lumbar osteochondroma [10].

Marrow and cortical continuity with the underlying parent bone defines the lesion [6] and this feature is better visualized on computed tomography scan [4]. MRI is useful to determine the extent of neurologic structures compromise and it identifies lesions that look suspicious of malignant transformation [6].

When symptomatic, the treatment of choice of osteochondromas is surgical resection. However, Gille et al. [2] recommend systematic surgical resection of all solitary spinal osteochondromas, given the risk of malignant transformation. The resection can be achieved in the majority of cases without spinal instrumentation because it rarely compromises the spinal stability, as osteochondromas show focal growth in the posterior elements. We have found only one case reported on which fusion and instrumentation surgery was necessary [5].

The most concerning complication of osteochondromas is malignant transformation, fortunately a rare complication. Chondrosarcoma of the spine represents 4–10% of all chondrosarcomas and 12% of all malignant tumors of the spine [15]; the frequency of degeneration is estimated at about 1% in solitary spinal osteochondromas [16]. Altay et al. [12] in a retrospective analysis of 627 cartilage-forming tumors revealed a rate of malignant transformation for solitary osteochondromas of 4,2% and a higher rate for multiple osteochondromas, namely, 9,2%. However, none of these tumors involve the spine. Malignant transformation leads to a chondrosarcoma in 90% of cases, which develops in the cartilage cap of the osteochondroma. The most consistent finding that may suggest malignancy might be a cap thickness >2 cm, but the diagnosis is only confirmed with a biopsy of the lesion [12, 17].

4. Conclusion

We report a case of a lumbar osteochondroma arising from the L5 spinous process, a rare cause of lumbar pain, especially in the 8th decade. Osteochondromas rarely involve the spine, but when they occur they can be asymptomatic or cause symptoms, like pain, radiculopathy or myelopathy, or, even, cosmetic deformation. The imagiologic exam of election for diagnosis is CT scan. When symptomatic the treatment of choice is surgical resection. The most concerning complication of osteochondromas is malignant transformation, fortunately a rare event.

Competing Interests

The authors declare that they have no conflict of interests.

References

[1] S. A. Qasem and B. R. Deyoung, "Cartilage-forming tumors," *Seminars in Diagnostic Pathology*, vol. 31, no. 1, pp. 10–20, 2014.

[2] O. Gille, V. Pointillart, and J.-M. Vital, "Course of spinal solitary osteochondromas," *Spine*, vol. 30, no. 1, pp. E13–E19, 2005.

[3] P. Gaetani, F. Tancioni, P. Merlo, L. Villani, G. Spanu, and R. Rodriguez y Baena, "Spinal chondroma of the lumbar tract: case report," *Surgical Neurology*, vol. 46, no. 6, pp. 534–539, 1996.

[4] E. Fiumara, T. Scarabino, G. Guglielmi, M. Bisceglia, and V. D'Angelo, "Osteochondroma of the L-5 vertebra: a rare cause of sciatic pain. Case report," *Journal of Neurosurgery*, vol. 91, no. 2, pp. 219–222, 1999.

[5] B. K. Choi, I. H. Han, W. H. Cho, and S. H. Cha, "Lumbar osteochondroma arising from spondylolytic L3 lamina," *Journal of Korean Neurosurgical Society*, vol. 47, no. 4, pp. 313–315, 2010.

[6] M. Thiart and H. Herbrst, "Lumbar osteochondroma causing spinal compression," *SA Orthopaedic Journal Winter*, vol. 9, no. 2, pp. 44–46, 2010.

[7] S. M. Kumar, B. K. Rai, S. S. Kumari, and V. C. Noel, "Solitary osteochondroma of L4 spinous process-a rare presentation," *Journal of Evolution of Medical and Dental Sciences*, vol. 2, no. 49, pp. 9520–9524, 2013.

[8] J. Xu, C.-R. Xu, H. Wu, H.-L. Pan, and J. Tian, "Osteochondroma in the lumbar intraspinal canal causing nerve root compression," *Orthopedics*, vol. 32, no. 2, p. 133, 2009.

[9] J. E. Carrera, P. A. Castillo, and O. M. Molina, "Osteocondroma de lámina lumbar y compresión radicular. Reporte de un caso," *Acta Ortopédica Mexicana*, vol. 21, no. 5, pp. 261–266, 2007.

[10] J. F. Fiechtl, J. L. Masonis, and S. L. Frick, "Spinal osteochondroma presenting as atypical spinal curvature: a case report," *Spine*, vol. 28, no. 13, pp. E252–255, 2003.

[11] S. Albrecht, J. S. Crutchfield, and G. K. SeGall, "On spinal osteochondromas," *Journal of Neurosurgery*, vol. 77, no. 2, pp. 247–252, 1992.

[12] M. Altay, K. Bayrakci, Y. Yildiz, S. Erekul, and Y. Saglik, "Secondary chondrosarcoma in cartilage bone tumors: report of 32 patients," *Journal of Orthopaedic Science*, vol. 12, no. 5, pp. 415–423, 2007.

[13] R. Louis, *Chirurgie du Rachis. Anatomie Chirurgicale et Voies d'Abord*, Springer, Berlin, Germany, 1998.

[14] E. G. Hassankhani, "Solitary lower lumbar osteochondroma (spinous process of L3 involvement): a case report," *Cases Journal*, vol. 2, no. 12, article 9359, 2009.

[15] C. Ruivo and M. A. Hopper, "Spinal chondrosarcoma arising from a solitary lumbar osteochondroma," *Journal of the Belgian Society of Radiology*, vol. 97, no. 1, pp. 21–24, 2014.

[16] D. C. Dahlin and K. K. Unni, *Bone Tumours*, Charles C. Thomas, Springfield, Ill, USA, 4th edition, 1986.

[17] E. Strovski, R. Ali, D. A. Graeb, P. L. Munk, and S. D. Chang, "Malignant degeneration of a lumbar osteochondroma into a chondrosarcoma which mimicked a large retropertioneal mass," *Skeletal Radiology*, vol. 41, no. 10, pp. 1319–1322, 2012.

5

Surgical Management of Intracanal Rib Head Dislocation in Neurofibromatosis Type 1 Dystrophic Kyphoscoliosis: Report of Two Cases and Literature Review

George I. Mataliotakis, Nikolaos Bounakis, and Enrique Garrido-Stratenwerth

Royal Hospital for Sick Children, Scottish National Spine Deformity Centre, Sciennes Road, Edinburgh EH9 1LF, UK

Correspondence should be addressed to George I. Mataliotakis; george.mataliotakis@gmail.com

Academic Editor: William B. Rodgers

There is still no consensus on the management of severe intracanal RH dislocation in neurofibromatosis type 1 dystrophic kyphoscoliosis. This study notes the early cord function impairment signs, reports a serious complication in a susceptible cord, identifies possible mechanisms of injury, and discusses the management of intracanal RH dislocation presented in the literature. First report is as follows: a 12-year-old female with cord compromise and preoperative neurology that underwent thoracotomy and anterior release. The RH was left in situ following a rib excision. During the posterior stage of the procedure she presented with complete loss of all IOM traces prior to any correction manoeuvres. The neurology recovered 72 h postop and the final correction and instrumented fusion were uneventfully completed 15 days postop. Second report is as follows: a 10-year-old male, whose only neurology was a provoked shock-like sensation to the lower limbs following direct pressure on the rib cage. He underwent an uneventful posterior RH excision and instrumented correction and posterior spinal fusion. In conclusion, any possible cord dysfunction sign should be sought during examination. Decompression of the spinal cord by resecting the impinging bony part, even in the absence of neurological symptoms, is advised before any attempt to release or correct the deformity.

1. Introduction

Neurofibromatosis type 1 (NF1), also known as von Recklinghausen's disease, is a single gene hamartomatous disease inherited by the autosomal dominant trait [1, 2]. The relentless deterioration of the short dystrophic curves, which leads to acute kyphosis and possible vertebral subluxation, mandates surgical stabilization [1, 3]. Intracanal rib head (RH) dislocation at the convex of the dystrophic curve may impinge on the cord and constitute another cause of neurology [3–9]. The "painful rib hump" sign caused by the RH dislocation has recently been described [8].

Even though there are recent reports of retraction of the RH away from the cord along with curve correction [2, 10, 11], there is still no consensus among authors that the excision of the dislocated RHs is indicated in symptomatic NF1-dystrophic curves [5, 8, 12, 13]. The preoperative identification of a "cord at risk," the susceptibility of the cord to intraoperative manipulations, and the sequence of an iatrogenic injury are not fully described yet.

We report two selected cases: a case of intraoperative neurological injury in a previously symptomatic patient with cord changes and a case of "hidden" neurology in an otherwise asymptomatic patient. The purpose of this study is to report a serious complication, identify a possible mechanism of injury, highlight the importance of early neurology, and discuss management of intraspinal RH dislocation.

2. Case 1

A 12-year-old premenarchal girl presented with back pain due to dystrophic NF1 left thoracic kyphoscoliosis (Figure 1(a)). She had bilateral brisk patellar reflexes and a left four beat ankle clonus. The patient reported shooting pain into her legs on deep forward bending. Preoperative MRI and CT scans revealed a flattened cord at the apex of the kyphosis with a penetrating left 6th RH adjacent to the cord without compression (Figures 1(b)–1(d)).

A combined fusion and posterior RH excision were planned with the aid of multimodal spinal cord monitoring.

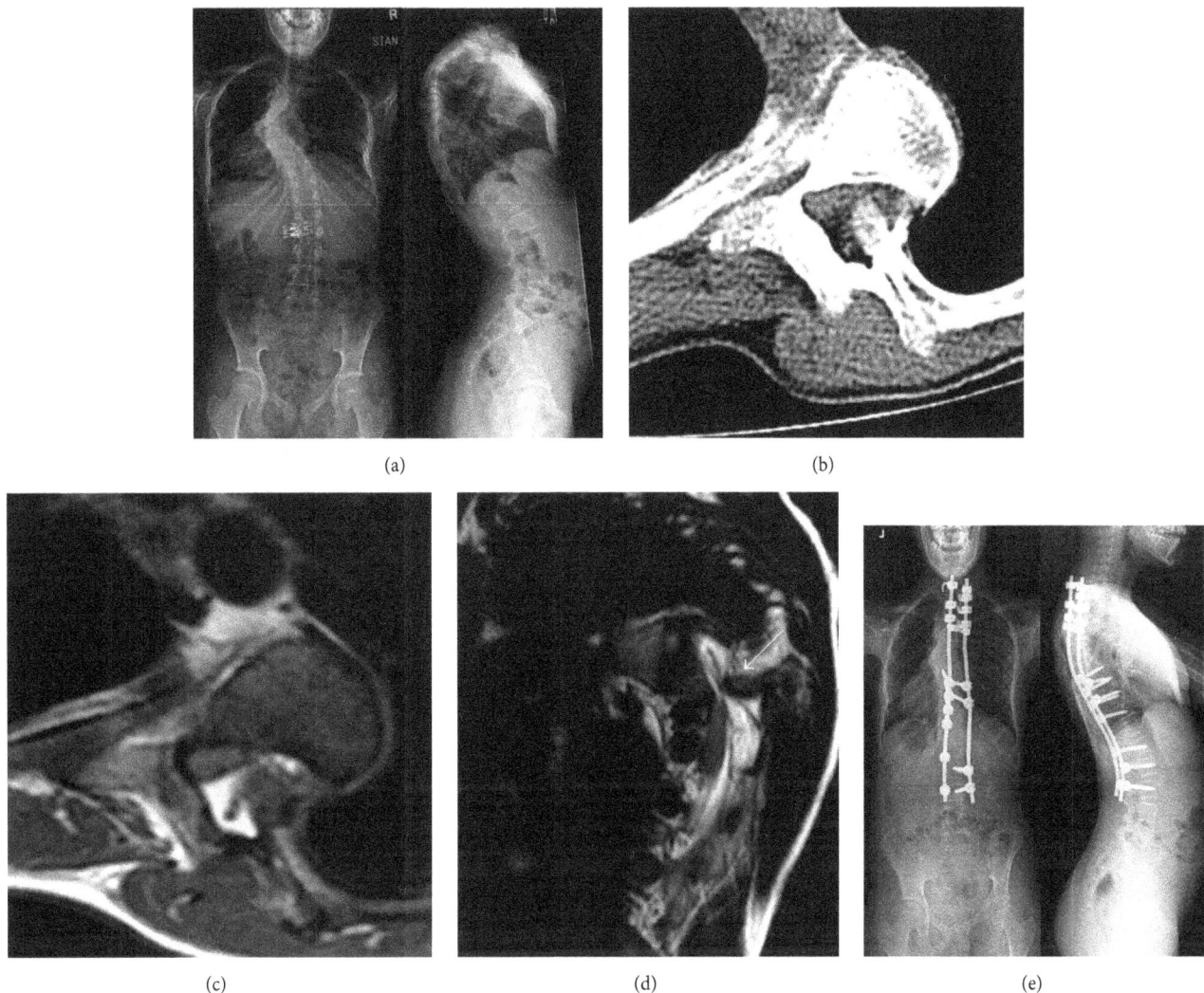

(a)   (b)

(c)   (d)   (e)

FIGURE 1: Preoperative whole spine AP and lateral X-ray (a). Preoperative CT (b) and axial T2 MRI (c) demonstrating the right 6th rib head intracanal dislocation and cord impingement. (d) Preoperative sagittal T2 MRI views demonstrating the rib head cord impingement and the flattening adjacent to the acute kyphosis (white arrow). Whole spine AP and lateral (e) X-rays 2 years postoperatively.

Following a thoracotomy the left 6th rib was excised, leaving the neck and head in situ. During the T4–T9 discectomies a transient loss of Motor Evoked Potentials (MEPs) occurred bilaterally in lower limbs, which responded to an increase in the mean arterial blood pressure. Somatosensory Evoked Potentials (SSEPs) remained normal.

Normal reference traces were present at the beginning of the second stage: posterior instrumented spinal fusion. After completion of the instrumentation and prior to correction manoeuvres all MEPs and SSEPs were lost completely. Following a laminectomy, the dislocated RH, which was not adherent to the dura but was impinging on the cord, was excised. Wake-up test showed no spontaneous movement in the lower limbs with good upper limbs movement.

Postoperative neurological examination showed grade 3 muscle power (MRC grading) in all muscle groups of the left lower limb. Right lower limb was normal. Fine touch and proprioception remained intact bilaterally. 48 h postop MRI scan showed no evidence of cord signal changes. 72 h postop

the patient regained normal muscle power and urinary continence.

Fifteen days postoperatively the patient underwent posterior correction of the deformity. The MEPs remained stable during the procedure. Postoperative radiographs evidenced a main thoracic curve of 45° (51% correction). Lateral radiographs and CT scan confirmed a correction of the thoracic kyphosis to 48° (36% correction). At 2-year follow-up (Figure 1(e)) there has been no significant loss of correction and the patient remains asymptomatic.

3. Case 2

A 10-year-old boy presented with a rapidly progressive spinal deformity and scapulae asymmetry, due to dystrophic NF1 sharp angular proximal thoracic kyphoscoliosis (Figure 2(a)). There was no neurologic deficit. Interestingly, the patient complained of discomfort only when lying on his right side with shock-like sensations to his lower limbs bilaterally. The

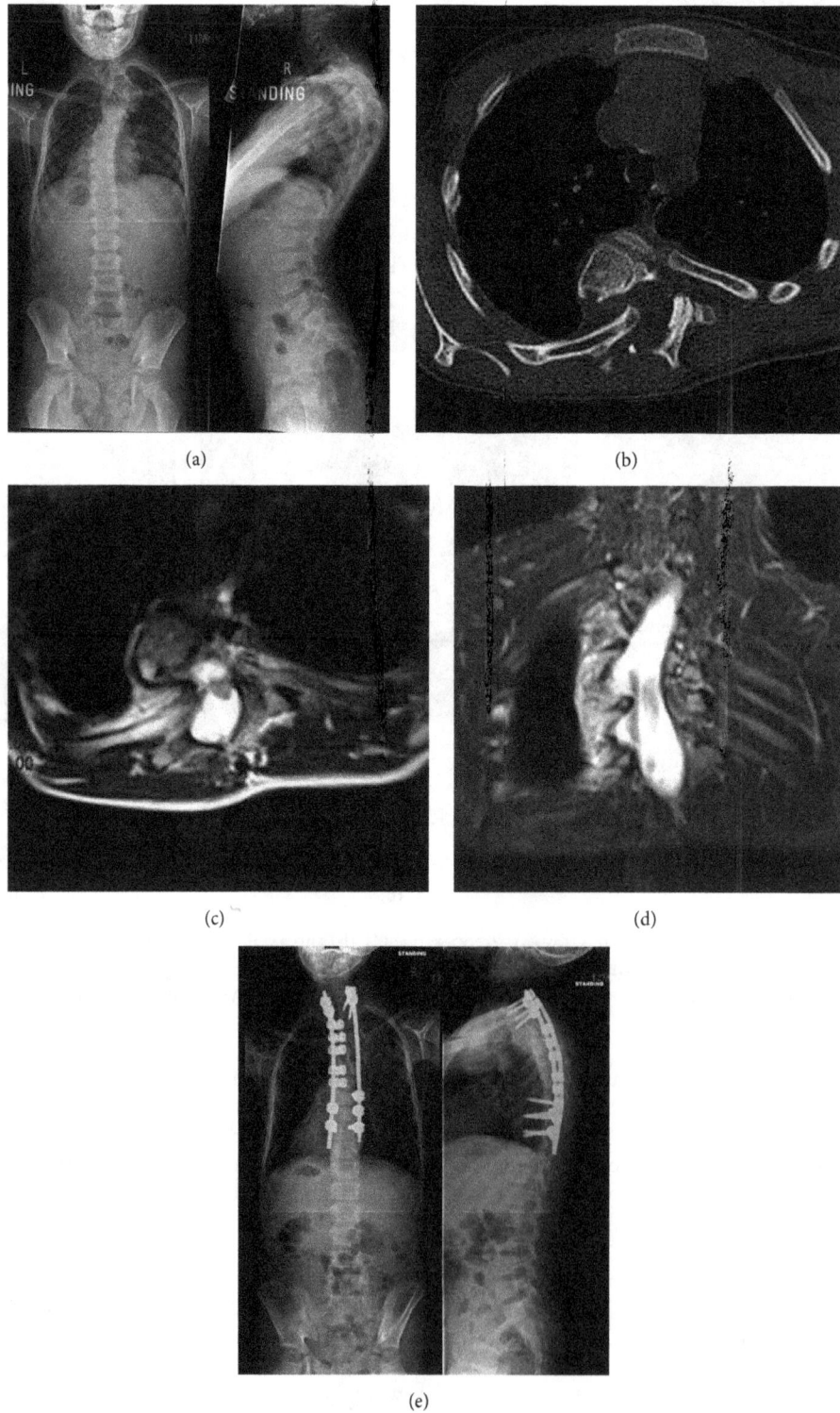

FIGURE 2: Preoperative whole spine AP and lateral X-ray (a). Preoperative CT scan (b) demonstrating the rib head intracanal dislocation. Preoperative sagittal T2 MRI axial (c) and coronal (d) views demonstrating the rib head in close proximity to the cord but without impingement. Postoperative whole spine AP and lateral X-rays (e).

CT/MRI imaging shows intracanal dislocation of the right 4, 5, and 6th ribs, with the 5th being in contact with the spinal cord and no cord-substance high signal present (Figures 2(b)–2(d)).

He underwent posterior resection of the 5th RH through a hemilaminectomy approach. Following alar/coronal ligament release, the RH was extracted with stable spinal cord monitoring traces. The posterior instrumented spinal fusion was then completed uneventfully (Figure 2(e)). A CTLSO was used postoperatively.

4. Discussion

The canal expansion due to dural ectasia is probably protective, regarding the early development of neurological symptoms [1]. Apart from possible neurofibromas, the acute kyphotic deformity and instability may lead to neurology compromise due to secondary cord injury [1–7, 9, 12, 14, 15].

The dislocation of the RH into the canal is caused by the insufficiency of the costovertebral/costotransverse articulation and medial-ward pressure by the thoracic cage [1–3]. It takes place through the enlarged neural foramina at the apex of the convexity of the curve [2]. The RH may impinge on the cord [3–9] and may cause neurology [3, 7–9]. Gkiokas et al. [8] described clearly the mobile RH, which causes neurology and pain in an otherwise neurologically intact patient, introducing the "painful rib hump" sign. Lhermitte's type phenomenon might represent early sign of cord irritation, manifesting as shock-like sensation to lower limbs [4, 12]. This was the only clinical finding on our 2nd case, indicating an unstable RH and possible early cord injury.

MRI with contrast is the imaging modality of choice for soft tissue lesions in NF and the T2W sequences may demonstrate the intraspinal RH dislocation [4]. However, there are reports where preoperative MRI failed to diagnose the intraspinal RH dislocation leading to postoperative neurological injury [5, 9, 15]. The CT scan can reliably demonstrate the intracanal RH dislocation because of better delineation of bony anatomy [3, 13]. The preoperative evaluation of the imaging should be cautious, as the RH and spine positions without gravitational forces may underestimate the degree of canal intrusion.

Surgical treatment is difficult due to excessive bleeding and the distorted anatomy. High pseudoarthrosis rates have been reported with posterior-only fusion in dystrophic scoliosis and therefore generous anteroposterior fusion has been advocated for curves exceeding 50° of kyphosis [16].

No consensus exists in the literature regarding the surgical sequence for the treatment of intraspinal RH dislocation and scoliosis correction.

A literature review reveals 16 publications with a total of 49 patients with NF1 and intraspinal dislocation of the rib (Table 1). Most of the patients were teenagers with a mean age of 13 years (average: 13.45 ± 5.72 years, range: 6–41 y) with almost 1 : 1 male to female ratio (25f : 23m). Neurological status was reported in 24 cases. Neurological deficits were present in 50% of the reported cases. Two or more ribs penetrating into the canal were presented into 43% of the nonsymptomatic patients and in 42% of the symptomatic

patients. In 47% (9/19) of the reported cases the RH was in close proximity or was impinging on the spinal cord. Six of the nine patients with a RH in close proximity to the spinal cord underwent resection. Of the three patients in whom the RH was not removed during scoliosis fusion, two patients developed delayed neurological deficits requiring subsequent decompression. The intraoperative monitoring traces were lost in the patient who had his RH left in situ and the distal rib resected [7].

Among all the reported cases with intracanal dislocation, 32 patients received PSF only; one had noninstrumented in situ PSF [5] and one had instrumented in situ PSF following previous correction by halo traction [6]. The in situ noninstrumented PSF led to lower limb weakness and paraparesis 6 weeks postoperatively with the authors not clarifying the cause of the neurology deterioration [5]. There were 19 staged operations with 11 of them being combined anterior and posterior. Of the 11 patients, 8 had ASF and 6 underwent the anterior procedure first.

RH excision is generally advised routinely in most of the case reports [3, 7, 14]. The posterior approach offers better visualisation than the unilateral exposure through an anterior approach [13].

Mao et al. [10] and Sun et al. [11] showed that spontaneous RH reduction occurred, following curve correction. Yalcin et al. [2] also observed under direct vision how the RH migrated out of the canal during scoliosis correction. They concluded that, in the presence of neurological symptoms or evidence of compression, resection of the rib prior to any surgical manipulation (release or correction) is necessary [2]. In asymptomatic patients with no evidence of spinal cord compression, RH excision was considered questionable. Yalcin et al. [2] suggested direct visualisation of the RH via hemilaminectomy during correction manoeuvres.

Abdulian et al. [6] offer a different point of view, advocating resection of every intracanal RH dislocation. In addition, the authors recommended rib shaft osteotomy in cases where the RH remains unresectable because of cord adhesions.

Similar to our case 1, in the report by Mukthar et al. [7] the spinal cord monitoring traces were lost following resection of the rib shaft and leaving the RH in situ. According to Leung et al. [17] a spinal cord at risk is more likely to demonstrate intraoperative monitoring changes and those changes are twice likely to be associated with postoperative neurological deficit. Cheh et al. [18] reported loss of MEPs in 21% of paediatric kyphosis correction which was attributed mainly to hypotension, overcorrection, or combination of the two and was completely reversed by increasing the mean arterial pressure or reducing the magnitude of correction. Shimizu et al. [19] in their recent animal study showed that severe kyphosis causes demyelination, reduced blood supply, and neuronal loss of anterior horn cells.

Several factors may have contributed to the transient neurological injury to herein reported case 1. Vascular insufficiency during the anterior discectomy stage may have caused the drop of the IOM traces, as they recovered after an increase in the mean arterial blood pressure. The RH was not removed during the anterior stage as this would result into greater haemorrhage and possible further secondary vascular insult

TABLE 1: Surgical management of intracanal rib head dislocation in neurofibromatosis type 1 dystrophic kyphoscoliosis.

Author	Age (range)/sex	Dislocated ribs [N of ribs (N of patients)]	Cord impingement	Other lesions present	Preoperative neurology	Operation details	Rib heads resection	Complications after 1st operation	Neurology recovery
Flood et al. 1986 [12]	13	>2	No	Yes	Knee and ankle clonus	Two-stage vertebral wedge resection with rib excision and fusion. Traction used perioperatively, PSF	Yes	NR	Residual clonus
Major and Huizenga 1988 [13]	13f	2	No	No	Transient loss of sensation below the waist and inability to move LL after fall on rib hump	Two-stage ASF with RH resection followed by segmental instrumented PSF	Yes	NR	n/a
	5f	2	No	No	No	Anterior interbody fusion with RH resection followed by segmental instrumented PSF	Yes	NR	n/a
	11m	1	No	No	No	Posterior fusion with RH resection	Yes	NR	n/a
Deguchi et al. 1995 [9]	12f	2	Yes	No	Weakness of the LL, difficulty walking with eventual paraparesis, hypesthesia below waist, ankle clonus, and knee/ankle HR; gradual	Laminectomy and proximal resection of the compression rib; two-stage combined ASF and instrumented PSF; dislocated RH was resected	Yes	NR	Yes
Dacher et al. 1995 [15]	10f	1	No	No	Bilateral ankle clonus and daytime micturition	Two-stage SF with CD instrumentation	NR	NR	Yes
Kamath et al. 1995 [20]	13m	1	No	Yes	No	Intraspinal RH resection with right T9/10 hemilaminectomy and instrumented PSF	Yes	NR	n/a
Khoshhal and Ellis 2000 [5]	16m	1	Yes	Yes	No	In situ noninstrumented PSF; revision: anterior decompression and RH resection 8 months postop due to residual neurology	No	Progressive LL weakness, spasticity, and being unable to walk	Residual HR
Legrand et al. 2003 [21]	13m	1	NR	NR	Hyperreflexia	PSF & ASF	No	NR	NR
	10f	2	NR	NR	No	NR	Yes	NR	n/a
	16m	1	NR	NR	Hypotonia	PSF & ASF	No	NR	Yes
	41f	2	NR	NR	Pyramidal tract syndrome	Halo traction and RH resection	Yes	NR	Yes
Mukhtar et al. 2005 [7]	10m	1	Yes	No	Back pain induced by movements; weakness and shock-like feeling in Rt LL on direct pressure of Rt side of torso; gradual	Posterior partial rib resection with RH left in situ; 2nd op: posterior in situ fusion (T6–T11)	No	Due to IOM changes the RH was left in situ and the rest of the Rib was excised	Yes

Table 1: Continued.

Author	Age (range)/sex	Dislocated ribs [N of ribs (N of patients)]	Cord impingement	Other lesions present	Preoperative neurology	Operation details	Rib heads resection	Complications after 1st operation	Neurology recovery
Gkiokas et al. 2006 [8]	13f	1	Yes	No	B/L Babinski, clonus, weakness in LL (foot drop), decreased sensation, HR, and daytime micturition; "painful rib hump" symptoms	Posterior decompression and resection of the RH, PSF	Yes	No	Yes
Yalcin et al. 2008 [2]	14m	2	No	Yes	No	Posterior laminectomy and PSF	Yes	No	n/a
	12f	2	Contact	Yes	No	Posterior laminectomy and PSF	No	No	n/a
	6m	2	No	NR	No	Anterior 5 level annulotomy and resection of T10 and T11 ribs; RH left in situ; growing rod construct	No	No	n/a
Cappella et al. 2008 [3]	14m	1	Yes	NR	Gradual weakness in lower limbs	Staged posterior instrumented and anterior SF with casting; revision: posterior decompression	No	Progression of deformity	Yes
	14m	2	No	Yes	Back pain, knee and ankle HR, and clonus and "painful rib hump" like symptoms	T4 laminectomy and posterior fusion and instrumentation	Yes	NR	NR
Ton et al. 2010 [4]	11f	1	Yes	No	No	Multilevel discectomies, T9 laminectomy, RH resection, and PSF	Yes	NR	n/a
	11m	1	No	No	No	T9 laminectomy, ASF, and PSF and 9th RH resection	Yes	NR	n/a
	9f	1	Yes	Yes	Back pain, R foot weakness, and B/L LL HR and clonus	Resection of neurofibroma and 6th RH, PSF, & ASF	Yes	NR	NR
Abdulian et al. 2011 [6]	14m	2	Yes	No	No	1st op: posterior T5 hemilaminectomy and T5/6 facetectomy, 2nd op: posterior T6 hemilaminectomy and T6/7 facetectomy; 3rd op: anterior T4–T9 release, and 4th op: T2–L3 instrumented PSF	Yes	The 2nd op was because the next intracanal protruding rib was missed	n/a

TABLE 1: Continued.

Author	Age (range)/sex	Dislocated ribs [N of ribs (N of patients)]	Cord impingement	Other lesions present	Preoperative neurology	Operation details	Rib heads resection	Complications after 1st operation	Neurology recovery
Krishnakumar and Renjitkumar 2012 [22]	1f	2	NR	NR	NR	PSF	Yes	NR	NR
Sun et al. 2013 [11]	13, 4f/2m	NR	NR	NR	No	SPOs and posterior correction with PSF	No	No	n/a
Mao et al. 2015 [10]*	13 (8–33), 10f:9m	1 (12), 2 (6), 3 (1)	NR	NR	No	The posterior correction could be alone or adjunct with perioperative traction and occasionally supplemented with SPO; the anterior stage could include anterior release or convex growth arrest or ASF. 13 posterior only and 6 anterior & posterior	No	NR	n/a

This table shows all published studies in the English literature to date, which are reporting on the management of intracanal rib head dislocation in neurofibromatosis type 1 dystrophic curves; level of evidence (LoE) V, * case series: (LoE) IV, PSF: posterior spinal fusion, RH: rib heads, and LL: lower limbs. Op: operation.

to the cord. Also, there is still no strong evidence in the literature to suggest a direct injury to the cord by a remaining RH stump. The subsequent prone position and the posterior facetectomies may have contributed to a degree of spinal instability and alteration of the kyphoscoliotic angle. Also, the change in alignment with translation of the spinal cord towards the convexity may have produced compression by the penetrating RH. Furthermore, the RH, having lost its lateral stabilizers due to the thoracotomy and rib resection, might have adopted a new medial position further impinging on the cord. Similar to our second case, it may be safer to relieve the cord from the RH compression, prior to any release or correction, which will change the relationships in the acute kyphos.

We postulate that the flail RH, left in the spinal canal following a rib-only resection, may be risky, because it loses the stability provided by the rib cage and because it may potentially change position. Secondly the loose RH will not reduce by ligamentotaxis during translational correction manoeuvres. In cases where the RH remains unresectable, because of cord adherence, translational correction manoeuvres should probably be avoided. We also believe that even asymptomatic cases without gross MRI cord signal changes should still be investigated for subtle signs of cord impairment, which might render it vulnerable during correction manoeuvres.

Even though the intracanal RH dislocation is a well-documented manifestation of the NF kyphoscoliosis, its severe form is not frequent enough for any conclusion to be supported by large number of cases. However, the conclusion is reasonable and is in line with the experience presented in all reports on the same topic in the literature. Preoperatively, we would suggest a thorough clinical investigation for cord impairment signs ("painful rib hump," Lhermitte's-like, etc.) and precise imaging for the intracanal RH position in relation to the cord. We would recommend excision of the RH, if in close proximity to the spinal cord, prior to attempting anterior spinal release or posterior correction manoeuvres. This sequence will also aid in the correct identification of the cause of a possible intraoperative IOM event.

5. Conclusion

Rib head intracanal dislocation is a dystrophic feature of patients with NF1 scoliotic curves. The protruding part of the rib although usually asymptomatic may cause neurological impairment by impinging on the spinal cord.

Provoked neurological signs should be sought during clinical examination in order to identify any cord dysfunction. CT and MRI scans should be performed to diagnose the extent of rib head penetration or cord involvement and to assist in surgical planning.

Decompression of the spinal cord by resecting the impinging bony part, even in the absence of neurological symptoms, is advised before any attempt to release or correct the deformity. This strategy seems to be the safest and will aid the surgeon and the neurophysiologist in discriminating the cause of possible positive IOM events during surgery.

Competing Interests

The authors did not receive grants or outside funding in support of their research or preparation of this paper. They did not receive payments or other benefits or a commitment or agreement to provide such benefits from a commercial entity. They have declared that no commercial entity paid, or directed, or agreed to pay or direct, any benefits to any research fund, foundation, educational institution, or other charitable or nonprofit organizations with which the authors are affiliated or associated.

References

[1] A. I. Tsirikos, A. Saifuddin, and M. H. Noordeen, "Spinal deformity in neurofibromatosis type-1: diagnosis and treatment," *European Spine Journal*, vol. 14, no. 5, pp. 427–439, 2005.

[2] N. Yalcin, E. Bar-on, and M. Yazici, "Impingement of spinal cord by dislocated rib in dystrophic scoliosis secondary to neurofibromatosis type 1: radiological signs and management strategies," *Spine*, vol. 33, no. 23, pp. E881–E886, 2008.

[3] M. Cappella, N. Bettini, E. Dema, M. Girardo, and S. Cervellati, "Late post-operative paraparesis after rib penetration of the spinal canal in a patient with neurofibromatous scoliosis," *Journal of Orthopaedics and Traumatology*, vol. 9, no. 3, pp. 163–166, 2008.

[4] J. Ton, R. Stein-Wexler, P. Yen, and M. Gupta, "Rib head protrusion into the central canal in type 1 neurofibromatosis," *Pediatric Radiology*, vol. 40, no. 12, pp. 1902–1909, 2010.

[5] K. I. Khoshhal and R. D. Ellis, "Paraparesis after posterior spinal fusion in neurofibromatosis secondary to rib displacement: case report and literature review," *Journal of Pediatric Orthopaedics*, vol. 20, no. 6, pp. 799–801, 2000.

[6] M. H. Abdulian, R. W. Liu, J. P. Son-Hing, G. H. Thompson, and D. G. Armstrong, "Double rib penetration of the spinal canal in a patient with neurofibromatosis," *Journal of Pediatric Orthopaedics*, vol. 31, no. 1, pp. 6–10, 2011.

[7] I. A. Mukhtar, M. Letts, and K. Kontio, "Spinal cord impingement by a displaced rib in scoliosis due to neurofibromatosis," *Canadian Journal of Surgery*, vol. 48, no. 5, pp. 414–415, 2005.

[8] A. Gkiokas, S. Hadzimichalis, E. Vasiliadis, M. Katsalouli, and G. Kannas, "Painful rib hump: a new clinical sign for detecting intraspinal rib displacement in scoliosis due to neurofibromatosis," *Scoliosis*, vol. 1, no. 1, article 10, pp. 1–4, 2006.

[9] M. Deguchi, N. Kawakami, H. Saito, K. Arao, K. Mimatsu, and H. Iwata, "Paraparesis after rib penetration of the spinal canal in neurofibromatous scoliosis," *Journal of Spinal Disorders*, vol. 8, no. 5, pp. 363–367, 1995.

[10] S. Mao, B. Shi, S. Wang et al., "Migration of the penetrated rib head following deformity correction surgery without rib head excision in dystrophic scoliosis secondary to type 1 Neurofibromatosis," *European Spine Journal*, vol. 24, no. 7, pp. 1502–1509, 2015.

[11] D. Sun, F. Dai, Y. Y. Liu, and J.-Z. Xu, "Posterior-only spinal fusion without rib head resection for treating type I neurofibromatosis with intracanal rib head dislocation," *Clinics*, vol. 68, no. 12, pp. 1521–1527, 2013.

[12] B. M. Flood, W. P. Butt, and R. A. Dickson, "Rib penetration of the intervertebral foraminae in neurofibromatosis," *Spine*, vol. 11, no. 2, pp. 172–174, 1986.

[13] M. R. Major and B. A. Huizenga, "Spinal cord compression by displaced ribs in neurofibromatosis. A report of three cases," *Journal of Bone and Joint Surgery—Series A*, vol. 70, no. 7, pp. 1100–1102, 1988.

[14] M. G. Lykissas, E. K. Schorry, A. H. Crawford, S. Gaines, M. Rieley, and V. V. Jain, "Does the presence of dystrophic features in patients with type 1 neurofibromatosis and spinal deformities increase the risk of surgery?" *Spine*, vol. 38, no. 18, pp. 1595–1601, 2013.

[15] J. N. Dacher, S. Zakine, M. Monroc, D. Eurin, J. Lechevallier, and P. Le Dosseur, "Rib displacement threatening the spinal cord in a scoliotic child with neurofibromatosis," *Pediatric Radiology*, vol. 25, no. 1, pp. 58–59, 1995.

[16] A. H. Crawford, "Neurofibromatosis," in *The Pediatric Spine: Principles and Practice*, S. L. Weinstein, Ed., pp. 471–490, Lippincott Williams & Wilkins, Philadelphia, Pa, USA, 2001.

[17] Y. L. Leung, M. Grevitt, L. Henderson, and J. Smith, "Cord monitoring changes and segmental vessel ligation in the 'at risk' cord during anterior spinal deformity surgery," *Spine*, vol. 30, no. 16, pp. 1870–1874, 2005.

[18] G. Cheh, L. G. Lenke, A. M. Padberg et al., "Loss of spinal cord monitoring signals in children during thoracic kyphosis correction with spinal osteotomy: why does it occur and what should you do?" *Spine*, vol. 33, no. 10, pp. 1093–1099, 2008.

[19] K. Shimizu, M. Nakamura, Y. Nishikawa, S. Hijikata, K. Chiba, and Y. Toyama, "Spinal kyphosis causes demyelination and neuronal loss in the spinal cord: a new model of kyphotic deformity using juvenile Japanese small game fowls," *Spine*, vol. 30, no. 21, pp. 2388–2392, 2005.

[20] S. V. Kamath, P. K. Kleinman, R. L. Ragland et al., "Intraspinal dislocation of the rib in neurofibromatosis: a case report," *Pediatric Radiology*, vol. 25, no. 7, pp. 538–539, 1995.

[21] B. Legrand, G. Filipe, A. Blamoutier, N. Khouri, and P. Mary, "Intraspinal rib penetration in four patients in neurofibromatosis vertebral deformities," *Revue de Chirurgie Orthopédique et Réparatrice de L'appareil Moteu*, vol. 89, no. 1, pp. 57–61, 2003.

[22] R. Krishnakumar and J. Renjitkumar, "Teaching Neuro*Images*: rib penciling and intraspinal dislocation of rib heads in type 1 neurofibromatosis," *Neurology*, vol. 78, no. 13, article e85, 2012.

6

Spontaneous Regression of Herniated Lumbar Disc with New Disc Protrusion in the Adjacent Level

Tayfun Hakan[1,2] and Serkan Gürcan[3]

[1]The Vocational School of Health Services, Okan University, 34959 Tuzla, Turkey
[2]Neurosurgery Clinic, International Kolan Hospital, Şişli, Istanbul, Turkey
[3]İstanbul Gelişim University, Avcılar, 34315 İstanbul, Turkey

Correspondence should be addressed to Tayfun Hakan; tayfunhakan@yahoo.com

Academic Editor: Ali F. Ozer

Spontaneous regression of herniated lumbar discs was reported occasionally. The mechanisms proposed for regression of disc herniation are still incomplete. This paper describes and discusses a case of spontaneous regression of herniated lumbar discs with a new disc protrusion in the adjacent level. A 41-year-old man was admitted with radiating pain and numbness in the left lower extremity with a left posterolateral disc extrusion at L5-S1 level. He was admitted to hospital with low back pain due to disc herniation caudally immigrating at L4-5 level three years ago. He refused the surgical intervention that was offered and was treated conservatively at that time. He had no neurological deficit and a history of spontaneous regression of the extruded lumbar disc; so, a conservative therapy, including bed rest, physical therapy, nonsteroidal anti-inflammatory drugs, and analgesics, was advised. In conclusion, herniated lumbar disc fragments may regress spontaneously. Reports are prone to advise conservative treatment for extruded or sequestrated lumbar disc herniations. However, these patients should be followed up closely; new herniation at adjacent/different level may occur. Furthermore, it is important to know which herniated disk should be removed and which should be treated conservatively, because disc herniation may cause serious complications as muscle weakness and cauda equine syndrome.

1. Introduction

Lumbar disc herniation continues to be a common health problem by decreasing the life quality and limiting the functions of the musculoskeletal system. Medical or surgical treatment can be chosen according to the clinical signs and symptoms of the patients. In some cases, spontaneous regression of herniated lumbar disc, protruded, extruded, or sequestrated, can be seen. It is a well-known phenomenon since Guinto et al. [1] demonstrated it as the first time in 1983. Examples of this rare condition, disappearance of herniated discs, were reported occasionally [2–4]. The symptoms of the patients may improve and they may return to their active life with the spontaneous absorption of the disc material. Spontaneous regression of lumbar disc herniation and a new disc protrusion in adjacent level is an exceptional condition that was reported only once in the literature [5]. Recurrence or reherniation of intervertebral disc is a common complication; but a new herniation in different segment without any recurrence is unusual. It is clear that the underlying mechanisms of disc herniation and resorption processes are very complex; as the factors cause a new disc herniation in adjacent level, the regeneration and/or reparation systems of the previously disturbed spine segment resist strongly reherniation.

Here, an additional case of a patient who experienced a new extruded lumbar disc herniation following the resorption of the previous herniation at the adjacent level is presented.

2. Case Presentation

A 41-year-old man was admitted with ten-day history of radiating pain and numbness in the left lower extremity.

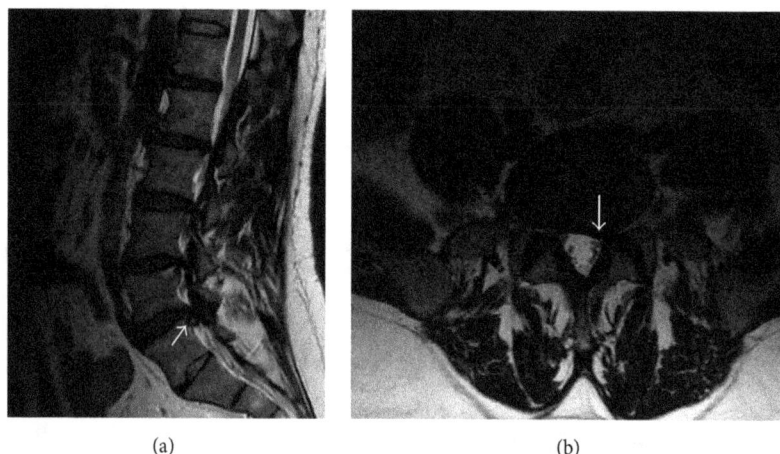

(a)   (b)

FIGURE 1: An extruded disc herniation that slightly migrated downward at L5-S1 level on T2 weighted sagittal (a) and axial (b) MR images after 3 years.

Neurological examination showed no abnormality except a positive left straight leg raising test. The Visual Analog Scale (VAS) for pain was noted as seven. Lumbar magnetic resonance imaging (MRI) revealed a left posterolateral disc extrusion at L5-S1 level (Figure 1). He said that he was admitted initially to another hospital with low back and radiating pain in both of his legs three years ago. According to him, his pain was nearly the same as that of the previous admission where he experienced low back and radiating pain in both of his legs three years ago; but he had low back and radiating pain only in his left leg for this time. Unfortunately, we were not able to reach his previous neurological records; but a huge extruded lumbar disc herniation that was caudally immigrating was found at L4-5 level when his initial MRI was examined (Figure 2). He had refused the surgical intervention that was offered and was treated conservatively with bed rest, nonsteroidal anti-inflammatory drugs, and analgesics nearly for three months at that time by our colleagues. He said that he was nearly symptom-free until the onset of new low back and left leg pain approximately for two and half years. The patient was a tradesman working on a table and defined no remarkable heavy physical stress upon a few months previous to his second involvement. A conservative therapy, including bed rest, physical therapy, nonsteroidal anti-inflammatory drugs, and analgesics was advised, because he had no neurological deficit and a history of spontaneous regression of the extruded lumbar disc.

3. Discussion

Lumbar disc herniation is one of the most common causes of low back pain and/or extremity radicular syndrome. Conservative management, including bed rest, oral anti-inflammatory and analgesics, spinal anesthetic blocks, and/or physical therapy, is recommended for treatment of lumbar disc herniations [6]. In the absence of symptom resolution in two months, or presence of cauda equine syndrome, muscle weakness, or progressive deficit while being medically managed, surgical intervention is advised [7]. The great potential

for regression of disc herniations has been occasionally reported [2, 4–6] and it leads to questioning of the choosing the treatment modality.

Although extensive documentations are found in the literature, the mechanisms proposed for regression of disc herniation are still incomplete [4, 8]. Dehydration within the nucleus pulposus and shrinkage, a mechanical retraction of herniated material back into the annulus fibrosus, and enzymatic degradation and phagocytic reduction via immunohistologic mediators are three popular mechanisms assumed in the literature. The second mechanism, mechanical retraction of the herniated disc, is a theoretical assumption expected to occur when the disc herniation protrudes through the annulus fibrosus by protecting anatomical relation. Third mechanism which has been studied by many authors depends on a series of inflammatory responses of autoimmune system, including neovascularization, production of matrix proteinase, increasing of cytokine levels, enzymatic degradation, and macrophage phagocytosis [1, 4, 6, 9, 10].

A mass of intervertebral disc herniation may be classified as protruded, extruded, or sequestrated that represents free fragments. Sequestrated and/or large disc fragments were found to be the most regressed herniations. [4, 6, 8]. Epidural vascular supply was suspected to be an important role for regression of the extruded disc fragments through the ruptured posterior longitudinal ligament. Splendiani et al. [11] reported that herniations with high signal intensity on T2 weighted MRI sequences and free fragment were regressed in 85.18% and 100% of the cases. However, in the presented study, the herniated disc was not a free fragment and it did not have high signal density, and it had a thick anatomical relation with the intervertebral disc material.

Gürkanlar et al. [5] reported spontaneous regression of two lumbar herniations at different levels and times in the same patient. The extruded L5-S1 disc was spontaneously regressed in three years and the extruded disc was regressed after one year. In the presented study, the new herniation has occurred in the inferior level after three years. In both of these cases, spine repaired and protected the previously

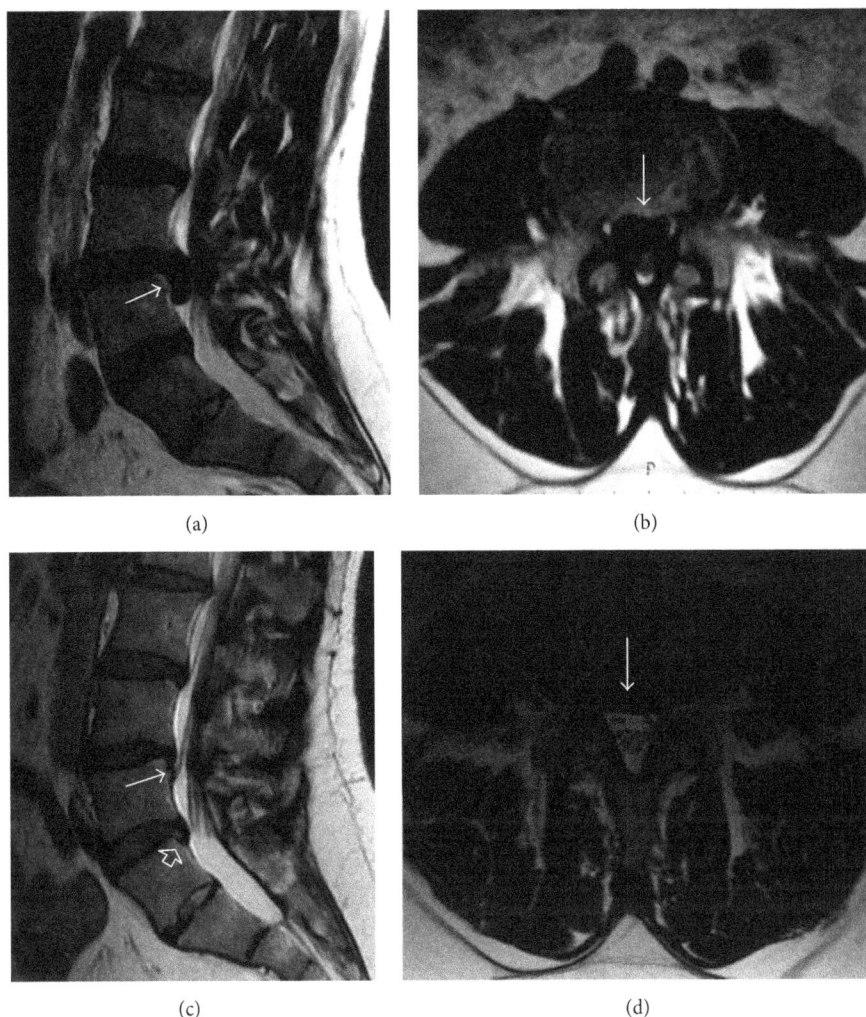

FIGURE 2: (a) A huge extruded disc herniation that migrated caudally (white arrow) at L4-5 level on T2 weighted sagittal lumbar MR images. (b) Axial view of the same disc, extruded disc occupying nearly half of the spinal canal. (c and d) The extruded disc has disappeared completely (white arrows) in sagittal and axial MR images after three years; the height of the disc space slightly decreased at L4-5 level and there was no sign of compression. The protrusion of L5-S1 disc (arrow head) that will be obvious in the left sagittal images.

herniated disc side so strongly that the factors leading to new herniations in adjacent levels did not affect them.

4. Conclusion

It is very important to know which herniated disk should be removed, because lumbar disc herniation is not purely innocent. Gene therapy, growth factor injection, cell-based therapies, and tissue engineering approaches are among the novel strategies developed for degeneration and regeneration problems of the intervertebral disc [12]. In the future, this sort of research for intervertebral disc regenerative therapies may contribute to understanding of the mechanisms underlying the regression of protruded disc herniation and may help choose the appropriate treatment for the patients. Until that time, it is still wise to wait for surgical treatment in patients with herniated lumber disc diseases that have nearly normal neurological findings and tolerable pain.

Competing Interests

The authors declared that there are no competing interests between them.

References

[1] F. C. Guinto Jr., H. Hashim, and M. Stumer, "CT demonstration of disk regression after conservative therapy," *American Journal of Neuroradiology*, vol. 5, no. 5, pp. 632–633, 1984.

[2] A. R. Gezici and R. Ergün, "Spontaneous regression of a huge subligamentous extruded disc herniation: short report of an illustrative case," *Acta Neurochirurgica*, vol. 151, no. 10, pp. 1299–1300, 2009.

[3] J. V. Martínez-Quiñones, J. Aso-Escario, F. Consolini, and R. Arregui-Calvo, "Spontaneous regression from intervertebral disc herniation. Propos of a series of 37 cases," *Neurocirugia*, vol. 21, no. 2, pp. 108–117, 2010.

[4] T. Orief, Y. Orz, W. Attia, and K. Almusrea, "Spontaneous resorption of sequestrated intervertebral disc herniation," *World Neurosurgery*, vol. 77, no. 1, pp. 146–152, 2012.

[5] D. Gürkanlar, A. Aciduman, H. Koçak, and A. Günaydin, "Spontaneous regression of lumbar disc herniations at different levels and times in a patient: A case report," *Turkish Neurosurgery*, vol. 15, no. 1, pp. 18–22, 2005.

[6] M. Macki, M. Hernandez-Hermann, M. Bydon, A. Gokaslan, K. McGovern, and A. Bydon, "Spontaneous regression of sequestrated lumbar disc herniations: literature review," *Clinical Neurology and Neurosurgery*, vol. 120, pp. 136–141, 2014.

[7] G. Rahmathulla and K. Kamian, "Lumbar disc herniations 'to operate or not' patient selection and timing of surgery," *Korean Journal of Spine*, vol. 11, no. 4, pp. 255–257, 2014.

[8] E. S. Kim, A. O. Oladunjoye, J. A. Li, and K. D. Kim, "Spontaneous regression of herniated lumbar discs," *Journal of Clinical Neuroscience*, vol. 21, no. 6, pp. 909–913, 2014.

[9] A. Geiss, K. Larsson, B. Rydevik, I. Takahashi, and K. Olmarker, "Autoimmune properties of nucleus pulposus: an experimental study in pigs," *Spine*, vol. 32, no. 2, pp. 168–173, 2007.

[10] A. Tsarouhas, G. Soufla, P. Katonis, D. Pasku, A. Vakis, and D. A. Spandidos, "Transcript levels of major MMPs and ADAMTS-4 in relation to the clinicopathological profile of patients with lumbar disc herniation," *European Spine Journal*, vol. 20, no. 5, pp. 781–790, 2011.

[11] A. Splendiani, E. Puglielli, R. De Amicis, A. Barile, C. Masciocchi, and M. Gallucci, "Spontaneous resolution of lumbar disk herniation: predictive signs for prognostic evaluation," *Neuroradiology*, vol. 46, no. 11, pp. 916–922, 2004.

[12] M. Molinos, C. R. Almeida, J. Caldeira, C. Cunha, R. M. Gonçalves, and M. A. Barbosa, "Inflammation in intervertebral disc degeneration and regeneration," *Journal of the Royal Society Interface*, vol. 12, no. 104, Article ID 20141191, 2015.

7

Open and Arthroscopic with Mini-Open Surgical Hip Approaches for Treatment of Pigmented Villonodular Synovitis and Concomitant Hip Pathology

Bridget Ellsworth[1] and Atul F. Kamath[2]

[1]*Perelman School of Medicine, University of Pennsylvania, Philadelphia, PA, USA*
[2]*Department of Orthopaedic Surgery, Perelman School of Medicine, University of Pennsylvania, Philadelphia, PA, USA*

Correspondence should be addressed to Atul F. Kamath; akamath@post.harvard.edu

Academic Editor: John Nyland

Background. Pigmented villonodular synovitis (PVNS) is a rare benign tumor affecting large joints and prompts excision to prevent local destruction of the joint. The purpose of this case report is to describe two differing surgical approaches for management of PVNS of the hip in patients requiring concomitant treatment for additional hip pathology. *Methods.* This report discusses the presentation, clinical and radiographic findings, and operative management of two contrasting cases of PVNS of the hip. Case 1 describes a 31-year-old female with localized PVNS in addition to a labral tear treated with arthroscopic labral repair followed by tumor excision via a mini-open incision. Case 2 describes a 29-year-old male with more diffuse PVNS in addition to a cam deformity managed with open surgical dislocation of the hip, tumor excision, and restoration of the femoral head/neck junction. *Results.* This report demonstrates two cases of successful excision of PVNS of the hip in addition to addressing concomitant hip pathology in both cases. *Conclusions.* Open surgical dislocation of the hip or arthroscopic surgery with a mini-open incision may be used in appropriately selected patients to successfully excise PVNS lesions in addition to addressing concomitant hip pathology.

1. Introduction

Pigmented villonodular synovitis (PVNS) is a rare benign proliferation of synovium involving the joints, bursae, or tendon sheaths [1]. PVNS is generally monoarticular and affects 1.8 patients per million per year; the hip is involved in 15% of cases [2, 3]. Although the origin of PVNS is unknown, it exhibits neoplastic characteristics such as chromosomal anomalies, local tissue invasion, and, rarely, malignant transformation [4]. PVNS may require early surgical excision to limit this local tissue invasion and subsequent joint destruction.

Lesional excision and synovectomy is the treatment of choice for PVNS and can be performed through an open or arthroscopic approach [3]. While the literature on surgical treatment of PVNS of the hip is limited and comprised mainly of case reports, recent studies suggest that arthroscopic techniques can be used safely in carefully selected patients

for the excision of PVNS tumors [5–7]. However, if exposure to the lesion is inadequate with arthroscopic techniques or additional hip pathology is present that cannot be addressed using arthroscopy alone, an open technique remains the preferred method of PVNS excision.

The unique aspect of this case report is that both described patients with PVNS lesions required additional treatment for hip pathology beyond tumor excision alone. The purpose of this article is to describe two differing surgical approaches for management of PVNS of the hip in patients requiring concomitant treatment for additional hip pathology. Case 1 describes a patient with PVNS and a labral tear treated with tumor excision through a mini-open incision following arthroscopic labral repair. Case 2 describes a patient with PVNS and a cam deformity managed with open surgical dislocation of the hip, tumor excision, and restoration of the femoral head/neck junction.

2. Case Report

2.1. Case 1. A 31-year-old woman with a history of right hip developmental dysplasia (DDH) presented with insidious onset of right hip pain, present for several years but significantly worsening over the year prior to presentation. The pain was exacerbated by prolonged sitting and walking and was associated with popping of the hip. Her physical exam was notable for a positive right anterior impingement sign and pain in the right groin exacerbated with log roll, Stinchfield, resisted psoas, and fan kick maneuvers.

Initial radiographs revealed right hip dysplasia and stigmata of femoroacetabular impingement (FAI), with the right hip exhibiting a cross-over sign (Figures 1(a) and 1(b)). Magnetic resonance (MRI) arthrogram revealed a tumor, 2.5 × 1.3 × 0.8 cm in dimension (anterior-posterior × transverse × craniocaudal) and of intermediate to low signal focus within the inferomedial aspect of the right hip joint. In addition, there was a complex tear of the anterior and anterosuperior acetabular labrum (Figure 1). The tumor raised suspicion for PVNS.

After discussion of the treatment options, the patient elected to undergo right hip arthroscopy with labral repair and possible mini-open incision for mass excision. The patient understood the likelihood of persistent dysplasia requiring osteotomy surgery at a later date after initial management of the tumor.

During the surgery, anterolateral and mid anterior portals were established with the right leg in traction. The labrum was repaired arthroscopically with suture anchor fixation.

The mass within the right hip joint was deemed inaccessible through the arthroscope and rather removed safely and en bloc via a separate mini-open incision along the Smith-Peterson interval. This approach has been described previously for treatment of FAI [8, 9]. An incision was made, starting approximately 2 cm lateral and 1 cm distal to the anterior-superior iliac spine, extending diagonally in line with the muscle belly of the tensor. This incision incorporated the previous mid-anterior portal established during arthroscopy.

The mass was located in the posterior-inferior aspect of the capsule. The nodular mass and stalk were excised sharply en bloc (Figure 2) and sent for formal pathologic analysis, which confirmed the presence of PVNS.

The capsule, fascia over the TFL, subcutaneous tissue, and skin were then closed in separate layers along with the portal sites. A sterile dressing was placed over the hip, and a HipRAP was applied for gentle compression. The patient's weight-bearing was protected postoperatively, and a labral repair hip arthroscopy physical therapy protocol was initiated, along with use of a continuous passive motion (CPM) machine.

2.2. Case 2. A 29-year-old male presented with left groin pain that began in adolescence but had been worsening over a two-year period. The pain was exacerbated with activities and was associated with locking and catching, with a history of a number of severe locking episodes in which he was unable to walk for several minutes. Physical exam was notable for pain in the left groin with passive hip rotation, as well as restrictions in range of motion. Outside hospital radiographs

were largely unremarkable but did reveal a left-sided cam deformity (Figure 3). A MRI revealed a multilobulated lesion measuring approximately 4.0 × 1.1 × 3.4 cm within the posterior/inferior aspect of the hip joint, with an associated large joint effusion (Figure 3). A computed tomography- (CT-) guided fine-needle aspiration was consistent with PVNS.

The patient elected to undergo a surgical dislocation of the left hip with mass excision and labral/chondral treatment, as an arthroscopic approach or anterior mini-open incision would likely not provide adequate circumferential hip access for excision of the large mass tethering the inferior femoral neck.

With the patient under general anesthesia, a surgical dislocation of the left hip was performed using the technique described by Ganz et al. [10] (Figure 4). The synovial mass was excised en bloc down to the stalk (Figure 4). The stalk was also excised and cauterized.

In addition to removal of the mass, the femoral head/neck junction was reshaped due to the presence of a cam deformity. Using a combination of osteotomes and a burr, the gentle waist of the femoral head and neck junction was reconstituted. Offset templates were used to verify extent of decompression needed. The retinacular vessels were identified and protected at all times, and gentle continuous irrigation was performed to exposed cartilage surfaces of the acetabulum and femur throughout. Bone wax was applied to the exposed bony surfaces after offset correction. The hip was reduced, and a very nice labral seal could be seen through the peripheral compartment.

The labrum was well reduced and stable onto the bony rim. The capsulotomy was closed without undue tension and with partial thickness (nonarticular sided) bites in interrupted fashion. The trochanteric flip osteotomy was reduced and fixed with screws. The trochanteric bursa was closed over the screws, and the subvastus approach to the femur was closed. The patient's weight-bearing was protected immediately postoperatively, and a surgical hip dislocation postoperative protocol was followed.

3. Discussion

The authors report two contrasting cases of PVNS of the hip in addition to concomitant hip pathology treated successfully using different approaches. While both lesions were located in the posterior-inferior aspect of the capsule, the patient's tumor in Case 1 was smaller and easily accessible via a mini-open approach following labral repair via hip arthroscopy, obviating the need for a larger incision. The patient's mass in Case 2 was larger and would have been difficult to visualize and excise using a minimally invasive approach. Furthermore, treatment of the large cam deformity could be performed concurrently through the open dislocation approach.

While PVNS is a benign lesion, it can be locally invasive and destructive and may require complete removal to minimize risk of recurrence. Thus, the patient in Case 2 elected for a more extensive procedure with surgical dislocation of the hip in order to ensure complete excision of the tumor.

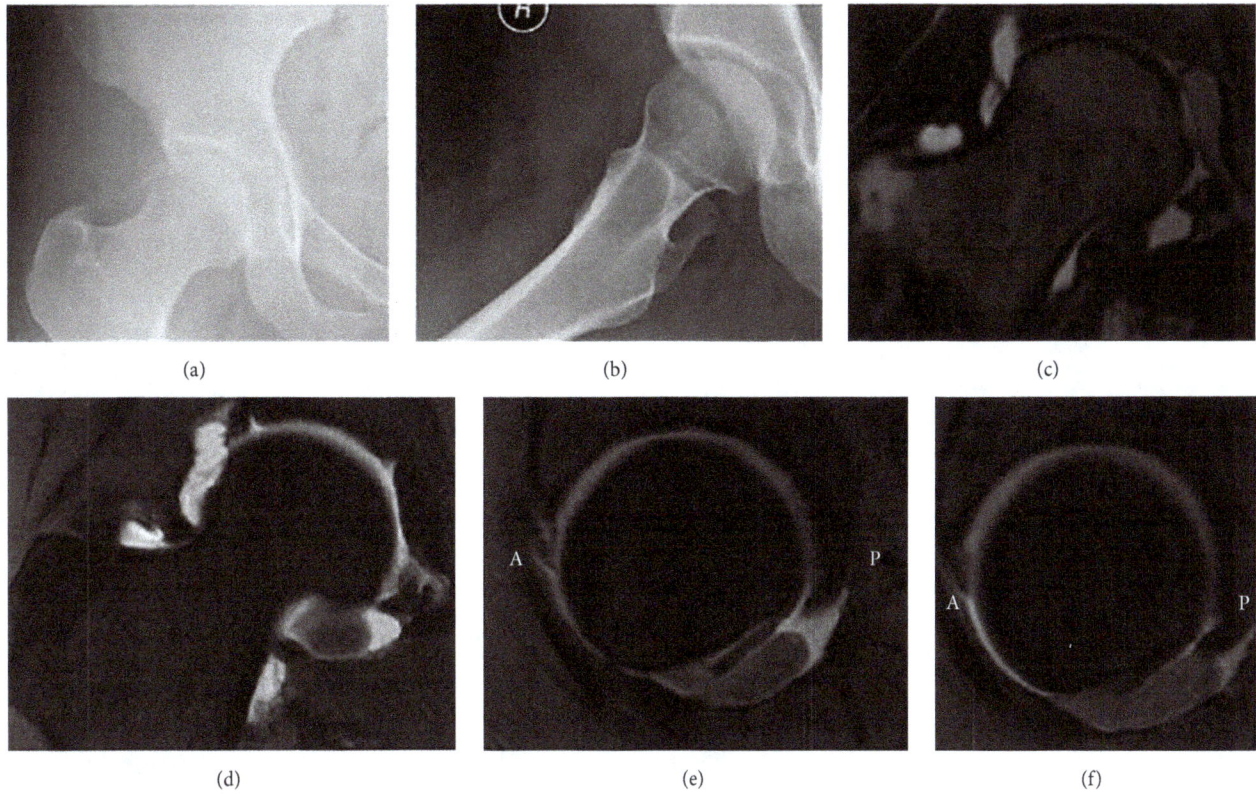

FIGURE 1: Preoperative anteroposterior (a) and frog-leg radiographs (b) of the right hip in Case 1 demonstrate developmental dysplasia of the hip and the presence of a cross-over sign. Preoperative coronal FIESTA 3D (c), coronal T1-weighted fat-saturated (d), and sagittal proton-density fat-saturated (e, f) magnetic resonance sequences with intra-articular contrast reveal the tumor, a 2.5 cm intermediate to low signal focus within the inferomedial aspect of the right hip joint, in addition to a complex tear of the right anterior and anterosuperior acetabular labrum. A = anterior; P = posterior.

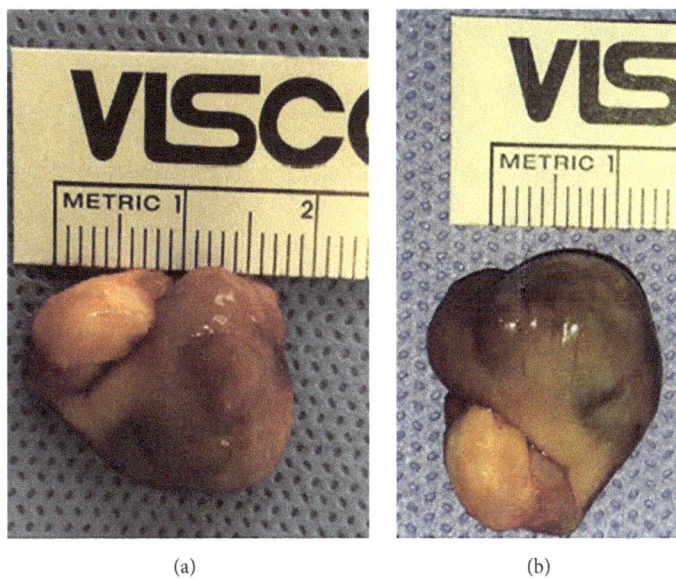

FIGURE 2: Gross pathology of PVNS from Case 1 (a, b), excised en bloc from the posterior-inferior aspect of the capsule and confirmed to be PVNS on formal pathological analysis.

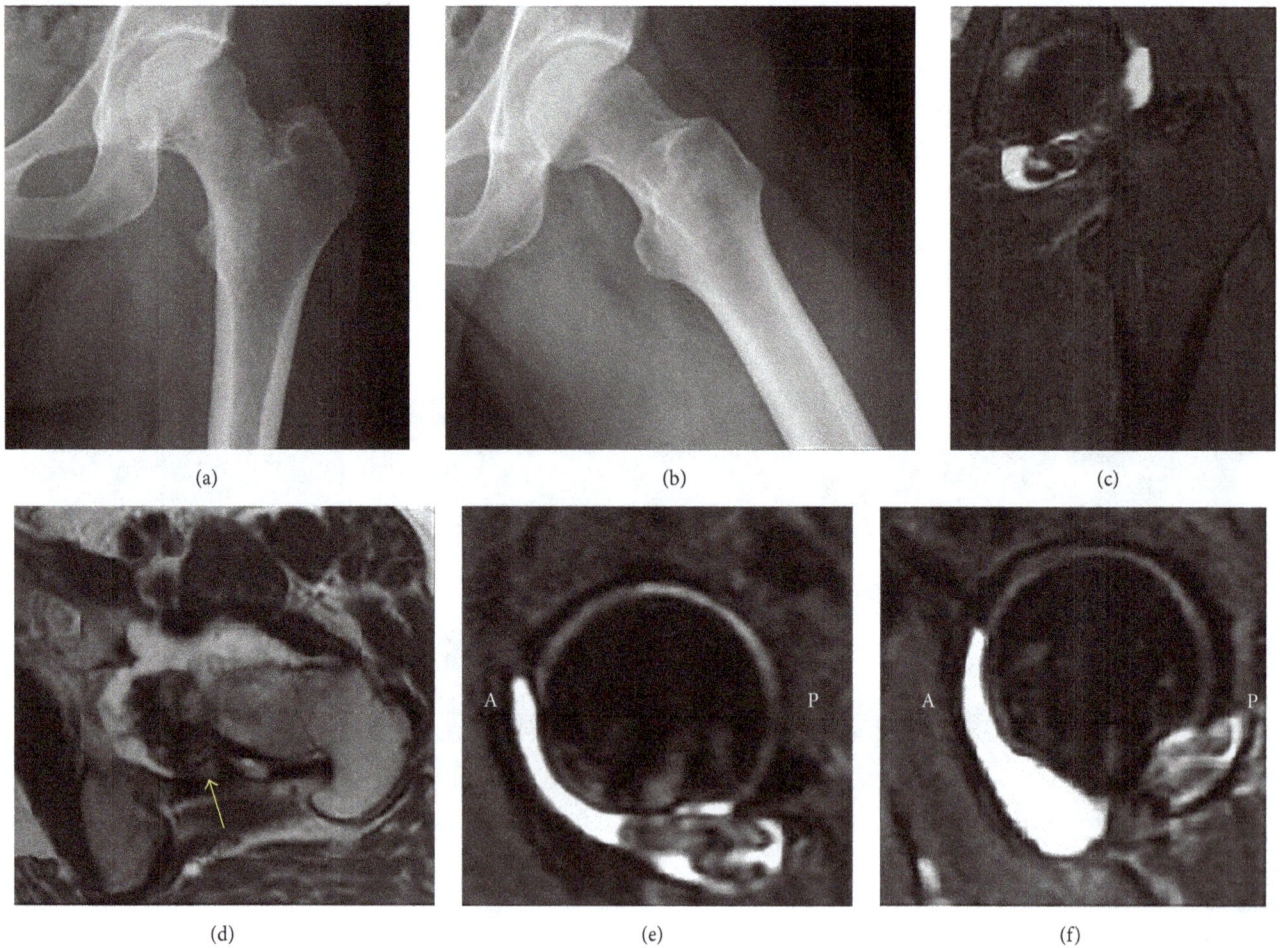

FIGURE 3: Preoperative anteroposterior (a) and frog-leg radiographs (b) of the left hip in Case 2 demonstrate a cam deformity. Preoperative coronal T2-weighted fat-saturated (c), axial T2-weighted (d), and sagittal T2-weighted fat-saturated (e, f) magnetic resonance sequences with intravenous contrast reveal a multilobulated low signal lesion (arrow in d) measuring approximately $4.0 \times 1.1 \times 3.4$ cm within the posterior/inferior aspect of the hip joint, with an associated large joint effusion. A = anterior; P = posterior.

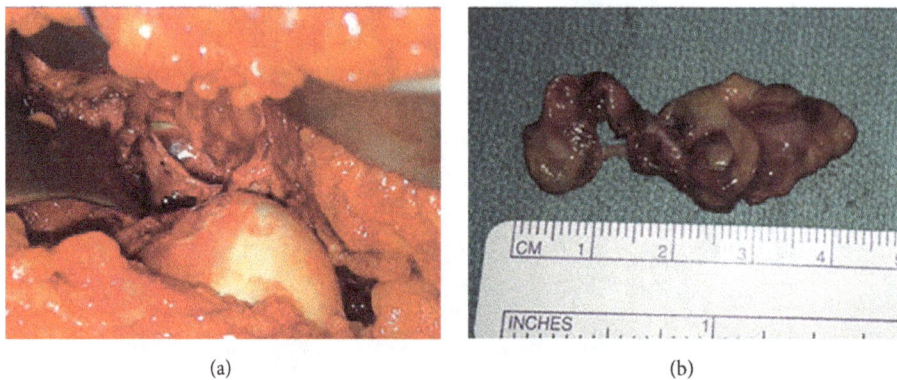

FIGURE 4: Intraoperative image of a surgical dislocation of the left hip in Case 2, which allowed for adequate exposure to visualize and excise the mass (a). Gross pathology of the tumor from the same case is depicted (b), excised en bloc from the posterior-inferior aspect of the capsule and confirmed to be PVNS on formal pathological analysis.

Additionally, both patients had concomitant hip pathology that required attention and treatment at the time of surgery.

This report demonstrates that PVNS of the hip must be managed on a case-by-case basis, as multiple factors, such as size and location of the lesion as well as additional hip pathology, can influence surgical management. A recent report by Shoji et al. describes two young patients (<30 years old) with advanced PVNS of the hip, both with evidence of radiographic joint-space narrowing at the time of presentation [11]. Instead of performing a combined synovectomy and arthroplasty, the authors opted for a joint-preserving procedure in these young patients. Both patients had areas of cartilage loss over weight-bearing aspects of the femoral head. In each patient they performed a synovectomy, a transtrochanteric rotational osteotomy (TRO) to transfer an area of femoral head with remaining cartilage to a weight-bearing area, and microfracture of areas with residual osteochondral lesions. In one patient autologous osteochondral transplantation (AOT) was also used for three areas of full-thickness cartilage defect. Both patients had similar good outcomes postoperatively at 2- and 2.5-year follow-up with no PVNS recurrence and minimal symptoms.

Both arthroscopic and open procedures have been successful in preventing recurrence of PVNS of the hip [3, 5]. However, Vastel et al. described a high rate of secondary osteoarthritis in patients treated for PVNS using an open approach with surgical dislocation of the hip [3]. This may be due to joint destruction already present at the time of PVNS diagnosis and unrelated to the surgical approach used. However, given this high rate of secondary osteoarthritis, there has been a recent push for minimally invasive approaches in the appropriate patient for treatment of PVNS. Byrd argued that while arthroscopy may not prevent the development of osteoarthritis depending on the damage already present at the time of surgery, it may prevent the need for two invasive procedures assuming the eventual need for arthroplasty [12].

However, due to limitations in exposure during arthroscopy, surgical dislocation of the hip is still required to excise certain lesions, especially large lesions in the posterior-inferior capsule, as in Case 2. As stated previously, many cases of PVNS already have significant secondary joint damage by the time of diagnosis and treatment. A recent systematic review by Levy et al. found a high revision rate in patients undergoing surgery for PVNS (about 1 in 4 patients) [13]. While this rate was similar for patients who had undergone synovectomy alone compared to a combined synovectomy and arthroplasty, the time to revision surgery was significantly shorter in those patients who had undergone synovectomy alone. Della Valle et al. reported follow-up data ranging from 2 to 23 years on 7 patients with PVNS [14]. They found a high rate of revision surgery in patients who had combined synovectomy and arthroplasty. Of 4 patients who underwent total hip arthroplasty (THA), 2 required revision arthroplasty due to aseptic loosening. However, none of the 4 patients with combined synovectomy and arthroplasty had a recurrence of PVNS. The one patient treated with synovectomy alone had recurrence of PVNS 9 years after synovectomy and underwent a repeat synovectomy and THA at that time. The patient in Case 2 elected to undergo mass excision with synovectomy alone while simultaneously addressing intra-articular pathology (cam lesion).

This case report demonstrates that patients with PVNS tumors and concomitant hip pathology may be successfully treated using multiple techniques. There are myriad factors that determine which technique should be used, but location and size of the lesion, additional hip pathology, surgeon experience and expertise, and patient preference should all play a role in the decision-making process. Further research is necessary to determine whether surgical approach to PVNS affects long-term outcomes and progression to secondary osteoarthritis.

4. Conclusion

Excision of PVNS of the hip is necessary to halt progression and local destruction of the joint. Patients with PVNS lesions of the hip may have additional hip pathology that must be addressed at the time of surgery. Open surgical dislocation of the hip or arthroscopic surgery with a mini-open incision may be used in appropriately selected patients to successfully excise PVNS lesions in addition to addressing concomitant hip pathology.

Disclosure

Work was performed at the University of Pennsylvania, Philadelphia, PA. There were no grants or external sources of funding utilized for this report.

Competing Interests

The authors declare that they have no competing interests.

References

[1] H. L. Jaffe, L. Lichtenstein, C. J. Sutro et al., "Pigmented villonodular synovitis, bursitis and tenosynovitis," *Archives of Pathology & Laboratory Medicine*, vol. 31, no. 3, pp. 731–765, 1941.

[2] B. W. Myers, A. T. Masi, and S. L. Feigenbaum, "Pigmented villonodular synovitis and tenosynovitis: a clinical epidemiologic study of 166 cases and literature review," *Medicine*, vol. 59, no. 3, pp. 223–238, 1980.

[3] L. Vastel, P. Lambert, G. De Pinieux, O. Charrois, M. Kerboull, and J.-P. Courpied, "Surgical treatment of pigmented villonodular synovitis of the hip," *The Journal of Bone & Joint Surgery—American Volume*, vol. 87, no. 5, pp. 1019–1024, 2005.

[4] H. Mankin, C. Trahan, and F. Hornicek, "Pigmented villonodular synovitis of joints," *Journal of Surgical Oncology*, vol. 103, no. 5, pp. 386–389, 2011.

[5] J. W. T. Byrd, K. S. Jones, and G. P. Maiers, "Two to 10 years' follow-up of arthroscopic management of pigmented villonodular synovitis in the hip: a case series," *Arthroscopy*, vol. 29, no. 11, pp. 1783–1787, 2013.

[6] F. McCormick, K. Alpaugh, B. Haughom, and S. Nho, "Arthroscopic T-capsulotomy for excision of Pigmented villonodular synovitis in the hip," *Orthopedics*, vol. 38, no. 4, pp. 237–239, 2015.

[7] S. Lee, M. S. Haro, A. Riff, C. A. Bush-Joseph, and S. J. Nho, "Arthroscopic technique for the treatment of pigmented villonodular synovitis of the hip," *Arthroscopy Techniques*, vol. 4, no. 1, pp. e41–e46, 2015.

[8] M. Ribas, C. Cardenas-Nylander, V. Bellotti, M. Tey, and O. Marin, "Mini-open technique for femoroacetabular impingement," *The Journal of Bone & Joint Surgery*, 2012, http://www.boneandjoint.org.uk/sites/default/files/Mini-open%20technique%20for%20femoroacetabular%20impingement.pdf.

[9] S. B. Cohen, R. Huang, M. G. Ciccotti, C. C. Dodson, and J. Parvizi, "Treatment of femoroacetabular impingement in athletes using a mini-direct anterior approach," *American Journal of Sports Medicine*, vol. 40, no. 7, pp. 1620–1627, 2012.

[10] R. Ganz, T. J. Gill, E. Gautier, K. Ganz, N. Krügel, and U. Berlemann, "Surgical dislocation of the adult hip," *Journal of Bone and Joint Surgery*, vol. 83, no. 8, pp. 1119–1124, 2001.

[11] T. Shoji, Y. Yasunaga, T. Yamasaki et al., "Transtrochanteric rotational osteotomy combined with intra-articular procedures for pigmented villonodular synovitis of the hip," *Journal of Orthopaedic Science*, vol. 20, no. 5, pp. 943–950, 2014.

[12] J. W. T. Byrd, "Synovial proliferative disorders," *Operative Techniques in Sports Medicine*, vol. 23, no. 3, pp. 231–240, 2015.

[13] D. M. Levy, B. D. Haughom, S. J. Nho, and S. Gitelis, "Pigmented villonodular synovitis of the hip: a systematic review," *The American Journal of Orthopedics*, vol. 45, no. 1, pp. 23–28, 2016.

[14] A. G. Della Valle, F. Piccaluga, H. G. Potter, E. A. Salvati, and R. Pusso, "Pigmented villonodular synovitis of the hip: 2- to 23-year follow up study," *Clinical Orthopaedics and Related Research*, no. 388, pp. 187–199, 2001.

8

Gluteal Compartment Syndrome Secondary to Pelvic Trauma

**Fernando Diaz Dilernia, Ezequiel E. Zaidenberg, Sebastian Gamsie,
Danilo E. R. Taype Zamboni, Guido S. Carabelli, Jorge D. Barla, and Carlos F. Sancineto**

Institute of Orthopaedics "Carlos E. Ottolenghi" Italian Hospital of Buenos Aires, C1199ACK Buenos Aires, Argentina

Correspondence should be addressed to Fernando Diaz Dilernia; ferdiaz18@hotmail.com

Academic Editor: Andreas Panagopoulos

Gluteal compartment syndrome (GCS) is extremely rare when compared to compartment syndrome in other anatomical regions, such as the forearm or the lower leg. It usually occurs in drug users following prolonged immobilization due to loss of consciousness. Another possible cause is trauma, which is rare and has only few reports in the literature. Physical examination may show tense and swollen buttocks and severe pain caused by passive range of motion. We present the case of a 70-year-old man who developed GCS after prolonged anterior-posterior pelvis compression. The physical examination revealed swelling, scrotal hematoma, and left ankle extension weakness. An unstable pelvic ring injury was diagnosed and the patient was taken to surgery. Measurement of the intracompartmental pressure was measured in the operating room, thereby confirming the diagnosis. Emergent fasciotomy was performed to decompress the three affected compartments. Trauma surgeons must be aware of the possibility of gluteal compartment syndrome in patients who have an acute pelvic trauma with buttock swelling and excessive pain of the gluteal region. Any delay in diagnosis or treatment can be devastating, causing permanent disability, irreversible loss of gluteal muscles, sciatic nerve palsy, kidney failure, or even death.

1. Introduction

Gluteal compartment syndrome (GCS) is extremely rare when compared to other anatomical regions, such as the forearm or the lower leg [1]. Several nontraumatic causes have been described. According to the literature, most cases present on patients with a history of drug abuse (alcohol or opioid intoxication) causing prolonged immobilization due to loss of consciousness [2–5]. Other causes such as anticoagulation, obesity, and incorrect position during orthopedic or urological surgeries with long operative time and epidural anesthesia have also been reported. However, GCS secondary to pelvic trauma has rarely been reported in the literature [6–8].

Clinical findings are similar to those of other compartment syndromes such as excessive pain (usually out of proportion to the injury), paresthesia, and tense compartments. Other possible findings range from sciatic nerve palsy to massive rhabdomyolysis (RM), acute kidney failure, multiple organ dysfunction syndrome, and even death. Most authors suggest an intracompartmental pressure threshold of 30 mmHg as the threshold for initiating treatment, but clinical diagnosis remains the best way for evaluating the patient. The measurement of gluteal compartment pressure may be especially helpful in unresponsive patients where symptoms like pain or paresthesias cannot be assessed. Image studies, such as MRI, CT scan, and ultrasound, are often omitted in order to avoid delays in treatment. The gold standard for treatment is emergent fasciotomy [9–11].

We present a case of gluteal compartment syndrome secondary to an anterior-posterior compression pelvic ring injury with a left sacroiliac dislocation and pubic symphysis diastasis without fracture.

2. Case Report

A 70-year-old Caucasian man with no prior medical history suffered a pelvic trauma after being run over by a truck, sustaining an anterior-posterior compression pelvic injury. Primary stabilization with pelvic external fixation and damage control was performed in another institution. Twelve hours after the accident, the patient was admitted to our emergency department.

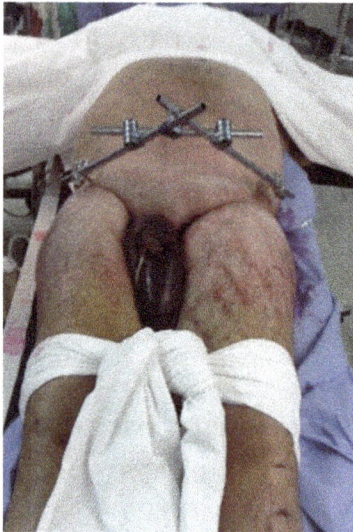

FIGURE 1: Clinical photograph showing skin marks of truck wheels on the left thigh, extensive scrotal hematoma, and swelling.

The patient was hemodynamically stable and responsive, complaining of pain on the lateral and posterior regions of the left buttock, accompanied by left ankle extension weakness. Physical examination revealed a truck wheel-shaped bruise on the left thigh, scrotal hematoma, and swelling (Figure 1). Left ankle extension showed active movement against gravity, with some weakness against resistance. Arterial pulses were intact, but sensory and motor deficits were consistent with left sciatic nerve palsy. Pelvic radiographs and computed tomography showed a traumatic disruption of the pelvic girdle without bony injury. Left sacroiliac dislocation and pubic symphysis diastasis were still evident despite the external fixation (Figure 2).

Admission laboratory results showed increased levels of creatine phosphokinase (CPK) and lactate dehydrogenase (LDH), suggesting muscle death and tissue damage. He subsequently lost left ankle flexion and extension, suggesting sciatic nerve palsy. One hour after his arrival and considering the clinical findings, diagnosis of GCS was made and urgent fasciotomy was indicated.

Prior to the surgery, an intracompartmental pressure of 46 mmHg was measured in the gluteus maximus compartment, confirming the diagnosis of gluteal compartment syndrome. Urgent fasciotomy was performed to decompress the three muscle compartments of the gluteal region (gluteus maximus, gluteus medius/minimus, and the fascia lata) (Figure 3). Vaccum assisted closure was applied for wound management.

Before surgery, the patient developed acute kidney failure with anuria along with increased serum values of urea and creatinine, requiring hemodialysis after the procedure. Once the patient was stable, open reduction and internal fixation by anterior and posterior approaches were performed. Laboratory markers (urea, CPK, Cr, and LDH) returned to normal values within the following month, after which the patient was discharged. Three months after initial trauma,

the patient recovered normal kidney function but continued with sciatic nerve palsy. At one-year follow-up, the patient persists with neurological deficit according to the Medical Research Council (MRC). He had 1/5 strength with testing of the anterior tibialis, musculus peroneus longus, and musculus peroneus brevis.

3. Discussion

Compartment syndrome (CS) is a surgical emergency caused by a microvascular phenomenon due to increase of the interstitial pressure in a nonexpandable musculoskeletal compartment. It results in soft tissue ischemia causing cellular hypoxia and death [9, 12]. Whitesides et al. reported that four-hour ischemia leads to irreversible muscle damage [2, 13]. Neurons are even more sensitive to hypoxia, and compromise of nervous tissue may occur in just 33 min [1, 13]. Other authors have reported that eight hours of muscle ischemia causes irreversible damage [13]. For this reason, early compartment syndrome identification remains the cornerstone, as a delay in the diagnosis can be disastrous for the patient and can lead to severe metabolic and neurological complications.

The incidence of compartment syndrome (CS) in the upper and lower limbs has been well documented but has rarely been reported in the literature as occurring in the gluteal region [1]. There are three compartments in this region, which in order of appearance (from lateral to medial) are as follows: tensor fasciae latae, gluteus medius and minimus, and finally gluteus maximus [1, 2, 6, 14]. The release of these three compartments is vital in the treatment of CS in the gluteal region [9].

The most common causes of GCS are related to prolonged local pressure on the gluteal muscles, usually from improper positioning during long surgical procedures or unconsciousness due to alcohol or drug abuse [2–5]. Obesity, unconsciousness, and epidural anesthesia are associated risk factors and can obscure the diagnosis. There are also some reports of GCS associated with the use of statins [15, 16], as a complication of hip surgery [17], intramuscular injections [18], Ehlers-Danlos syndrome [19], infection [20], superior gluteal artery rupture, sickle cell disease, and trauma, with the latter rarely being associated with this pathology [6–8]. Henson et al. performed a systematic review and found seven articles with a total of 28 cases [21]. Causes included prolonged immobilization (50%), post-total joint arthroplasty with epidural anesthesia (21%), trauma (21%), and necrotizing fasciitis (7%) [21].

Measurement of compartment pressures (CP) may be helpful, especially in unconscious patients. Normal intracompartmental pressure is 0–8 mmHg in adults. Pain and paresthesias appear with a pressure above 20–30 mmHg [22]. Pressures greater than 30 mmHg are suggestive of CS and fasciotomy is indicated [14]. Despite this, there is no consensus in the literature about the threshold that is an indication for surgery. If there is clinical suspicion, surgical intervention must be performed immediately [14]. Early treatment with fasciotomy considerably improves the chances for full recovery [10, 11].

In late stages of the GCS, ischemic changes occur in the sciatic nerve [23]. Symptoms progress through paresthesias,

(a)

(b)

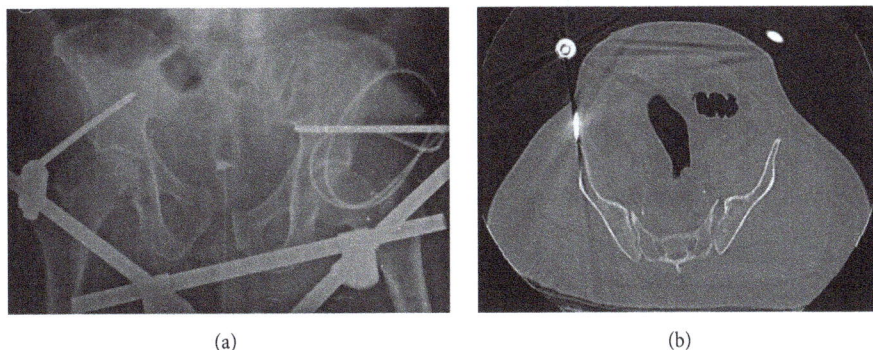

FIGURE 2: (a) Anteroposterior radiograph of the pelvis showing pubic symphysis diastasis. (b) CT scan axial view confirms pelvic ring injury due to sacroiliac joint subluxation without bone involvement.

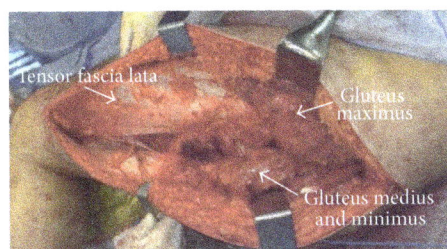

FIGURE 3: Intraoperative image showing the urgent fasciotomy and the decompression of the three gluteal compartments (tensor fascia lata, gluteus minimus and medius, and the gluteus maximus) with distal extension through the left tight.

paresis, anesthesia, and, finally, palsy with loss of peripheral pulses [24]. In the pelvis, the sciatic nerve runs between the gluteus maximus and the pelvis external rotator complex, making it susceptible to compression by swelling of the gluteal muscles. This may result in a compression-induced neuropathy [25]. Hargens et al. showed that the time required to produce peripheral nerve compromise is inversely proportional to intracompartmental pressure [26]. More than half of the patients suffer neurological symptoms due to sciatic nerve damage and symptoms persist if the treatment is delayed [3]. This hypothesis could explain the sciatic nerve palsy sequelae that our patient suffered, which could have probably been related to delayed diagnosis and treatment.

Another possible complication of the GCS is crush syndrome, also known as traumatic rhabdomyolysis or Bywater's syndrome. Crush syndrome is the systemic consequence of severe rhabdomyolysis characterized by significantly elevated values of creatinine and urea, with myoglobin present in the urine and hyperkalemia. The necrotic muscle causes cellular death with release of myoglobin and potassium to the extracellular space and blood stream. The resulting hyperkalemia causes acidosis, and myoglobin deposits in the distal renal tubules, which may result in acute kidney failure [9, 27–29]. The treatment for crush syndrome must be aggressive in order to prevent further kidney damage, and the treatment includes fluid resuscitation and urine alkalinization [10].

GCS is an extremely rare condition that can be easily overlooked, especially in obese or unconscious patients. Due to patient responsiveness in the present case, the swelling and tautness were easily recognized and diagnosed immediately, allowing a prompt treatment. However, it is possible that the 12-hour delay in the patient's arrival to our institution may have been the cause of complications such as kidney failure and sciatic nerve palsy.

Trauma surgeons must be aware of the possibility of GCS in patients who have an acute pelvic trauma with swelling and excessive pain of the gluteal region. It has a high morbidity rate and must be kept in mind in the differential diagnosis for patients with pelvic trauma. Any delay in diagnosis or treatment can be devastating, causing permanent disability, irreversible loss of gluteal muscles, sciatic nerve palsy, or even end-stage kidney failure. This case highlights the importance of early diagnosis and treatment of this uncommon condition.

Ethical Approval

All investigations were conducted in conformity with ethical principles of research.

Disclosure

All authors certify that their institution has approved the reporting of this case.

Competing Interests

All authors declare that there are no competing interests regarding the publication of this paper.

Acknowledgments

The study was performed at the Italian Hospital of Buenos Aires, Argentina.

References

[1] G. Hayden, M. Leung, and J. Leong, "Gluteal compartment syndrome," *ANZ Journal of Surgery*, vol. 76, no. 7, pp. 668–670, 2006.

[2] N. M. Mustafa, A. Hyun, J. S. Kumar, and L. Yekkirala, "Gluteal compartment syndrome: A case report," *Cases Journal*, vol. 2, no. 11, article no. 190, 2009.

[3] S. Iizuka, N. Miura, T. Fukushima, T. Seki, K. Sugimoto, and S. Inokuchi, "Gluteal compartment syndrome due to prolonged immobilization after alcohol intoxication: a case report," *Tokai Journal of Experimental and Clinical Medicine*, vol. 36, no. 2, pp. 25–28, 2011.

[4] J. E. Hynes and A. Jackson, "Atraumatic gluteal compartment syndrome," *Postgraduate Medical Journal*, vol. 70, no. 821, pp. 210–212, 1994.

[5] K. D. Osteen and S. H. Haque, "Bilateral gluteal compartment syndrome following right total knee revision: a case report," *The Ochsner Journal*, vol. 12, no. 2, pp. 141–144, 2012.

[6] B. C. Taylor, C. Dimitris, A. Tancevski, and J. L. Tran, "Gluteal compartment syndrome and superior gluteal artery injury as a result of simple hip dislocation: a case report," *The Iowa Orthopaedic Journal*, vol. 31, pp. 181–186, 2011.

[7] R. J. Brumback, "Traumatic rupture of the superior gluteal artery, without fracture of the pelvis, causing compartment syndrome of the buttock. A case report," *Journal of Bone and Joint Surgery A*, vol. 72, no. 1, pp. 134–137, 1990.

[8] G. Belley, B. P. Gallix, A. M. Derossis, D. S. Mulder, and R. A. Brown, "Profound hypotension in blunt trauma associated with superior gluteal artery rupture without pelvic fracture," *Journal of Trauma—Injury, Infection and Critical Care*, vol. 43, no. 4, pp. 703–705, 1997.

[9] S. L. Hill and J. Bianchi, "The gluteal compartment syndrome," *The American Surgeon*, vol. 63, no. 9, pp. 823–826, 1997.

[10] R. J. Gaines, C. J. Randall, K. L. Browne, D. R. Carr, and J. G. Enad, "Delayed presentation of compartment syndrome of the proximal lower extremity after low-energy trauma in patients taking warfarin," *American Journal of Orthopedics*, vol. 37, no. 12, pp. E201–E204, 2008.

[11] P. F. Lachiewicz and H. A. Latimer, "Rhabdomyolysis following total hip arthroplasty," *The Journal of Bone & Joint Surgery—British Volume*, vol. 73, no. 4, pp. 576–579, 1991.

[12] V. Kumar, K. Saeed, A. Panagopoulos, and P. J. Parker, "Gluteal compartment syndrome following joint arthroplasty under epidural anaesthesia: a report of 4 cases," *Journal of Orthopaedic Surgery*, vol. 15, no. 1, pp. 113–117, 2007.

[13] T. E. Whitesides, H. Hirada, and K. Morimoto, "The response of skeletal muscle to temporary ischaemia: an experimental study," *The Journal of Bone & Joint Surgery—American Volume*, vol. 53, pp. 1027–1028, 1971.

[14] R. Keene, J. M. Froelich, J. C. Milbrandt, and O. B. Idusuyi, "Bilateral gluteal compartment syndrome following robotic-assisted prostatectomy," *Orthopedics*, vol. 33, no. 11, p. 852, 2010.

[15] S. Flamini, C. Zoccali, E. Persi, and V. Calvisi, "Spontaneous compartment syndrome in a patient with diabetes and statin administration: a case report," *Journal of Orthopaedics and Traumatology*, vol. 9, no. 2, pp. 101–103, 2008.

[16] M. J. Ramdass, G. Singh, and B. Andrews, "Simvastatin-induced bilateral leg compartment syndrome and myonecrosis associated with hypothyroidism," *Postgraduate Medical Journal*, vol. 83, no. 977, pp. 152–153, 2007.

[17] V. S. Pai, "Compartment syndrome of the buttock following a total hip arthroplasty," *Journal of Arthroplasty*, vol. 11, no. 5, pp. 609–610, 1996.

[18] T. Klockgether, M. Weller, T. Haarmeier, B. Kaskas, G. Maier, and J. Dichgans, "Gluteal compartment syndrome due to rhabdomyolysis after heroin abuse," *Neurology*, vol. 48, no. 1, pp. 275–276, 1997.

[19] T. P. Schmalzried and J. J. Eckardt, "Spontaneous gluteal artery rupture resulting in compartment syndrome and sciatic neuropathy: report of a case in Ehlers-Danlos syndrome," *Clinical Orthopaedics and Related Research*, no. 275, pp. 253–257, 1992.

[20] Y. Kontrobarsky and J. Love, "Gluteal compartment syndrome following epidural analgesic infusion with motor blockage," *Anaesthesia Intensive Care*, no. 25, pp. 696–698, 1997.

[21] J. T. Henson, C. S. Roberts, and P. V. Giannoudis, "Gluteal compartment syndrome," *Acta Orthopaedica Belgica*, vol. 75, no. 2, pp. 147–152, 2009.

[22] S. J. Mubarak, C. A. Owen, A. R. Hargens, L. P. Garetto, and W. H. Akeson, "Acute compartment syndromes: diagnosis and treatment with the aid of the wick catheter," *Journal of Bone and Joint Surgery—Series A*, vol. 60, no. 8, pp. 1091–1095, 1978.

[23] V. David, J. Thambiah, F. H. Y. Kagda, and V. P. Kumar, "Bilateral gluteal compartment syndrome: a case report," *The Journal of Bone & Joint Surgery—American Volume*, vol. 87, no. 11, pp. 2541–2545, 2005.

[24] T. P. Schmalzried, W. C. Neal, and J. J. Eckardt, "Gluteal compartment and crush syndromes: a report of three cases and review of the literature," *Clinical Orthopaedics and Related Research*, no. 277, pp. 161–165, 1992.

[25] R. J. Bleicher, H. F. Sherman, and B. A. Latenser, "Bilateral gluteal compartment syndrome," *Journal of Trauma-Injury, Infection and Critical Care*, vol. 42, no. 1, pp. 118–122, 1997.

[26] A. R. Hargens, J. S. Romine, J. C. Sipe et al., "Peripheral nerve conduction block by high muscle compartment syndrome," *The Journal of Bone & Joint Surgery, Series A*, vol. 61, pp. 192–200, 1979.

[27] F. M. Rommel, R. L. Kabler, and J. J. Mowad, "The crush syndrome: a complication of urological surgery," *Journal of Urology*, vol. 135, no. 4, pp. 809–811, 1986.

[28] S. J. Mubarak and C. A. Owen, "Compartmental syndrome and its relation to the crush syndrome: a spectrum of disease. A review of 11 cases of prolonged limb compression," *Clinical Orthopaedics and Related Research*, no. 113, pp. 81–89, 1975.

[29] H. Yoshioka, "Gluteal compartment syndrome: a report of 4 cases," *Acta Orthopaedica*, vol. 63, no. 3, pp. 347–349, 1992.

9

Scedosporium prolificans Septic Arthritis and Osteomyelitis of the Hip Joints in an Immunocompetent Patient

Luca Daniele, Michael Le, Adam Franklin Parr, and Lochlin Mark Brown

Department of Orthopaedics, Gold Coast Health Service, Gold Coast University Hospital, 1 Hospital Blvd., Southport, QLD 4215, Australia

Correspondence should be addressed to Michael Le; michael.93le@gmail.com

Academic Editor: Mark K. Lyons

Scedosporium prolificans, also known as *Scedosporium inflatum*, is a fungus widespread in soil, sewage, and manure. This species is highly virulent and is an emerging opportunistic pathogen found in penetrating injuries in immunocompromised patients. Here we report on an immunocompetent patient with bilateral hip *S. prolificans*-associated osteomyelitis and septic arthritis caused by intentional penetrating trauma. The condition was refractory to initial antimicrobial suppression and surgical irrigation and debridement. Successful outcome was achieved after incorporating a bilateral two-stage total-hip-arthroplasty with Voriconazole-loaded cement and spacer.

1. Introduction

Scedosporium prolificans, also known as *Scedosporium inflatum*, is a fungus ubiquitous in soil, sewage, potted plants, and manure [1]. This species is an emerging opportunistic pathogen found in penetrating injuries in immunocompromised patients [2]. *S. prolificans* infections are resistant to most currently available antifungals thus making treatment options challenging [3]. It was first described in 1984 after isolation from a bone biopsy specimen in an area of osteomyelitis [4]. Treatment of *S. prolificans* infections is complicated by its resistance to most currently available antifungals [3]. Disseminated infections occur more commonly in immunocompromised individuals [5] while localized infections presenting as septic arthritis and osteomyelitis are more common in immunocompetent patients.

2. Case Presentation

A 47-year-old male with background history of bilateral hip osteoarthritis presented to the Emergency Department in February 2016 with a one-month history of progressive bilateral groin pain and four-day history of inability to bear weight on the left side. The pain was worse on the left and radiated towards the knees bilaterally. The patient was otherwise well and denied a history of fevers or other constitutional symptoms. Prior to presentation, he was privately managed for five months with multiple intra-articular hip HCLA injections by a radiologist. This provided good effect for four months until one month prior to presentation.

On examination, the patient had hyperaesthesia on palpation over the greater trochanter and groin region. Passive and active movement of both hips were painful with restricted ranges of motion in all directions bilaterally. Neurovascular status was intact. Initial laboratory results revealed a raised CRP (105) with unremarkable FBC, U&E, and LFTs. Neurovascular status was intact. Initial laboratory results revealed a raised CRP (105) with unremarkable FBC, U&E, and LFTs. 24-hour blood cultures, *Chlamydia trachomatis*, gonorrhoea, rheumatoid factor, and anticyclic citrullinated peptide in consideration of rheumatic and infective causes were negative.

Ultrasound guided aspiration of the left hip revealed haemoserous fluid and scant leukocytes but was negative for crystals and bacteria. Interim bone scan (Figure 1) and MRI (Figure 2) showed a probable focus of osteomyelitis within the left anterior inferior iliac spine (AIIS) and small bilateral

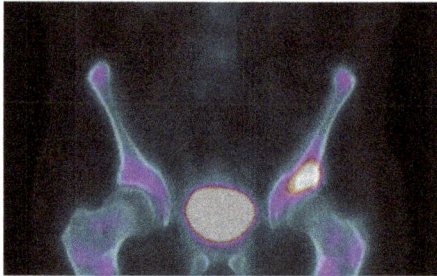

FIGURE 1: Delayed-phase SPECT/CT displaying increased activity in the left AIIS extending to the superior acetabular rim.

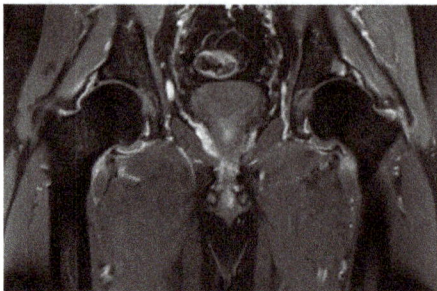

FIGURE 2: T2 weighted MRI demonstrating a hyperintense focus in the left superior acetabular rim and hip effusion and capsular edema consistent with osteomyelitis and septic arthritis.

effusions concerning for superimposed septic arthritis. Bone scintigraphy confirmed activity at the left AIIS (Figure 2). Despite being commenced on IV flucloxacillin, ciprofloxacin, and vancomycin, a low-grade fever developed over the following days. A left hip washout revealed cloudy fluid and exudate with reactive appearance of labrum and capsule. Cultures returned a positive result for S. prolificans after five days necessitating the commencement of Voriconazole and Terbinafine.

Following initial improvements, the patient developed worsening left groin pain and rising CRP. A second washout and MRI suggested ongoing left septic arthritis and associated osteomyelitis with contralateral concerning pathology in the right hip. A subsequent bilateral hip washout, left head core decompression, and acetabulum debridement were performed on day 28. Repeat MRI demonstrated worsening left septic arthritis and acetabular osteomyelitis despite ongoing surgical debridement, lavage, and medical therapy. All left-sided intraoperative samples returned positive for S. prolificans while right-sided specimens remained negative to date.

Departmental decision was made to perform a two-stage left total-hip-arthroplasty. The first stage initially involved aggressive acetabular debridement, lavage and reaming. An acetabular cup loaded with 200 mg Voriconazole in Palacos cement and similarly loaded cement spacer were implanted (Figure 3). Prior to home discharge with regular Voriconazole, the patient was mobilising with pain score of 0 on the left and minimal pain on the right side. However, due to interval radiological changes (Figure 4) and right-sided pain at

follow-up, a first-stage right hip arthroplasty was performed (Figure 5). The patient is currently seven months after left and 6 months after right first-stage total-hip-arthroplasty. Progression to second-stage total-hip-arthroplasty will be considered following a disease-free period of at least twelve months.

3. Discussion

Scedosporium prolificans, also known as *Scedosporium inflatum*, is an emerging opportunistic pathogen found in penetrating injuries in immunocompromised patients [2]. Treatment of *S. prolificans* infections is complicated by its resistance to most currently available antifungals [3]. Disseminated infections occur more commonly in immunocompromised individuals [5] while localized infections presenting as septic arthritis and osteomyelitis are more common in immunocompetent patients. We believe the repeated HCLA injections provided a point of entry and a locally immune-deficient environment for the infection to take hold. Corticosteroids may induce an immunosuppressed environment as they inhibit the accumulation of inflammatory cells, phagocytosis, and production of neutrophils and prevent the synthesis and secretion of inflammatory mediators [6, 7]. Previous literature has suggested that the local immunosuppressive effects associated with invasive steroid treatments such as HCLA injection may influence and increase the susceptibility to infection [8]. Thus, any factors which could potentially inhibit the ability of joint to withstand infection should be minimized [8]. This is also in light of the possibility of infection being introduced at the time of invasive therapy. Several case reports of septic arthritis and/or osteomyelitis have appeared in published literature. Here we report on an immunocompetent patient with bilateral hip *S. prolificans*-associated osteomyelitis and septic arthritis treated with a two-stage total-hip-arthroplasty incorporating Voriconazole-loaded cement and spacer.

Although treatment is difficult, localized infections have previously showed response to antifungal therapy and surgical debridement. A recent systematic review included 23 reported cases of *S. prolificans*-associated osteoarticular infections in both immunocompetent or immunocompromised patients [9]. Our review of the English literature revealed 14 case reports of *S. prolificans* infection of the joints (Table 1) in only immunocompetent patients. Reports have seen success with older antifungal agents including Amphotericin B, Ketoconazole, Miconazole, nystatin, 5-fluorocytosine, and fluconazole [3, 10, 11]. Three previous reports have demonstrated satisfactory results with newer antifungal agents Terbinafine/Voriconazole in immunocompetent patients with septic arthritis [12–15]. Another report has shown success in an 8-year-old immunocompetent patient using Hexadecylphosphocholine with Voriconazole/Terbinafine [16]. In vitro synergistic effects have been reported with Voriconazole and Terbinafine, reducing the minimum inhibitory concentration for *S. prolificans* [17, 18]. However, there remains no consensus for the duration of treatment with the Voriconazole/Terbinafine combination for septic arthritis and osteomyelitis caused by *S. prolificans*. Regardless of that,

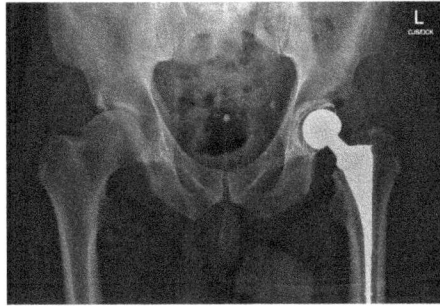

FIGURE 3: Postoperative radiograph demonstrating first-stage cemented total hip replacement with 48/32 mm Stryker RimFit Ace-tabular cup and size 9 Biomet Simplex cement spacer.

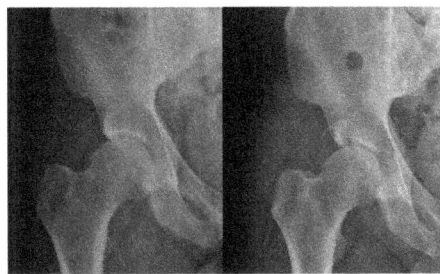

FIGURE 4: Plain radiograph showing progressive osteolysis of the superior right acetabular rim consistent with chronic infection.

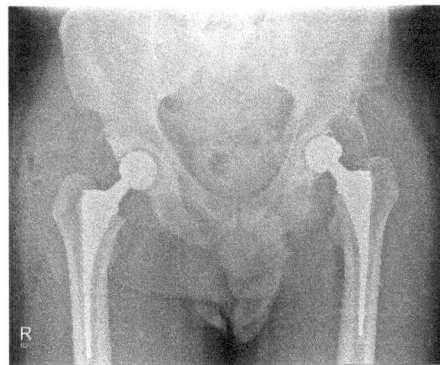

FIGURE 5: Postoperative radiograph demonstrating bilateral first-stage cemented total hip replacement.

irrigation and surgical debridement are vital components in the eradication of infections in all cases. In cases unresponsive to antifungal treatment and surgical debridement, arthrodesis [15] alongside radical excisions and amputations has been necessitated [19].

This is the first described case to our knowledge of *S. prolificans*-associated septic arthritis and osteomyelitis treated using a two-stage hip arthroplasty with Voriconazole-loaded cement and spacer. Studies have confirmed that Voriconazole is stable at high temperatures and therefore suitable to be used with Palacos cement [20]. Previous studies have suggested that the elution of Voriconazole from bone cement would be able to maintain a minimum inhibitory concentration for *S. prolificans* [21]. Higher antimicrobial content has been shown to increase cement porosity and thus elution. However,

concern exists as load-bearing strength potential of cement and hardening time is consequently reduced. This affects the time required for spacer preparation. Therefore, a balance between these factors needs to be considered.

The objective in this case, to permanently eradicate the infection and restore function to the patient, was successful. This case therefore highlights the need to consider alternative avenues before undertaking more drastic measures such as arthrodesis or amputation for *S. prolificans* septic arthritis and osteomyelitis.

Consent

Informed consent was obtained from the patient for the publication of this case report.

TABLE 1: Reported *Scedosporium prolificans*-associated osteomyelitis and/or septic arthritis infections from penetrating trauma in immuno-competent patients.

Age/gender	Location	Mechanism of introduction	Site/presentation	Treatments used	Final Outcome	Author/Year
6/M	North America	Penetrating injury	Foot osteomyelitis	Surgical debridement, Amphotericin B, Ketoconazole, Miconazole,	Improvement	Taj-Aldeen et al. 2015 [9]
3/M	South America	Trauma	Knee septic arthritis	Surgery, Ketoconazole, Amphotericin B, Ketoconazole, intra-articular Amphotericin B, intra-articular Miconazole	Amputation	Wilson et al. 1990 [19]
5/M	North America	Penetrating trauma from thorn	Knee septic arthritis	Surgery, Amphotericin B 5-FC, intra-articular Amphotericin B, Miconazole, Ketoconazole	Improvement	Wilson et al. 1990 [19]
54/M	North America	Trauma from axe	Knee arthritis	Surgery, Amphotericin B, Ketoconazole; Miconazole	Improvement	Wilson et al. 1990 [19]
6/M	North America	Penetrating injury from nail	Foot osteomyelitis	Surgical debridement	Improvement	Wilson et al. 1990 [19]
6/M	North America	Penetrating injury from nail	Foot osteomyelitis	Surgery, Amphotericin B, Ketoconazole	Improvement	Wilson et al. 1990 [19]
35/M	North America	Penetrating injury/IV drug use	Hip septic arthritis	Joint drainage, Amphotericin B, 5-fluorocytosine	Improvement	Wilson et al. 1990 [19]
11/M	Australia	Laceration	Ankle septic arthritis	Surgical debridement, Amphotericin B, Itraconazole	Improvement	Wood et al. 1992 [11]
5/M	North America	Penetrating injury from nail	Foot osteomyelitis	Surgical debridement, polyhexamethylene, biguanide, Voriconazole, caspofungin	Improvement	Steinbach et al. 2003 [3]
9/M	Sweden	Penetrating injury from thorn	Knee osteomyelitis	Surgical debridement, cefuroxime, Amphotericin B, Itraconazole, Voriconazole	Improvement with arthrodesis	Studahl et al. 2003 [15]
5/M	Australia	Ankle abrasion due to trauma	Ankle septic arthritis	Surgical debridement, Amphotericin B, Itraconazole, Terbinafine, Voriconazole	Improvement	Dalton et al. 2006 [13]
8/F	Australia	Trauma from tractor	Hip osteomyelitis and hip septic arthritis	Surgical debridement, Hexadecylphosphocholine, Terbinafine, Voriconazole	Improvement	Kesson et al. 2009 [16]
4/M	United Kingdom	Penetrating injury from thorn	Foot osteomyelitis	Surgical debridement, Voriconazole, Terbinafine	Improvement	Bhagavatula et al. 2014 [14]
54/M	Australia	Penetrating injury from HCLA injections	Hip osteomyelitis and hip septic arthritis	2-stage total-hip-arthroplasty with Voriconazole-loaded cement and spacer, Voriconazole, Terbinafine	Improvement	Daniele et al. 2016

Competing Interests

The authors declare that there is no conflict of interests regarding the publication of this paper.

References

[1] K. J. Cortez, E. Roilides, F. Quiroz-Telles et al., "Infections caused by *Scedosporium* spp.," *Clinical Microbiology Reviews*, vol. 21, no. 1, pp. 157–197, 2008.

[2] J. Meletiadis, J. W. Mouton, J. F. G. M. Meis, and P. E. Verweij, "Combination chemotherapy for the treatment of invasive infections by *Scedosporium prolificans*," *Clinical Microbiology and Infection*, vol. 6, no. 6, pp. 336–337, 2000.

[3] W. J. Steinbach, W. A. Schell, J. L. Miller, and J. R. Perfect, "Scedosporium prolificans osteomyelitis in an immunocompetent child treated with voriconazole and caspofungin, as well as locally applied polyhexamethylene biguanide," *Journal of Clinical Microbiology*, vol. 41, no. 8, pp. 3981–3985, 2003.

[4] D. Malloch and I. Salkin, *A New Species of Scedosporium Associated with Osteomyelitis in Humans*, Mycotaxon, 1984.

[5] B. P. Howden, M. A. Slavin, A. P. Schwarer, and A. M. Mijch, "Successful control of disseminated *Scedosporium prolificans* infection with a combination of voriconazole and terbinafine," *European Journal of Clinical Microbiology and Infectious Diseases*, vol. 22, no. 2, pp. 111–113, 2003.

[6] P. Creamer, "Intra-articular corticosteroid treatment in osteoarthritis," *Current Opinion in Rheumatology*, vol. 11, no. 5, pp. 417–421, 1999.

[7] E. Ayhan, H. Kesmezacar, and I. Akgun, "Intraarticular injections (corticosteroid, hyaluronic acid, platelet rich plasma) for the knee osteoarthritis," *World Journal of Orthopaedics*, vol. 5, no. 3, pp. 351–361, 2014.

[8] S. Kaspar and J. D. V. de Beer, "Infection in hip arthroplasty after previous injection of steroid," *Journal of Bone and Joint Surgery—Series B*, vol. 87, no. 4, pp. 454–457, 2005.

[9] S. J. Taj-Aldeen, B. Rammaert, M. Gamaletsou et al., "Osteoarticular infections caused by non-*Aspergillus* filamentous fungi in adult and pediatric patients: a systematic review," *Medicine*, vol. 94, no. 50, Article ID e2078, 2015.

[10] M. Malekzadeh, G. D. Overturf, S. B. Auerbach, L. Wong, and M. Hirsch, "Chronic, recurrent osteomyelitis caused by *Scedosporium inflatum*," *The Pediatric Infectious Disease Journal*, vol. 9, no. 5, pp. 357–359, 1990.

[11] G. M. Wood, J. G. McCormack, D. B. Muir et al., "Clinical features of human infection with scedosporium inflatum," *Clinical Infectious Diseases*, vol. 14, no. 5, pp. 1027–1033, 1992.

[12] I. B. Gosbell, V. Toumasatos, J. Yong, R. S. Kuo, D. H. Ellis, and R. C. Perrie, "Cure of orthopaedic infection with *Scedosporium prolificans*, using voriconazole plus terbinafine, without the need for radical surgery," *Mycoses*, vol. 46, no. 5-6, pp. 233–236, 2003.

[13] P. A. Dalton, W. J. Munckhof, and D. W. Walters, "Scedosporium prolificans: an uncommon cause of septic arthritis," *ANZ Journal of Surgery*, vol. 76, no. 7, pp. 661–663, 2006.

[14] S. Bhagavatula, L. Vale, J. Evans, C. Carpenter, and R. A. Barnes, "Scedosporium prolificans osteomyelitis following penetrating injury: a case report," *Medical Mycology Case Reports*, vol. 4, no. 1, pp. 26–29, 2014.

[15] M. Studahl, T. Backteman, F. Stålhammar, E. Chryssanthou, and B. Petrini, "Bone and joint infection after traumatic implantation of Scedosporium prolificans treated with voriconazole and surgery," *Acta Paediatrica, International Journal of Paediatrics*, vol. 92, no. 8, pp. 980–982, 2003.

[16] A. M. Kesson, M. C. Bellemore, T. J. O'Mara, D. H. Ellis, and T. C. Sorrell, "*Scedosporium prolificans* osteomyelitis in an immunocompetent child treated with a novel agent, hexadecylphospocholine (miltefosine), in combination with terbinafine and voriconazole: a case report," *Clinical Infectious Diseases*, vol. 48, no. 9, pp. 1257–1261, 2009.

[17] "In vitro synergy between terbinafine and voriconazole against Scedosporium *prolificans*," in *Proceedings of the 42nd Interscience Conference on Antimicrobial Agents and Chemotherapy*, R. Perrie and D. Ellis, Eds., San Diego, Calif, USA, 2002.

[18] J. Meletiadis, J. F. G. M. Meis, J. W. Mouton et al., "In vitro activities of new and conventional antifungal agents against clinical *Scedosporium* isolates," *Antimicrobial Agents and Chemotherapy*, vol. 46, no. 1, pp. 62–68, 2002.

[19] C. M. Wilson, E. J. O'Rourke, M. R. McGinnis, and I. F. Salkin, "Scedosporium inflatum: clinical spectrum of a newly recognized pathogen," *Journal of Infectious Diseases*, vol. 161, no. 1, pp. 102–107, 1990.

[20] J. J. Deelstra, D. Neut, and P. C. Jutte, "Successful treatment of *Candida albicans*–infected total hip prosthesis with staged procedure using an antifungal-loaded cement spacer," *Journal of Arthroplasty*, vol. 28, no. 2, pp. 374.e5–374.e8, 2013.

[21] C. Grimsrud, R. Raven, A. W. Fothergill, and H. T. Kim, "The in vitro elution characteristics of antifungal-loaded PMMA bone cement and calcium sulfate bone substitute," *Orthopedics*, vol. 34, no. 8, pp. e378–e381, 2011.

10

Myelopathy due to Spinal Extramedullary Hematopoiesis in a Patient with Polycythemia Vera

Shuhei Ito,[1] **Nobuyuki Fujita,**[1] **Naobumi Hosogane,**[2] **Narihito Nagoshi,**[1]
Mitsuru Yagi,[1] **Akio Iwanami,**[1] **Kota Watanabe,**[1] **Takashi Tsuji,**[3] **Masaya Nakamura,**[1]
Morio Matsumoto,[1] **and Ken Ishii**[1]

[1]*Department of Orthopaedic Surgery, Keio University School of Medicine, Tokyo, Japan*
[2]*Department of Orthopaedic Surgery, National Defence Medical College, Saitama, Japan*
[3]*Department of Orthopaedic Surgery, Fujita Health University School of Medicine, Aichi, Japan*

Correspondence should be addressed to Nobuyuki Fujita; nfujita@a7.keio.jp

Academic Editor: Paolo Perrini

Extramedullary hematopoiesis (EMH) occasionally occurs in patients exhibiting hematological disorders with decreased hematopoietic efficacy. EMH is rarely observed in the spinal epidural space and patients are usually asymptomatic. In particular, in the patients with polycythemia vera, spinal cord compression due to EMH is extremely rare. We report a case of polycythemia vera, in which operative therapy proved to be an effective treatment for myelopathy caused by spinal EMH.

1. Introduction

Extramedullary hematopoiesis (EMH) occasionally occurs in patients exhibiting hematological disorders with decreased hematopoietic efficacy, such as myelofibrosis, thalassemia, and polycythemia vera. The condition most commonly occurs at sites involved in embryonal hematopoiesis such as liver, spleen, and lymph nodes [1–3]. EMH is rarely observed in the spinal epidural space and patients are usually asymptomatic. Spinal cord compression due to EMH is extremely rare. The diagnosis relies on the history of hematological disorders, magnetic resonance imaging (MRI) findings of soft tissue masses that lead to spinal cord compression, and histological examination.

Polycythemia vera is a bone marrow disease marked by the excessive production of red blood cells and is occasionally accompanied by an increased number of white blood cells and platelets. We report a case of polycythemia vera with spinal cord compression caused by spinal EMH, in which operative therapy proved to be an effective treatment for myelopathy.

2. Case Presentation

A 55-year-old woman had been diagnosed as having polycythemia vera in 2005 and followed up by a hematologist at another hospital. In 2012, she developed walking difficulty with progressive numbness and weakness in both legs, which started 3 months after radiation therapy for splenomegaly. She was seen at a nearby clinic, and MRI revealed an epidural lesion in the thoracic spine. At the initial visit to our hospital, cranial nerve examination and strength of the upper limbs were normal; however, both lower limbs were weak with power of 4/5 in iliopsoas, quadriceps, and hamstrings. Deep tendon reflexes were normal, and Babinski sign was negative. Sensation to touch and pain below navel was 5/10. The Japanese Orthopedic Association (JOA) score for thoracic myelopathy was 6/11. Blood test showed increased red blood cell count (19,900/μL), hemoglobin level (17.6 g/dL), and reduced platelet count (74,000 μL). Radiograph finding of the thoracic spine was normal. MRI of the thoracic spine showed an epidural mass extending from the fifth to the tenth thoracic vertebra (Figure 1). The lesion appeared isointense

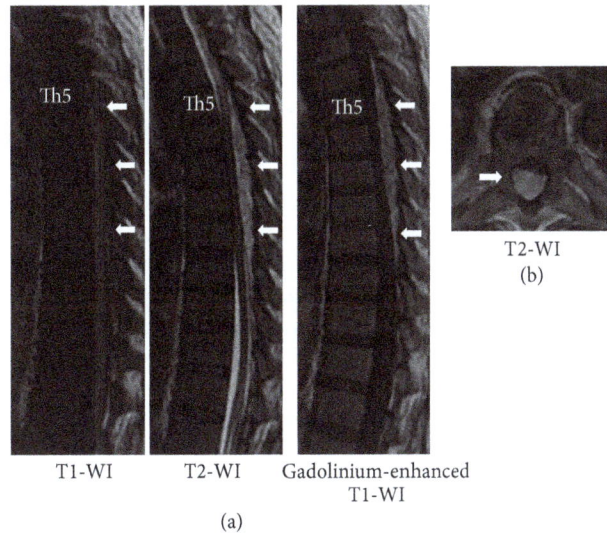

FIGURE 1: Preoperative MRI showed an epidural mass extending from the fifth to the tenth thoracic vertebra canal. (a) Sagittal plane. (b) Axial plane (Th7).

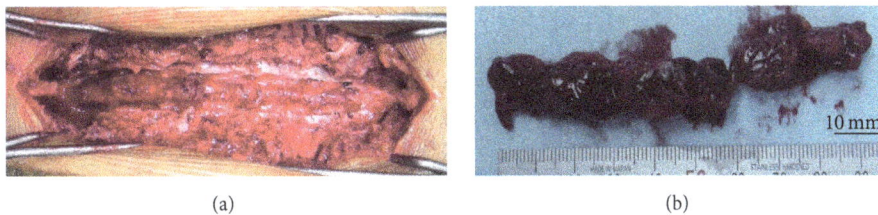

FIGURE 2: Photograph of the thoracic epidural mass. (a) The dorsal epidural mass is continuous from the fifth to the tenth thoracic vertebra canal after laminectomy. (b) The thoracic epidural mass specimen is reddish brown and hematoma like in appearance.

on T1-weighted images (WI) and hyperintense on T2-WI and showed heterogeneous enhancement after gadolinium administration. The spinal cord was compressed by the posterior epidural mass.

Because her neurological symptoms were progressively getting worse, posterior decompression surgery was performed from the fourth to the ninth thoracic vertebra with intraoperative transfusion of platelets. The laminal arch of vertebrae from the fourth to the ninth thoracic spine was removed, and the reddish brown continuous mass was excised (Figure 2). The mass was not adhered to the dura mater and was easily removed. The operation time was 185 min, and the estimated blood loss was 1250 g. Histological examination confirmed the diagnosis of EMH because of the presence of hematopoietic cells differentiated into mature myelopoietic, erythropoietic, and megakaryocytic cells (Figure 3). Furthermore, immunohistochemical analysis of surgical sample was performed by using glycophorin A (DAKO, clone: JC159, 1 : 400) for erythroblasts, CD41 (Calbiochem, clone: 283.16B7, 1 : 2000) for megakaryocytes, and MPO (DAKO, rabbit polyclonal, 1 : 500) for granulocytes (Figure 4). These results also clearly supported the diagnosis of EMH. Immediately after surgery, she was able to walk and the leg numbness and weakness were resolved. She was not given postoperative radiation therapy and chemotherapy. A year

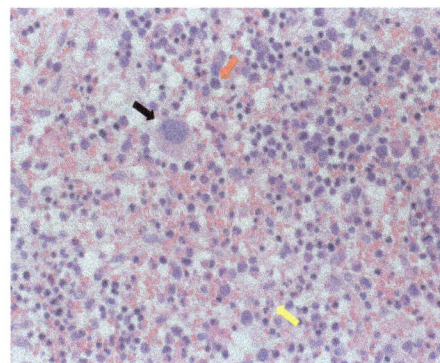

FIGURE 3: Histology of the epidural mass. Hematoxylin and eosin staining. Arrows suggest hematopoietic cells. Black, megakaryocytic; red, erythropoietic; yellow, myelopoietic. Magnification ×40.

after the surgery, there were no clinical or radiological signs of recurrence (Figure 5).

3. Discussion

Gatto et al. first reported a case of spinal EMH in 1954 [4]. Spinal lesions have been reported to occur in 11%–15%

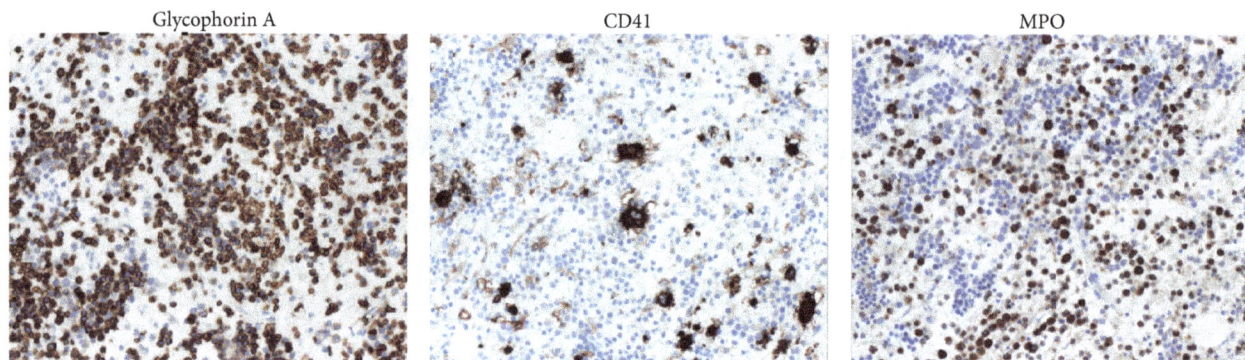

FIGURE 4: Immunohistochemistry of the epidural mass. High expression of cell surface markers for erythroblasts (glycophorin A), megakaryocytes (CD41), and granulocytes (MPO) was observed. Magnification ×40.

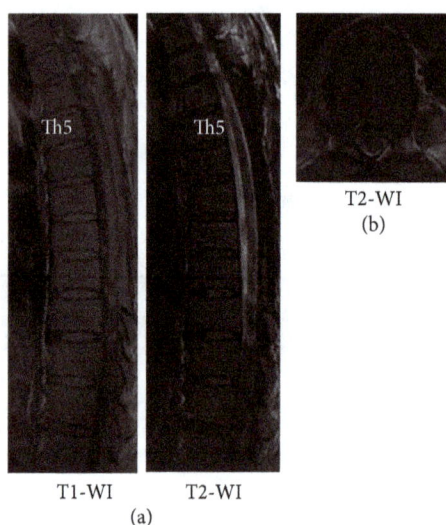

FIGURE 5: MRI taken one year later shows no recurrence. (a) Sagittal plane. (b) Axial plane.

of EMH (male-to-female ratio of 2.5 : 1) and predominantly affect the thoracic spine [5–8]. Furthermore, 80% of all patients are asymptomatic; patients with myelopathy are uncommon [9]. In a study by Koch et al., spinal lesions of EMH were observed only in 0.6% of a total of 510 cases [10]. With respect to spinal cord compression due to spinal EMH, the most common underlying cause has been reported to be thalassemia according to a previous study of 42 patients [5, 6].

Polycythemia vera is a bone marrow disease marked by excessive production of red blood cells and is often accompanied by an increased number of white blood cells and platelets. The disorder is frequently observed in middle-aged and older men [11, 12]. The physical findings are nonspecific but may include an enlarged liver or spleen, plethora, or gouty nodules. It is often accompanied with circulatory disorders and coagulation abnormalities. Phlebotomy and chemotherapy are used to decrease blood thickness [13]. To the best of our knowledge, in polycythemia vera, myelopathy caused by spinal EMH is extremely rare with only 11 reported cases identified [12, 14, 15].

History of hematological disorders that could present with EMH is important for the diagnosis of spinal EMH.

Moreover, MRI is useful as a diagnostic imaging modality. These masses appear as isointense signals on T1-WI and high-intensity signals on T2-WI and are often enhanced by gadolinium administration. Differential diagnosis includes lymphoma, metastatic spinal tumors, and epidural hematoma. A definitive diagnosis can be made by the identification of three hematopoietic cell elements on biopsy specimens or surgical samples.

The main treatment for myelopathy caused by spinal EMH is radiation or surgical decompression, and both therapies offer relatively good clinical outcomes [8, 16]. Although EMH has a relatively high radio-sensitivity and reduction of spinal lesions can be expected with the radiation, recurrence has been reported in some cases [17, 18]. In polycythemia vera, only two cases were previously reported to be treated by decompression surgery without radiation; however both of them showed no improvement of the symptoms [12]. On the other hand, in the present case, decompression surgery could achieve improvement of the symptoms without recurrence, indicating that surgical treatment may be also effective on the polycythemia vera patient with myelopathy due to spinal EMH. In cases of hematological disorders, including polycythemia vera, the platelet counts may be decreased; therefore, special care must be taken for perioperative bleeding when performing surgical treatment including laminectomy and excision of the EMH masses. In our case, intraoperative bleeding was 1250 g despite intraoperative transfusion of platelets. Previous reports have described surgical treatment combined with radiation therapy; however, in the present case, postoperative radiation therapy was not considered necessary as EMH masses were almost completely dissected during operation and the symptoms improved immediately after surgery. No recurrence was observed one year after the surgery as confirmed by MRI examination.

Taken together, occurrence of myelopathy and paralysis in patients with polycythemia vera should prompt investigators to confirm the presence of spinal EMH by immediate spinal MRI. If EMH is observed within the spinal column, a treatment strategy involving radiation therapy, surgery, or a combination of both should be considered. Patients with severe myelopathy or paralysis should be treated by early decompression surgery.

Competing Interests

The authors declare that they have no competing interests.

References

[1] Y. Ohta, H. Shichinohe, and K. Nagashima, "Spinal cord compression due to extramedullary hematopoiesis associated with polycythemia vera," *Neurologia Medico-Chirurgica*, vol. 42, no. 1, pp. 40–43, 2002.

[2] E. Orphanidou-Vlachou, C. Tziakouri-Shiakalli, and C. S. Georgiades, "Extramedullary hemopoiesis," *Seminars in Ultrasound, CT and MRI*, vol. 35, no. 3, pp. 255–262, 2014.

[3] N. De Klippel, M. F. Dehou, C. Bourgain, R. Schots, J. De Keyser, and G. Ebinger, "Progressive paraparesis due to thoracic extramedullary hematopoiesis in myelofibrosis. Case report," *Journal of Neurosurgery*, vol. 79, no. 1, pp. 125–127, 1993.

[4] R. Landolfi, M. A. Nicolazzi, A. Porfidia, and L. Di Gennaro, "Polycythemia vera," *Internal and Emergency Medicine*, vol. 5, no. 5, pp. 375–384, 2010.

[5] F. Dore, P. Cianciulli, S. Rovasio et al., "Incidence and clinical study of ectopic erythropoiesis in adult patients with thalassemia intermedia," *Annali Italiani di Medicina Interna*, vol. 7, no. 3, pp. 137–140, 1992.

[6] S. Issaragrisil, A. Piankijagum, and P. Wasi, "Spinal cord compression in thalassemia. Report of 12 cases and recommendations for treatment," *Archives of Internal Medicine*, vol. 141, no. 8, pp. 1033–1036, 1981.

[7] I. S. Martina and P. A. van Doorn, "Spinal cord compression due to extramedullary haematopoiesis in thalassaemia: a case report and review of the literature," *Journal of Neurology*, vol. 243, no. 4, pp. 364–366, 1996.

[8] T. A. Mattei, M. Higgins, F. Joseph, and E. Mendel, "Ectopic extramedullary hematopoiesis: evaluation and treatment of a rare and benign paraspinal/epidural tumor," *Journal of Neurosurgery: Spine*, vol. 18, no. 3, pp. 236–242, 2013.

[9] K. Parsa and A. Oreizy, "Nonsurgical approach to paraparesis due to extramedullary hematopoiesis. Report of two cases," *Journal of Neurosurgery*, vol. 82, no. 4, pp. 657–660, 1995.

[10] C. A. Koch, C.-Y. Li, R. A. Mesa, and A. Tefferi, "Nonhepatosplenic extramedullary hematopoiesis: associated diseases, pathology, clinical course, and treatment," *Mayo Clinic Proceedings*, vol. 78, no. 10, pp. 1223–1233, 2003.

[11] K. Garg, P. Chandra, P. Singh, and M. Singh, "Long segment spinal epidural extramedullary hematopoiesis," *Surgical Neurology International*, vol. 4, no. 1, article no. 161, 2013.

[12] I. C. Scott and C. H. Poynton, "Polycythaemia rubra vera and myelofibrosis with spinal cord compression," *Journal of Clinical Pathology*, vol. 61, no. 5, pp. 681–683, 2008.

[13] I. Gatto, V. Terrana, and L. Biondi, "Compression of the spinal cord due to proliferation of bone marrow in epidural space in a splenectomized person with Cooley's disease," *Haematologica*, vol. 38, pp. 61–75, 1954.

[14] P. P. Piccaluga, C. Finelli, E. Vigna et al., "Paraplegia due to a paravertebral extramedullary haemopoiesis in a patient with polycythaemia vera," *Journal of Clinical Pathology*, vol. 60, no. 5, pp. 581–582, 2007.

[15] J. M. Baehring, "Cord compression caused by extramedullary hematopoiesis within the epidural Space," *Journal of Neuro-Oncology*, vol. 86, no. 2, pp. 173–174, 2008.

[16] R. Haidar, H. Mhaidli, and A. T. Taher, "Paraspinal extramedullary hematopoiesis in patients with thalassemia intermedia," *European Spine Journal*, vol. 19, no. 6, pp. 871–878, 2010.

[17] N. Kambara, K. Toyoda, and H. Tanaka, "A case of recurrent epidural extramedullary hematopoiesis complicated with myelofibrosis," *Orthopedics & Traumatology*, vol. 61, no. 3, pp. 509–512, 2012.

[18] M. Goerner, S. Gerull, E. Schaefer, M. Just, M. Sure, and P. Hirnle, "Painful spinal cord compression as a complication of extramedullary hematopoiesis associated with β-thalassemia intermedia," *Strahlentherapie und Onkologie*, vol. 184, no. 4, pp. 224–226, 2008.

11

A Fatal Sepsis Caused by Hyaluronate Knee Injection: How Much the Medical History and the Informed Consent Might Be Important?

F. Manfreda,[1] G. Rinonapoli,[1,2] A. Nardi,[2] P. Antinolfi,[2] and A. Caraffa[1,2]

[1]*Department of Orthopedics and Traumatology, University of Perugia, Perugia, Italy*
[2]*Division of Orthopedics and Trauma Surgery, Santa Maria della Misericordia Hospital, Perugia, Italy*

Correspondence should be addressed to F. Manfreda; francesco.manfreda@libero.it

Academic Editor: Bayram Unver

The incidence of Osteoarthritis (OA) is gradually increasing worldwide due to two main reasons: longer life expectation and increased functional demand. Several treatment options have been proposed for this disease. Conservative treatment has the goal to improve the quality of life, reduce pain, and prevent the progression of the disease. Hyaluronate viscosupplementation is one of the most used infiltrative treatments for OA, but, despite its common use, clinical efficacy is still under question. Though adverse reactions for this medical option are actually rare, septic arthritis is a very scaring complication. We present a case report of a 59-year-old man who has been submitted to only one knee hyaluronate injection and consequently reported a severe septic arthritis and systemic sepsis, which lead to the death of the patient. We recommend producing correct guidelines for a clean aseptic procedure of injection to obtain proper consensus from the patient and to pay attention to his clinical history and comorbidities before acting any kind of invasive treatment, including joint injection.

1. Introduction

Knee Osteoarthritis (OA) is one of the commonest orthopedic pathologies [1] whose prevalence is increasing worldwide. This burden will continue to increase in the general population [2]; actually, it gives functional deficits in 10% of individuals over the age of 55 years [3]. Several treatments for OA have been proposed during the years in a very large range of strategies [4], including interventions to increase tolerance for functional activity, improve quality of life, prevent the disease, and stop its progression [5]. Among them, intra-articular injection is one of the most used treatments in order to reduce symptoms, both in early and in the severe stages of the disease [6].

Viscosupplementation with intra-articular hyaluronic acid was approved as a conservative option for OA in 1997 by FDA (Food and Drug Administration) [7, 8]. Important benefits for this kind of treatment have been proven in the last years: a recent Cochrane review found overall benefits of viscosupplementation in comparison to placebo for pain, function, and patient global assessment scores [9]. But there are also some other clinical trials and reviews that report fewer or inconsistent beneficial effects [10, 11].

In general, an excellent safety profile for this treatment method has been widely shown, with few common adverse events, such as mild injection site pain and swelling [12–16]. However, there are several adverse effects that may occur in either poor injection technique or patients with preexisting morbidities [17, 18]. While periarticular complications are the most common, with an incidence until 43%, intraarticular adverse reacts (2%–10%) and in particular infections (0,001%–0,072%) are the most dangerous [19].

In this report, we describe a case of a man who received an intra-articular hyaluronate injection for knee OA and developed a severe articular infection and systemic sepsis.

2. Case Presentation

The patient is a 59-year-old male affected by bilateral knee OA. He has already been subjected to surgical intervention of total hip arthroplasty for Hip OA. Past medical features included a severe obesity, with a body mass index higher than 32, chronic bronchial asthma treated with steroid drugs, and systemic arterial hypertension treated with β-blockers. VAS score corresponded to 8-9.

Knee X-rays had shown specific characters of articular OA that we could categorize as grade 3 of disease according to Kellgren-Lawrence scale [20].

His right knee pain was difficult to control with conservative measures, including NSAIDs and narcotics. Oral steroid drugs were improved by his family physician in order to get pain relief but with no benefits.

So he was submitted to an intra-articular hyaluronate injection, without immediate complications. A high molecular weight hyaluronic acid has been used (about 1200 kDa). Cleaning technique was employed prior to the treatment, including the use of antiseptic solution and sterile gloves; sterile infiltrative practice in clean condition has been conducted.

About 48 hours after that, he reported a severe fever, at about 102.2 Fahrenheit/39° Celsius. Antipyretic drugs did not decrease body temperature and in a few hours his general clinical conditions got worse.

72 hours after the injection, he was hospitalized. The input diagnosis was septic shock, which was quickly treated with adequate antibiotic and support therapy. CRP and ESR values reported a gradual reduction and the shock had a quick remission.

Blood and knee synovial fluid cultures had clear and dramatic positive results for two different atypical microorganisms: multiresistant *Escherichia Coli* and multiresistant *Klebsiella*.

Specific antibiogram had shown sensitivity to very few antibiotics for this kind of bacteria. A combination of Vancomycin (500 mg I.V., 4 times a day) and Cephalosporin (Ceftriaxone 2 gr I.V., twice daily) was used for the full treatment.

Anyway, twelve days after admission, the patient presented a complete flaccid paralysis. An encephalic and spinal MRI was performed, showing a septic involvement of more than two vertebrae, in particular from C5 to C7, and the corresponding cervical spinal cord (Figure 1).

The patient was mainly assisted by the Spinal Unit of our hospital which cooperated with the orthopedic team.

Neurologists performed a proper evaluation of spinal function by the ASIA Standard Neurological Classification of Spinal Cord Injury [21]: results were inauspicious. In fact, he did not report any positive response to stimulation and paralysis was complete and permanent.

He has been treated with an intensive rehabilitation program for several weeks.

Meanwhile, he presented a fistula in the proximal region of the leg. So, a new knee X-ray and an MRI were conducted: a severe septic arthritis of the knee and osteomyelitis of tibia and femur were confirmed (Figure 2).

Surgical debridement of the knee and the leg was performed in order to reduce their septic involvement.

Despite his rehab program, the patient did not report any neurological improvements; at a 5-week follow-up, a new cephalic and cervical MRI showed worse conditions: septic

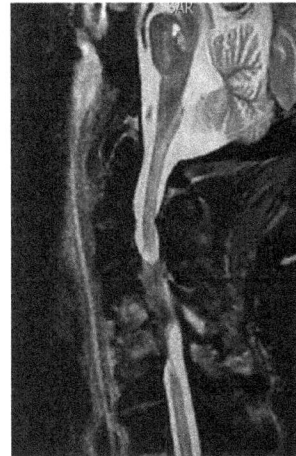

FIGURE 1: Septic involvement of cervical spine and spinal cord.

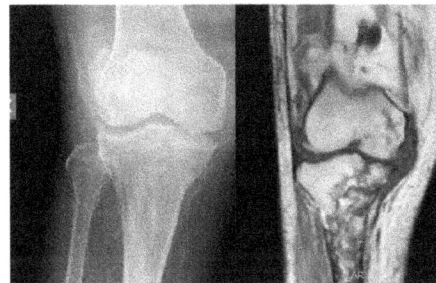

FIGURE 2: X-ray and MRI showing both knee septic arthritis and tibial and femur osteomyelitis.

features have been found in cerebral ventricles, and spinal disease became larger than before: almost the full cervical spine (C2–C7) was involved by the infection (Figure 3).

The higher spinal cord involvement has made self-contained breathing impossible. Thus, the patient started artificial breathing.

At about four months from the entrance to the hospital, breath complications arose, which led to a poor prognosis. The patient died because of severe acquired pneumonia, caused by *Pseudomonas aeruginosa*.

3. Discussion

As mentioned, sodium hyaluronate injection has been proven to be quite safe, with low incidence of adverse reaction [16, 22]. Septic arthritis is a rare but potentially fatal [8, 23–25] severe complication after an intra-articular injection. Although injective practice is conducted in sterile ways, the incidence of joint infection is estimated to be 0,01%–0,072% [19]. In scientific literature, there are several reports about infections for this kind of treatment [8, 16–26]. The causative bacteria could be aerobic, anaerobic, or mixed flora; *S. Aureus* is the most common [27]. Risk factors for joint infections include immunosuppression, diabetes, trauma, and operative infections. Sodium hyaluronate injection is contraindicated if skin disease or current infection is present at the injection

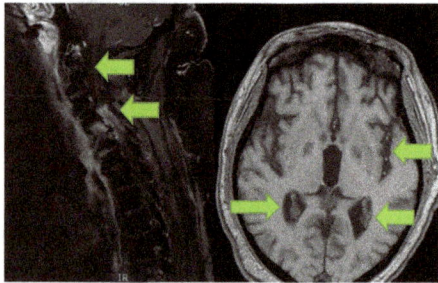

FIGURE 3: Cephalic and cervical MRI showing septic collections in cerebral ventricles and cervical spinal cord.

site, but there is no mention of contraindication for viscosupplementation in immunosuppressed patients or patients with underlying malignancy [8, 28].

Our patient was used to take steroid drugs for his chronic asthma, and there is strong evidence about a connection between chronic steroid therapy with both immunosuppression and increase of atypical infection [29, 30]. He was affected by two uncommon bacteria for joints that presented resistance to several antibiotics, with poor sensibility to Vancomycin and Cephalosporin. Antibiotic resistance has caused a poor response to therapy. So we could think that chronic steroids, which had been increased to relieve pain, could have caused an atypical infection. This could have been also the cause of rapid spreading of infection from joint to bloodstream.

Then, there is strong evidence about increased risk of infection in case of obesity [31, 32]; our patient was not used to practicing any sport activity and he had a very high BMI.

Actually, we do not know exactly how bacteria have been inoculated in his joint. Maybe, even if skin was safe, it might have been the source of inoculation in this immunodepressive condition.

Clinical history of patients should be accurately examined in order to decide proper treatment options related to comorbidities and to evaluate risks of complications related to invasive action.

Another important issue concerns informed consensus. American College of Rheumatology and Italian Consensus of Rheumatology agree about the need of obtaining clear consensus by patients who will be submitted to a joint injection or an arthrocentesis [33, 34]. It should be acquired both orally and in writing, generally after explaining what are the risks and benefits of such action.

We think that a proper and accurate evaluation of the clinical history of patients and the acquirement of clear consensus are essential for every kind of medical action towards patients. Joint injection, too, should indeed be considered an invasive treatment.

Clean careful practice is recommended by using sterile gloves, sterile materials, and clean procedure. Then, it should be noted that there are no international common agreements about guidelines for implementation of clean and aseptic technique [8].

Apart from complications, the debate about long-term effectiveness of intra-articular hyaluronate for OA is always open [9, 11, 35–38].

Several studies show overall benefits for this kind of treatment: it could be considered a viable option in younger patients with less severe disease [9, 35, 36], though some other systematic reviews did not succeed in proving efficacy of hyaluronate joint injection for regression of articular damage [11, 37, 38].

4. Conclusion

The overall incidence of side effects of hyaluronate acid intra-articular injection is lower than 3% [19]. Even if adverse events are quite rare, septic arthritis could be a life-threatening complication. We have presented a case report that underlines the importance of the accurate evaluation of clinical history and comorbidities and the need of clear informed consensus for every invasive treatment, including joint injection. Furthermore, we recommend clear internationally accepted guidelines for clean methods regarding intra-articular injections.

Competing Interests

The authors declare that they have no competing interests.

References

[1] G. S. Dulay, C. Cooper, and E. M. Dennison, "Knee pain, knee injury, knee osteoarthritis & work," *Best Practice and Research: Clinical Rheumatology*, vol. 29, no. 3, pp. 454–461, 2015.

[2] Y. Zhang and J. M. Jordan, "Epidemiology of osteoarthritis," *Rheumatic Disease Clinics of North America*, vol. 34, no. 3, pp. 515–529, 2008.

[3] T. Y. Ammar, T. A. P. Pereira, S. L. L. Mistura, A. Kuhn, J. I. Saggin, and O. V. Lopes Júnior, "Viscosupplementation for treating knee osteoarthrosis: review of the literature," *Revista Brasileira de Ortopedia*, vol. 50, no. 5, pp. 489–494, 2015.

[4] S. P. Yu and D. J. Hunter, "Managing osetoarthritis," *Australian Prescriber*, vol. 38, no. 4, pp. 115–119, 2015.

[5] D. J. Hunter, "Lower extremity osteoarthritis management needs a paradigm shift," *British Journal of Sports Medicine*, vol. 45, no. 4, pp. 283–288, 2011.

[6] A. Migliore, E. Bizzi, J. Herrero-Beaumont, R. J. Petrella, R. Raman, and X. Chevalier, "The discrepancy between recommendations and clinical practice for viscosupplementation in osteoarthritis: mind the gap!," *European Review for Medical and Pharmacological Sciences*, vol. 19, no. 7, pp. 1124–1129, 2015.

[7] B. A. McArthur, C. J. Dy, P. D. Fabricant, and A. Gonzalez Della Valle, "Long term safety, efficacy, and patient acceptability of hyaluronic acid injection in patients with painful osteoarthritis of the knee," *Patient Preference and Adherence*, vol. 2012, no. 6, pp. 905–910, 2012.

[8] S. Virupannavar and C. Guggenheim, "A Patient with fatal necrotizing fasciitis following the use of intra-articular sodium hyaluronate injections: a case report," *Case Reports in Medicine*, vol. 2013, Article ID 531794, 4 pages, 2013.

[9] N. Evaniew, N. Simunovic, and J. Karlsson, "Cochrane in CORR®: viscosupplementation for the treatment of osteoarthritis of the knee," *Clinical Orthopaedics and Related Research*, vol. 472, no. 7, pp. 2028–2034, 2014.

[10] S. P. Yu and D. J. Hunter, "Managing osteoarthritis," *Australian Prescriber*, vol. 38, no. 4, pp. 115–119, 2015.

[11] A. W. S. Rutjes, P. Jüni, B. R. da Costa, S. Trelle, E. Nüesch, and S. Reichenbach, "Viscosupplementation for osteoarthritis of the knee: a systematic review and meta-analysis," *Annals of Internal Medicine*, vol. 157, no. 3, pp. 180–191, 2012.

[12] T. E. Clegg, D. Caborn, and C. Mauffrey, "Viscosupplementation with hyaluronic acid in the treatment for cartilage lesions: a review of current evidence and future directions," *European Journal of Orthopaedic Surgery and Traumatology*, vol. 23, no. 2, pp. 119–124, 2013.

[13] J. F. R. Hammesfahr, A. B. Knopf, and T. Stitik, "Safety of intra-articular hyaluronates for pain associated with osteoarthritis of the knee," *American journal of orthopedics (Belle Mead, N.J.)*, vol. 32, no. 6, pp. 277–283, 2003.

[14] M. M. Cohen, R. D. Altman, R. Hollstrom, C. Hollstrom, C. Sun, and B. Gipson, "Safety and efficacy of intra-articular sodium hyaluronate (Hyalgan®) in a randomized, double-blind study for osteoarthritis of the ankle," *Foot and Ankle International*, vol. 29, no. 7, pp. 657–663, 2008.

[15] P. Jüni, S. Reichenbach, S. Trelle et al., "Efficacy and safety of intraarticular hylan or hyaluronic acids for osteoarthritis of the knee: a randomized controlled trial," *Arthritis & Rheumatism*, vol. 56, no. 11, pp. 3610–3619, 2007.

[16] C. Peterson and J. Hodler, "Adverse events from diagnostic and therapeutic joint injections: a literature review," *Skeletal Radiology*, vol. 40, no. 1, pp. 5–12, 2011.

[17] P. Courtney and M. Doherty, "Joint aspiration and injection," *Best Practice and Research: Clinical Rheumatology*, vol. 19, no. 3, pp. 345–369, 2005.

[18] F. G. O'Connor, "Common injections in sports medicine: general principles and specific techniques," in *Sports Medicine: Just the Facts*, F. G. O'Connor, Ed., pp. 426–433, McGraw-Hill Medical, New York, NY, USA, 2005.

[19] M. B. Stephens, A. I. Beutler, and F. G. O'Connor, "Musculoskeletal injections: a review of the evidence," *American Family Physician*, vol. 78, no. 8, pp. 971–976, 2008.

[20] J. H. Kellgren, M. JeVrey, and J. Ball, *Atlas of Standard Radiographs,* vol. 2, Blackwell Scientific, Oxford, UK, 1963.

[21] American Spinal Injury Association, "Standard neurological classification of spinal cord injury," *Continuum*, vol. 17, no. 3, pp. 644–645, 2011.

[22] D. H. Neustadt, "Long-term efficacy and safety of intra-articular sodium hyaluronate (Hyalgan®) in patients with osteoarthritis of the knee," *Clinical and Experimental Rheumatology*, vol. 21, no. 3, pp. 307–311, 2003.

[23] A. Lim, D. Speers, and C. Inderjeeth, "Cladophialophora (Xylohypha) bantiana—an unusual cause of septic arthritis," *Rheumatology*, vol. 52, no. 5, pp. 958–959, 2013.

[24] T. Konkel, T. Schaberg, H. Dölle, and M. Schulte, "SIRS and ARDS as a result of drug injection in the shoulder region," *Unfallchirurg*, vol. 111, no. 6, pp. 448–454, 2008.

[25] M.-L. Kortelainen and T. Särkioja, "Fatal complications of intramuscular and intra-articular injections," *Zeitschrift für Rechtsmedizin*, vol. 103, no. 7, pp. 547–554, 1990.

[26] J. Bento-Rodrigues, F. Judas, J. Pedrosa Rodrigues et al., "Necrotizing faciitis after shoulder mobilization and intra-articular infiltration with betametasone," *Acta Medica Portuguesa*, vol. 26, no. 4, pp. 456–459, 2013.

[27] S. Trouillet-Assant, L. Lelièvre, P. Martins-Simões et al., "Adaptive processes of Staphylococcus aureus isolates during the progression from acute to chronic bone and joint infections in patients," *Cellular Microbiology*, vol. 18, no. 10, pp. 1405–1414, 2016.

[28] *Hyalgan*, Fidia Pharma, Parsippany, NJ, USA, 2011.

[29] W. H. Reinhart, "Corticosteroid therapy," *Praxis*, vol. 94, no. 7, pp. 239–243, 2005.

[30] J. J. Rinehart, S. P. Balcerzak, A. L. Sagone, and A. F. LoBuglio, "Effects of corticosteroids on human monocyte function," *Journal of Clinical Investigation*, vol. 54, no. 6, pp. 1337–1343, 1974.

[31] Y. M. Arabi, S. I. Dara, H. M. Tamim et al., "Clinical characteristics, sepsis interventions and outcomes in the obese patients with septic shock: an international multicenter cohort study," *Critical Care*, vol. 17, no. 2, article R72, 2013.

[32] S. Thelwall, P. Harrington, E. Sheridan, and T. Lamagni, "Impact of obesity on the risk of wound infection following surgery: results from a nationwide prospective multicentre cohort study in England," *Clinical Microbiology and Infection*, vol. 21, no. 11, pp. 1008.e1–1008.e8, 2015.

[33] M. C. Hochberg, R. D. Altman, K. T. April et al., "American College of Rheumatology 2012 recommendations for the use of nonpharmacologic and pharmacologic therapies in osteoarthritis of the hand, hip, and knee," *Arthritis Care and Research*, vol. 64, no. 4, pp. 465–474, 2012.

[34] L. Punzi, M. A. Cimmino, L. Frizziero et al., "Italian Society of Rheumatology (SIR) recommendations for performing arthrocentesis," *Reumatismo*, vol. 59, no. 3, pp. 227–234, 2007.

[35] N. Bellamy, J. Campbell, V. Robinson, T. Gee, R. Bourne, and G. Wells, "Viscosupplementation for the treatment of osteoarthritis of the knee," *The Cochrane Database of Systematic Reviews*, no. 2, Article ID CD005321, 2006.

[36] W. Zhang, G. Nuki, R. W. Moskowitz et al., "OARSI recommendations for the management of hip and knee osteoarthritis. Part III: changes in evidence following systematic cumulative update of research published through January 2009," *Osteoarthritis and Cartilage*, vol. 18, no. 4, pp. 476–499, 2010.

[37] P. Jüni, A. W. Rutjes, B. R. da Costa, and S. Reichenbach, "Viscosupplementation for osteoarthritis of the knee," *Annals of Internal Medicine*, vol. 158, no. 1, p. 75, 2013.

[38] E. Ayhan, H. Kesmezacar, and I. Akgun, "Intraarticular injections (corticosteroid, hyaluronic acid, platelet rich plasma) for the knee osteoarthritis," *World Journal of Orthopaedics*, vol. 5, no. 3, pp. 351–361, 2014.

12

Traumatic Periprosthetic Acetabular Fracture Treated with One-Stage Exchange and Bone Reconstruction Using a Synthetic Bone Graft Substitute

Jan Svacina

Department of Orthopaedic Surgery, Bodden-Kliniken Ribnitz-Damgarten GmbH, 18311 Ribnitz-Damgarten, Germany

Correspondence should be addressed to Jan Svacina; svacinadr@hotmail.com

Academic Editor: Federico Canavese

A case of a traumatic periprosthetic acetabular fracture in an elderly patient, which was treated by one-stage hip exchange with implantation of an antiprotrusio cage and reconstruction of the acetabular bone loss with an injectable calcium sulphate/hydroxyapatite bone graft substitute, is reported. The paste-like bone graft substitute was injected through the holes of the antiprotrusio cage. After a setting time of 15 minutes, a low-profile cup was cemented onto the cage using polymethylmethacrylate and a new stem was inserted. The patient was encouraged to ambulate three days postoperatively weight-bearing as tolerated. At the one-year follow-up visit the patient was ambulatory and full weight-bearing without any walking aids. The follow-up radiographs demonstrated stable position and articulation of the revision hip arthroplasty with no signs of loosening of the antiprotrusio cage. However, the most interesting finding was that the bone graft substitute had remodelled to a great extent into bone. This calcium sulphate/hydroxyapatite composite shows high osteoconductive potential and can be used to regenerate bone stock in revision arthroplasty.

1. Introduction

Periprosthetic acetabular fractures are rare injuries, but their incidence is rising due to increased prevalence of total hip arthroplasty [1]. They can occur intraoperatively during the insertion of the acetabular component [2] or postoperatively as a result of osteolytic pelvic lesions [3] or periprosthetic insufficiency fractures [4]. Only a few reports about traumatic periprosthetic fractures of the acetabulum and their management are available in the literature [3, 5].

We present the case of a traumatic periprosthetic acetabular fracture (central protrusion fracture) treated by one-stage exchange using a Burch-Schneider antiprotrusio cage and bone reconstruction with a calcium sulphate/hydroxyapatite bone graft substitute.

2. Case Presentation

An 84-year-old male was admitted to hospital after a fall, complaining of pain at his left hip and inability to walk. Seven weeks before a cementless total hip arthroplasty (T.O.P.

cup, polyethylene inlay, ceramic head 32 M, Link, Hamburg, Germany, and AL 2000 shaft, size 8, Speetec Implantate GmbH, Langelsheim, Germany) had been implanted due to severe osteoarthritis of the left hip. No complications had occurred after surgery or during rehabilitation.

The clinical and X-ray examinations revealed a periprosthetic acetabular fracture with dislocation of the loosened cup into the small pelvis (Figure 1). The patient was hemodynamically stable. The fracture was assessed as central protrusion fracture and the fracture type classified as IV.6 B3 (UCS classification for periprosthetic fractures) [6]. According to the classification and recommendation of Peterson II and Lewallen [7], for this type II fracture (loosening of the THA cup-component) we planned a surgical revision with exchange of the loosened cup, additional fracture augmentation, and bone reconstruction with a synthetic bone graft substitute. Informed consent of the patient was obtained.

Surgery was performed four days after admission. The patient was placed on a radiolucent table in supine position. The anterior-lateral approach of the initial surgery was used.

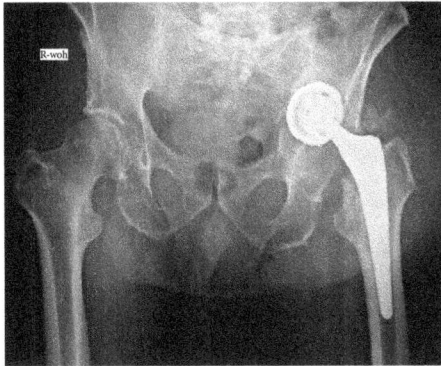

FIGURE 1: Radiograph of pelvis (deep) after fall: periprosthetic acetabular fracture (type IIIa acetabular defect according to Paprosky et al. [20]).

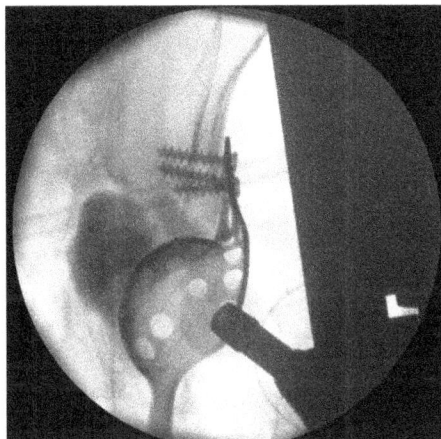

FIGURE 2: Fluoroscopy during surgery: acetabular fracture reduced, Burch-Schneider antiprotrusio cage implanted, and CERAMENT|BVF injected behind the cage.

The loosened cup and the femoral stem were removed. The fracture was reduced and a Burch-Schneider antiprotrusio cage (size 50, Zimmer, Freiburg im Breisgau, Germany) implanted. The significant acetabular bone loss was filled with 18 mL CERAMENT™|BONE VOID FILLER (Bonesupport, Lund, Sweden) under fluoroscopic control (Figure 2). This paste-like calcium sulphate/hydroxyapatite bone graft substitute was injected through the holes of the Burch-Schneider cage. After a setting time of 15 minutes, a low-profile cup (size 48, Longevity, Durasul PE, with a ceramic head 32 M, Zimmer, Freiburg im Breisgau, Germany) was cemented using polymethylmethacrylate (PMMA). Finally, a new stem (AL 2000, size 9, Speetec Implantate GmbH, Langelsheim, Germany) was inserted in a press-fit technique. The patient received a total of five erythrocyte concentrates, two intraoperatively and three postoperatively. The postoperative course was event-free. X-ray confirmed correct position of the antiprotrusio cage and the revision THA (Figure 3). The incision healed *per primam intentionem* without prolonged wound drainage. Diclofenac 75 mg (Ratiopharm GmbH, Ulm, Germany) orally once a day was used as prevention

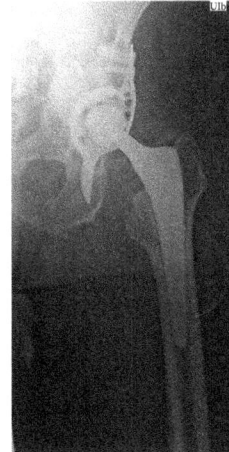

FIGURE 3: Radiograph of left hip a.p. (supine) on the second day postoperatively.

of heterotopic ossifications. The patient was encouraged to ambulate three days postoperatively weight-bearing as tolerated, first with the support of a walking frame and then with a rollator-walker. At postoperative day 17 the patient was discharged and a week later rehabilitation started in an inpatient setting.

2.1. Follow-Up at One Year. At the one-year follow-up visit the patient was ambulatory and full weight-bearing without any walking aids. Extension/flexion of the left hip was 0°-0°-80° and external/internal rotation 20°-0°-10°.

The X-rays at follow-up demonstrated correct position and articulation of the revision THA with no signs of loosening of the Burch-Schneider cage. The bone graft substitute had remodelled to a great extent into trabecular bone (Figure 4). However, heterotopic ossifications (HO) had formed around the hip joint (Arcq classification grade II, Booker classification grade III) [8, 9].

2.2. Follow-Up at Two Years and Eight Months. At the 2-year follow-up examination the patient was ambulatory using a walking stick (Figure 5). He was independent with self-care in his house and had no pain during standing and sitting. His gait was slow and limping with minor pain in the left hip.

Extension/flexion of the left hip was 0°-20°-70°, abduction/adduction 40°-0°-10°, and external/internal rotation 10°-0°-10° (Figure 6). The patient was satisfied with the result of the revision surgery and in general emotionally well.

Radiographically, complete remodelling of CERAMENT|BONE VOID FILLER is now displayed (Figure 7). No signs of loosening of the antiprotrusio cage or movement of the revision THA were found.

The HO had increased; the joint seemed to be completely encased (Arcq classification grade II, Booker classification grade III) [8, 9].

3. Discussion

Only a few cases of periprosthetic acetabular fractures have been reported [2, 7, 10]. Two types of periacetabular fractures

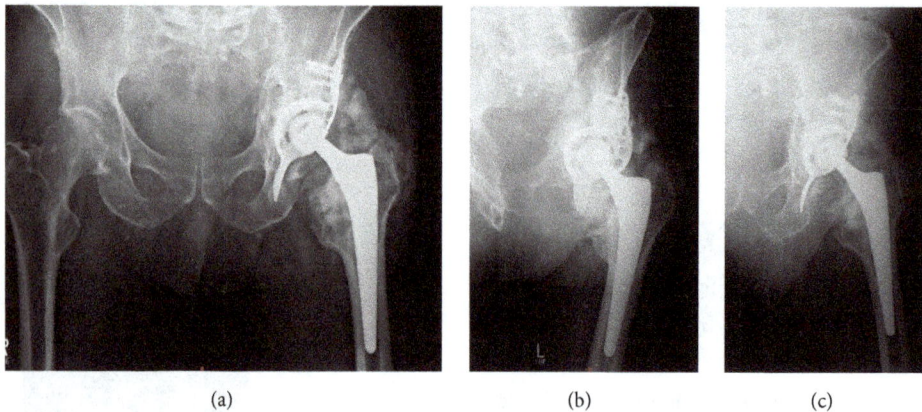

(a)   (b)   (c)

FIGURE 4: Follow-up X-ray (a.p., obturator and ala-view) one year postoperatively.

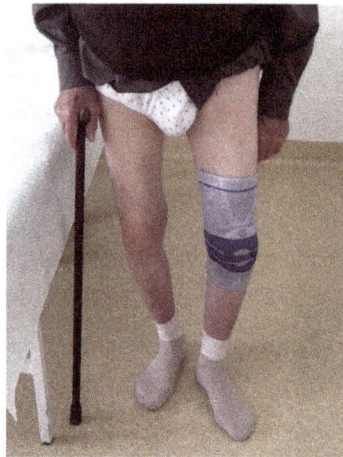

FIGURE 5: Two years and eight months after surgery. Patient is ambulatory using a walking stick.

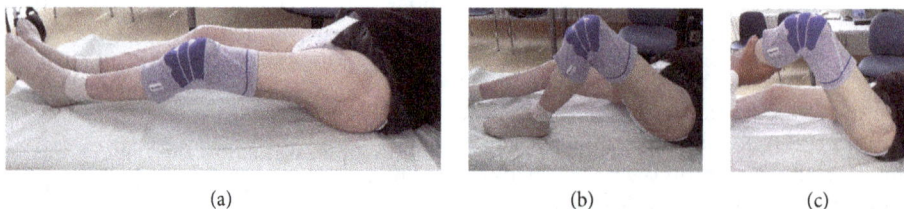

(a)   (b)   (c)

FIGURE 6: Clinical examination two years and eight months postoperatively. Extension/flexion of the left hip 0°-20°-70°, abduction/adduction 40°-0°-10°, and rotation 10°-0°-10°.

should be distinguished: (I) with well-fixed cup-component and (II) with loosening of the THA cup-component. In situation one, a conservative approach is usually recommended [7]. However, to ensure early mobilisation and reduce cup loosening at follow-up, Gras et al. recently advocated a navigated percutaneous screw fixation technique of periprosthetic acetabular fractures [11].

A preoperative CT scan would have been beneficial in our case to describe the fracture and to exclude a pelvic discontinuity, which would have needed additional fixation of the posterior acetabular column.

Risk factors for a periprosthetic acetabular fracture are age, osteoporosis, female gender, overreaming of the

acetabulum, and use of a cementless cup. In our case, we were faced with a type two fracture with loosening of the cup-component. In a revision surgery all components of the THA were removed, the acetabular fracture was reduced, and an antiprotrusio cage, a cemented cup, and an uncemented stem were implanted. This approach has been described before, combined with cancellous allograft to treat the acetabular bone loss [12]. We used the injectable calcium sulphate/hydroxyapatite bone graft substitute CERAMENT|BONE VOID FILLER to reconstruct the bony defect. This material had remodelled into bone to a great extent at the X-ray follow-up after one year (Figure 8). The remodelling was almost complete after two years and eight

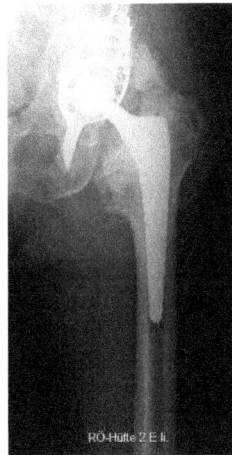

FIGURE 7: Follow-up X-ray of left hip a.p. two years and eight months postoperatively.

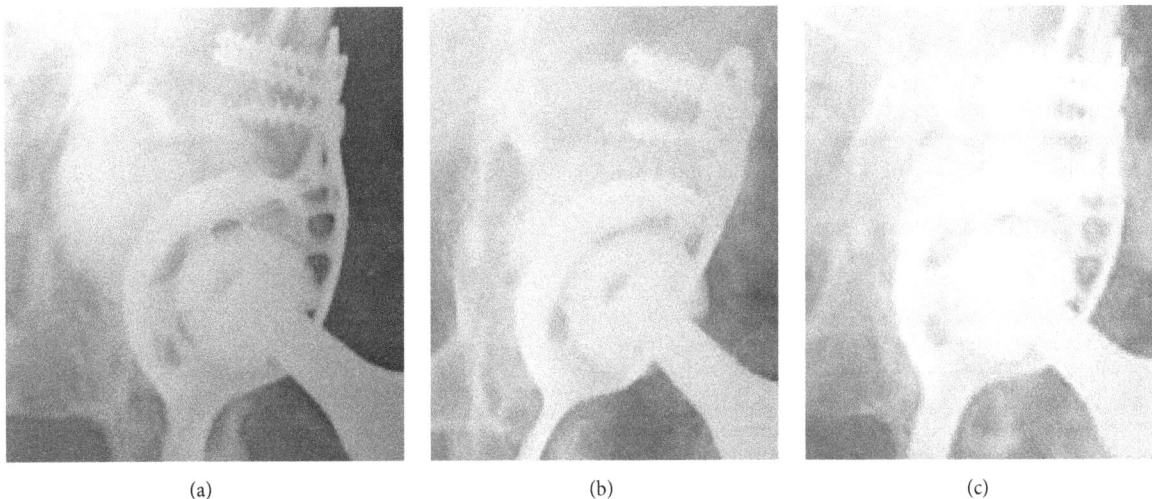

(a)   (b)   (c)

FIGURE 8: Enlargement of the a.p. X-rays of the left hip: at (a) two days, (b) one year, and (c) two years and eight months postoperatively: continuing remodelling of CERAMENT|BONE VOID FILLER into bone.

months. Other bone graft substitutes tend to be resorbed too early (e.g., calcium sulphate) [13] to allow bone regeneration or do not remodel into bone after several years (e.g., calcium phosphate) [14]. The combination of 60% calcium sulphate and 40% hydroxyapatite seems to fulfil the criterion of equal resorption and new bone formation at the same pace [15]. The advantages of remodelling are the prevention of foreign body reaction or infection and induction of new bone stock, which may be required in further hip revision surgery.

In the reported case, the range of motion of the left hip is significantly reduced by HO, which has developed despite the prophylactic use of Diclofenac. HO has been reported in about 10% of primary THA [16], but usually without any limitation of the range of motion. The genesis of HO is still not completely understood [17]. Risk factors are joint arthroplasty, spinal cord injury, traumatic brain injury, blast trauma, elbow and acetabular fractures, and thermal injury [17]. In addition to drug prophylaxis, usually with Indomethacin, prophylactic radiation can be used to prevent

HO. The bone graft substitute used is osteoconductive, but in contrast to growth factors not osteoinductive. An increased rate of HO has not been previously reported in the use of this bone graft substitute [18, 19] and is the subject of a current case series in acetabular revision surgery.

Competing Interests

The author declares no competing interests regarding the publication of this paper.

References

[1] C. J. Della Valle, N. G. Momberger, and W. G. Paprosky, "Periprosthetic fractures of the acetabulum associated with a total hip arthroplasty," *Instructional Course Lectures*, vol. 52, pp. 281–290, 2003.

[2] P. F. Sharkey, W. J. Hozack, J. J. Callaghan et al., "Acetabular fracture associated with cementless acetabular component

insertion: a report of 13 cases," *Journal of Arthroplasty*, vol. 14, no. 4, pp. 426–431, 1999.

[3] J. Sánchez-Sotelo, B. J. McGrory, and D. J. Berry, "Acute periprosthetic fracture of the acetabulum associated with osteolytic pelvic lesions: a report of 3 cases," *Journal of Arthroplasty*, vol. 15, no. 1, pp. 126–130, 2000.

[4] P. Andrews, R. L. Barrack, and W. H. Harris, "Stress fracture of the medial wall of the acetabulum adjacent to a cementless acetabular component," *Journal of Arthroplasty*, vol. 17, no. 1, pp. 117–120, 2002.

[5] P. Harvie, R. Gundle, and K. Willett, "Traumatic periprosthetic acetabular fracture: life threatening haemorrhage and a novel method of acetabular reconstruction," *Injury*, vol. 35, no. 8, pp. 819–822, 2004.

[6] C. P. Duncan and F. S. Haddad, "The Unified Classification System (UCS): improving our understanding of periprosthetic fractures," *Bone and Joint Journal*, vol. 96, no. 6, pp. 713–716, 2014.

[7] C. A. Peterson II and D. G. Lewallen, "Periprosthetic fracture of the acetabulum after total hip arthroplasty," *The Journal of Bone & Joint Surgery—American Volume*, vol. 78, no. 8, pp. 1206–1213, 1996.

[8] M. Arcq, "Die paraartikulären Ossifikationen—eine Komplikation der Totalhüftendoprothese des Hüftgelenks," *Archiv für Orthopädische und Unfall-Chirurgie*, vol. 77, pp. 108–131, 1973.

[9] A. F. Brooker, J. W. Bowerman, R. A. Robinson, and L. H. Riley Jr., "Ectopic ossification following total hip replacement. Incidence and a method of classification," *The Journal of Bone and Joint Surgery—American Volume*, vol. 55, no. 8, pp. 1629–1632, 1973.

[10] M. Chatoo, J. Parfitt, and M. F. Pearse, "Periprosthetic acetabular fracture associated with extensive osteolysis," *Journal of Arthroplasty*, vol. 13, no. 7, pp. 843–845, 1998.

[11] F. Gras, I. Marintschev, K. Klos, A. Fujak, T. Mückley, and G. O. Hofmann, "Navigated percutaneous screw fixation of a periprosthetic acetabular fracture," *Journal of Arthroplasty*, vol. 25, no. 7, pp. 1169. e1–1169. e4, 2010.

[12] I. D. Gelalis, A. N. Politis, C. M. Arnaoutoglou, N. Georgakopoulos, D. Mitsiou, and T. A. Xenakis, "Traumatic periprosthetic acetabular fracture treated by acute one-stage revision arthroplasty. A case report and review of the literature," *Injury*, vol. 41, no. 4, pp. 421–424, 2010.

[13] M. Sidqui, P. Collin, C. Vitte, and N. Forest, "Osteoblast adherence and resorption activity of isolated osteoclasts on calcium sulphate hemihydrate," *Biomaterials*, vol. 16, no. 17, pp. 1327–1332, 1995.

[14] M. Bohner, "Calcium orthophosphates in medicine: from ceramics to calcium phosphate cements," *Injury*, vol. 31, supplement 4, pp. D37–D47, 2000.

[15] M. Nilsson, J.-S. Wang, L. Wielanek, K. E. Tanner, and L. Lidgren, "Biodegradation and biocompatability of a calcium sulphate-hydroxyapatite bone substitute," *The Journal of Bone & Joint Surgery—British Volume*, vol. 86, no. 1, pp. 120–125, 2004.

[16] D. S. Edwards, S. A. R. Barbur, A. M. J. Bull, and G. J. Stranks, "Posterior mini-incision total hip arthroplasty controls the extent of post-operative formation of heterotopic ossification," *European Journal of Orthopaedic Surgery and Traumatology*, vol. 25, no. 6, pp. 1051–1055, 2015.

[17] K. Ranganathan, S. Loder, S. Agarwal et al., "Heterotopic ossification: basic-science principles and clinical correlates," *The Journal of Bone and Joint Surgery—American Volume*, vol. 97, no. 13, pp. 1101–1111, 2015.

[18] A. Abramo, M. Geijer, P. Kopylov, and M. Tägil, "Osteotomy of distal radius fracture malunion using a fast remodelling bone substitute consisting of calcium sulphate and calcium phosphate," *Journal of Biomedical Materials Research—Part B Applied Biomaterials*, vol. 92, no. 1, pp. 281–286, 2010.

[19] R. Iundusi, E. Gasbarra, M. D'Arienzo, A. Piccioli, and U. Tarantino, "Augmentation of tibial plateau fractures with an injectable bone substitute: CERAMENT™. Three year follow-up from a prospective study," *BMC Musculoskeletal Disorders*, vol. 16, article 115, 2015.

[20] W. G. Paprosky, P. G. Perona, and J. M. Lawrence, "Acetabular defect classification and surgical reconstruction in revision arthroplasty. A 6-year follow-up evaluation," *The Journal of Arthroplasty*, vol. 9, no. 1, pp. 33–44, 1994.

13

Acute Pectoralis Major Rupture Captured on Video

Alejandro Ordas Bayon,[1] **Enrique Sandoval,**[1] **and María Valencia Mora**[2]

[1]*Department of Orthopedic Surgery, Hospital Universitario Severo Ochoa, Avenida de Orellana SN, 28914 Leganés, Spain*
[2]*Department of Orthopedic Surgery, Hospital Universitario Fundación Jiménez Díaz, Avenida Reyes Católicos 2, 28040 Madrid, Spain*

Correspondence should be addressed to Alejandro Ordas Bayon; ordastrauma@gmail.com

Academic Editor: Pedro Carpintero

Pectoralis major (PM) ruptures are uncommon injuries, although they are becoming more frequent. We report a case of a PM rupture in a young male who presented with axillar pain and absence of the anterior axillary fold after he perceived a snap while lifting 200 kg in the bench press. Diagnosis of PM rupture was suspected clinically and confirmed with imaging studies. The patient was treated surgically, reinserting the tendon to the humerus with suture anchors. One-year follow-up showed excellent results. The patient was recording his training on video, so we can observe in detail the most common mechanism of injury of PM rupture.

1. Introduction

PM ruptures are rare. Their incidence is rising due to the great number of weight-training injuries. They affect almost exclusively men aged between 20 and 40 years and, in some cases, they are associated with the use of anabolic steroids [1].

It is exceptional to capture on video the exact moment of PM rupture. To our knowledge, there are no videos showing the PM rupture during the eccentric phase of the bench press, which represents the most common mechanism of injury.

We present a typical acute case of PM rupture, surgically treated, with excellent final outcomes.

2. Case Presentation

A 29-year-old male presented with pain in the left axillary area and ecchymosis preceded by a snap while lifting 200 kg in bench press three days earlier. He admitted a previous history of anabolic steroid use, with the last consumption being six months earlier.

Physical examination revealed an extensive hematoma and swelling in the medial side of the left upper arm and absence of the anterior axillary fold with pain in that area. Shoulder range of motion, both passive and active, was complete.

Patient had recorded the training exercise so we could observe the injury. He was laying down on the bench press with an assistant by his head, and he was being recorded from his left side. He was lifting exactly 212.5 kg, and during the third repetition, at the beginning of the eccentric phase, the loss of the natural contour and immediate medial retraction of the PM muscle can be observed (video 1 in Supplementary Material available online at http://dx.doi.org/10.1155/2016/2482189).

Plain radiographs did not show any abnormality. To determine the extension and localization of the rupture, ultrasound (US) and magnetic resonance imaging (MRI) studies were performed. US were interpreted as a probable partial tear of the left PM tendon, while MRI reported on a rupture of PM muscle at myotendinous junction with medial retraction of the inferior portion of the muscle belly.

The patient was treated surgically, thirteen days after the injury. Under general anesthesia on a beach chair position, we performed a modified deltopectoral approach. A rupture affecting the musculotendinous junction was confirmed intraoperatively. The medial stump was identified and controlled with a total of three threads in a Krackow fashion from three corresponding suture anchors. Three holes were drilled lateral to the bicipital groove just where the native footprint was located. The three threads were firmly tightened passing the sutures through the drilled holes with the arm adducted and tied with simple knots.

The patient was postoperatively immobilized in a sling. The second week after surgery, he was allowed to start a passive range of motion; on the third month, he started with resisted motion exercises. On the fourth month, he had returned back to his normal physical activity. In the last follow-up, one year after surgery, he did not mention any pain and was satisfied with the aesthetic. The range of motion regarding the affected shoulder was normal and he had started performing some weightlifting, nevertheless not lifting so much weight as before.

3. Discussion

There are about four hundred cases reported in the literature of PM ruptures. Most of them belong to the last decade, which suggests that PM injuries and those associated with weightlifting are becoming more frequent, in relation to the significant increase in weight-training injuries reported in the last twenty years [1–5] and probably with a concurrent increment in anabolic steroid use [6].

Most cases occur in young active men [2], probably due to the lower elasticity of male tendons, lower tendon to muscle diameter, and an apparent affinity of male for high-energy activities; however, this has not been demonstrated [7].

Anatomically, PM muscle has a triangular-like shape and it origins in the medial clavicle, anterior sternum, first to sixth costal cartilage, and aponeurosis of the oblique external muscle of the abdomen. Its muscular belly has two heads or portions: a clavicular head and a sternal head. The sternal head is also subdivided into another seven segments, although they are not constant. Both heads converge in short, wide, flattened, and bifascicular tendon inserting in the humerus, lateral to the bicipital groove. The two fascicles or layers of the tendon are one anterior, formed by the clavicular head and the more superior segments of the sternal head, and one posterior, formed by the inferior segments of the sternal head. It is remarkable that the clavicular head is shorter than any other of the sternal segments but the two last two segments, S6 and S7, are about 1 to 2 cm shorter than the segments above and the angle of lateral attachment is greater also in these two segments [8, 9].

The main function of the PM muscle is to adduct and internally rotate the shoulder, although it also participates in flexion through the clavicular head [10]. It is a powerful muscle, highly developed in athletes, and its rupture has been related with anabolic steroid use [7, 9, 11].

The most common mechanism of injury is an indirect trauma, during the eccentric phase of the bench press exercise, when the shoulder is abducted, extended, and externally rotated [2, 3, 12]. In this position, PM disrupts in a predictable sequence, being the most inferior segments of the sternal head the first to fail, due to the relative shorter length and greater lateral attachment angle, which generates bigger tensions. The most superior segments of the sternal head and the clavicular head follow the disruption [10]. This can be observed in our video.

Pochini et al. [13] reported on a rupture of pectoralis major captured on video, occurring between the transition between eccentric and concentric phases during a bench press contest in a powerlifting athlete, who also had an anabolic steroid consumption history. It is probable that steroid use leads to abnormal muscle hypertrophy and tendinopathy [14] and thus rupture happens in concentric phase when lifting extremely high weight.

Diagnosis is based on a compatible history and physical examination [3, 15, 16]. Findings as pain in the medial side of the upper arm, swelling and ecchymosis, asymmetry, and weakness with adduction and internal rotation are common, but the most useful sign is the absence of the anterior axillary fold evidenced by resisted adduction or passive abduction of the affected arm [12].

Simple X-rays must be taken to rule out the infrequent cases of bony avulsion. MRI is the preferred imaging technique to determine rupture extension and localization [15]. US requires a more experienced operator, although it can be used if the diagnosis is not clear or when there is an unacceptable delay to MRI [12].

Nowadays the classification system proposed by ElMaraghy and Devereaux [1] is the most complete one. It includes injury timing, acute versus chronic; location, muscle, tendon, bony, avulsion; and extension, width and thickness.

Treatment options vary, depending on patient and injury type. Factors that must be considered are pain, range of motion, adduction weakness or power decrease, aesthetical defect, occupation, and activity level [2, 7, 11, 17]. Conservative treatment is limited to low-demanding patients and partial-tendon or muscle-fibers ruptures [18]. It consists of immobilization, analgesics, ice, and physiotherapy [12]. A prospective study, level 2 of evidence, stated the poor outcomes of conservative treatment in athletes [19].

Many surgical techniques have been described to repair PM ruptures, including tendon-to-tendon suture, bone trough repair, anchor sutures, transosseous sutures, and tendon reinsertion to clavipectoral fascia [20, 21]. In most cases, direct repair to bone is possible with either a transosseous or a suture-anchor repair [15]. Early surgical treatment has demonstrated better outcomes than conservative [3, 7, 18, 22], especially in active patients [11, 17–19, 23]. A meticulous surgical technique and specific rehabilitation programs have been shown to play a more important role in outcomes than a delay in surgery [15, 16, 24, 25]. In case of chronic ruptures, autografts or allografts may be necessary [15]. Surgical complications include infection, heterotopic ossification, injury to the long head of the biceps, neurovascular injuries, and rerupture (0–7.7%) [12]. In an experimental study [26], the majority of failures occurred through the suture used for tendon repair, especially regarding suture-anchor repairs compared with bone trough group.

Postoperatively an individualized rehabilitation protocol is essential. Immediately after surgery, immobilization with sling allowing only shoulder passive motion until the third-fourth week is recommended [22]. Active assisted motion is started between third and sixth weeks, progressing then to active motion [15]. Shoulder is protected from normal life activities for four to six months postoperatively.

4. Conclusions

Pectoralis major ruptures occur more frequently during the eccentric phase of bench press in young male adults because, in this position, the more inferior segments of the muscle are overloaded. Although videos of PM ruptures during eccentric phase can be found, they are not published in recognized medical literature. Our purpose of this paper is to provide access to it to health care professionals as well as bringing a small and helpful review of anatomy, diagnosis, imaging, treatment possibilities, and postoperative management.

Disclosure

Level of evidence is V.

Competing Interests

The authors declare that there are no competing interests regarding the publication of this paper.

Acknowledgments

The authors thank Teresa Quintano for her technical support with the video editing, Miguel Ángel García García, Juliana Marín Ocampo, Rodrigo Díez Tafur, and Juan Luis Jiménez Alarcón for clinical support, and Francisco Forriol and Luis Moraleda for their extensive reviews.

References

[1] A. W. ElMaraghy and M. W. Devereaux, "A systematic review and comprehensive classification of pectoralis major tears," *Journal of Shoulder and Elbow Surgery*, vol. 21, no. 3, pp. 412–422, 2012.

[2] K. Bak, E. A. Cameron, and I. J. P. Henderson, "Rupture of the pectoralis major: a meta-analysis of 112 cases," *Knee Surgery, Sports Traumatology, Arthroscopy*, vol. 8, no. 2, pp. 113–119, 2000.

[3] K. Hasegawa and J. M. Schofer, "Rupture of the pectoralis major: a case report and review," *Journal of Emergency Medicine*, vol. 38, no. 2, pp. 196–200, 2010.

[4] Z. Y. Kerr, C. L. Collins, and R. D. Comstock, "Epidemiology of weight training-related injuries presenting to United States emergency departments, 1990 to 2007," *The American Journal of Sports Medicine*, vol. 38, no. 4, pp. 765–771, 2010.

[5] J. Petilon, C. I. Ellingson, and J. K. Sekiya, "Pectoralis major muscle ruptures," *Operative Techniques in Sports Medicine*, vol. 13, no. 3, pp. 162–168, 2005.

[6] M. E. Westerman, C. M. Charchenko, M. J. Ziegelmann, G. C. Bailey, T. B. Nippoldt, and L. Trost, "Heavy testosterone use among bodybuilders," *Mayo Clinic Proceedings*, vol. 91, no. 2, pp. 175–182, 2016.

[7] V. Äärimaa, J. Rantanen, J. Heikkilä, I. Helttula, and S. Orava, "Rupture of the pectoralis major muscle," *American Journal of Sports Medicine*, vol. 32, no. 5, pp. 1256–1262, 2004.

[8] L. Fung, B. Wong, K. Ravichandiran, A. Agur, T. Rindlisbacher, and A. Elmaraghy, "Three-dimensional study of pectoralis major muscle and tendon architecture," *Clinical Anatomy*, vol. 22, no. 4, pp. 500–508, 2009.

[9] S. W. Wolfe, T. L. Wickiewicz, J. T. Cavanaugh, and P. Shirley, "Ruptures of the pectoralis major muscle. An anatomic and clinical analysis," *The American Journal of Sports Medicine*, vol. 20, no. 5, pp. 587–593, 1992.

[10] D. C. Ackland, P. Pak, M. Richardson, and M. G. Pandy, "Moment arms of the muscles crossing the anatomical shoulder," *Journal of Anatomy*, vol. 213, no. 4, pp. 383–390, 2008.

[11] R. G. Kakwani, J. J. Matthews, K. M. Kumar, A. Pimpalnerkar, and N. Mohtadi, "Rupture of the pectoralis major muscle: surgical treatment in athletes," *International Orthopaedics*, vol. 31, no. 2, pp. 159–163, 2007.

[12] M. T. Provencher, K. Handfield, N. T. Boniquit, S. N. Reiff, J. K. Sekiya, and A. A. Romeo, "Injuries to the pectoralis major muscle: diagnosis and management," *The American Journal of Sports Medicine*, vol. 38, no. 8, pp. 1693–1705, 2010.

[13] A. C. Pochini, B. Ejnisman, C. V. Andreoli et al., "Exact moment of tendon of pectoralis major muscle rupture captured on video," *British Journal of Sports Medicine*, vol. 41, no. 9, pp. 618–619, 2007.

[14] G. Kanayama, J. DeLuca, W. P. Meehan et al., "Ruptured tendons in anabolic-androgenic steroid users: a cross-sectional cohort study," *The American Journal of Sports Medicine*, vol. 43, no. 11, pp. 2638–2644, 2015.

[15] U. Butt, S. Mehta, L. Funk, and P. Monga, "Pectoralis major ruptures: a review of current management," *Journal of Shoulder and Elbow Surgery*, vol. 24, no. 4, pp. 655–662, 2015.

[16] J. F. Quinlan, M. Molloy, and B. J. Hurson, "Pectoralis major tendon ruptures: when to operate," *British Journal of Sports Medicine*, vol. 36, no. 3, pp. 226–228, 2002.

[17] A. A. Schepsis, M. W. Grafe, H. P. Jones, and M. J. Lemos, "Rupture of the pectoralis major muscle: outcome after repair of acute and chronic injuries," *American Journal of Sports Medicine*, vol. 28, no. 1, pp. 9–15, 2000.

[18] J. E. McEntire, W. E. Hess, and S. S. Coleman, "Rupture of the pectoralis major muscle. A report of eleven injuries and review of fifty-six," *The Journal of Bone & Joint Surgery—American Volume*, vol. 54, no. 5, pp. 1040–1046, 1972.

[19] A. de Castro Pochini, B. Ejnisman, C. V. Andreoli et al., "Pectoralis major muscle rupture in athletes: a prospective study," *The American Journal of Sports Medicine*, vol. 38, no. 1, pp. 92–98, 2010.

[20] J. Liu, J.-J. Wu, C.-Y. Chang, Y.-H. Chou, and W.-H. Lo, "Avulsion of the pectoralis major tendon," *American Journal of Sports Medicine*, vol. 20, no. 3, pp. 366–368, 1992.

[21] G. S. Samitier, A. I. Marcano, and K. W. Farmer, "Pectoralis major transosseous equivalent repair with knotless anchors: technical note and literature review," *International Journal of Shoulder Surgery*, vol. 9, no. 1, pp. 20–23, 2015.

[22] G. Merolla, F. Campi, P. Paladini, and G. Porcellini, "Surgical approach to acute pectoralis major tendon rupture," *Il Giornale di Chirurgia*, vol. 30, no. 1-2, pp. 53–57, 2009.

[23] A. De Castro Pochini, C. V. Andreoli, P. S. Belangero et al., "Clinical considerations for the surgical treatment of pectoralis major muscle ruptures based on 60 cases: a prospective study and literature review," *American Journal of Sports Medicine*, vol. 42, no. 1, pp. 95–102, 2014.

[24] M. Guity, A. S. Vaziri, H. Shafiei, and A. Farhoud, "Surgical treatment of pectoralis major tendon rupture (outcome assessment)," *Asian Journal of Sports Medicine*, vol. 5, no. 2, pp. 129–135, 2014.

[25] G. Merolla, P. Paladini, F. Campi, and G. Porcellini, "Pectoralis major tendon rupture. Surgical procedures review," *Muscles, Ligaments and Tendons Journal*, vol. 2, no. 2, pp. 96–103, 2012.

[26] S. J. Rabuck, J. L. Lynch, X. Guo et al., "Biomechanical comparison of 3 methods to repair pectoralis major ruptures," *American Journal of Sports Medicine*, vol. 40, no. 7, pp. 1635–1640, 2012.

14

Technical Innovation Case Report: Ultrasound-Guided Prolotherapy Injection for Insertional Achilles Calcific Tendinosis

Benjamin K. Buchanan, Jesse P. DeLuca, and Kyle P. Lammlein

Primary Care Sports Medicine Department, Fort Belvoir Community Hospital, Fort Belvoir, VA, USA

Correspondence should be addressed to Benjamin K. Buchanan; bbsportsmed@gmail.com

Academic Editor: Johannes Mayr

We describe the use of ultrasound guidance for hyperosmolar dextrose (prolotherapy) injection of the distal calcaneal tendon specifically just anterior to identified enthesophytes in patients with insertional Achilles calcific tendinosis refractory to conservative treatment. This specific technique has not to our knowledge been described or used in literature previously.

1. Introduction

Insertional Achilles tendinosis is a common chronic overuse injury in both athletes and nonathletes alike. Symptoms can last anywhere from weeks to years and cause significant difficulties in daily activities. Treatments can range widely from rest, NSAIDs, topical medications, physical therapy, various injections, and in extreme cases surgical intervention.

Recently, there has been growing interest in prolotherapy injections for this condition [1–3]. Prolotherapy is a relatively safe procedure, with no evidence that points towards decreased tensile strength or increased risk of tendon rupture [2, 4]. One study evaluated radiographic evidence of tendon repair under ultrasonography after prolotherapy treatment that showed reductions in size and severity of hypoechoic regions and intratendinous tears as well as improvements in neovascularity [3]. Evidence is conflicting currently as to the clinical efficacy as well as proper technique of prolotherapy injections for insertional Achilles tendinosis [2]. Thus, further studies are warranted to evaluate the effectiveness of prolotherapy for this condition. This limited technical innovation report is specifically interested in a subset of the previously mentioned patient group who have ultrasound evidence of calcific findings or enthesopathy of the Achilles tendon. The aim of this report is to provide specific ultrasound technique guidance as well as a basis to further evaluate the long term

reduction in pain specifically in patients with the diagnosis of insertional Achilles calcific tendinosis.

2. Materials and Methods

2.1. Ultrasound-Guided Technique. From August 2014 to March 2016, patients presenting to the Primary Care Sports Medicine Department complaining of heel pain, found to have insertional Achilles calcific tendinosis, unresponsive to conservative treatment (i.e., eccentric exercises, Alfredson protocol, rest, and nonsteroidal anti-inflammatory drugs) were treated with an ultrasound-guided prolotherapy technique as described below. Institutional review board approval was obtained for this study and informed consent was obtained from all patients.

2.1.1. Preparation. The patient is placed in the prone position. A towel or pillow is placed under the distal tibia or hung off the side of the table to allow the foot to hang freely in neutral position. The skin overlying the heel should be cleaned and prepared in a sterile manner. We used alcohol based swabs. A nerve block can be performed but most patients do well with a topical spray such as ethyl chloride spray.

2.1.2. Survey Scan. The soft tissues and tendons of the hind foot (Achilles and Plantaris) along with the posterior surface

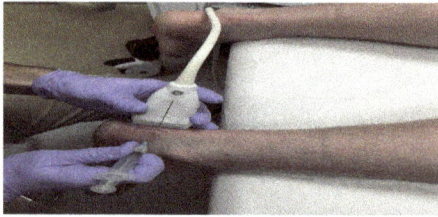

FIGURE 1: Photograph of sonographically guided prolotherapy injection procedure on 42-year-old male with chronic insertional Achilles calcific tendinosis shows simultaneous use of ultrasound probe and 25-gauge needle to target significant sonographic features.

of the calcaneus should be examined in longitudinal and transverse views. A linear or small footprint high frequency (7–12 MHz) ultrasound probe is used. The probe is held on the dorsal aspect of the Achilles tendon over the insertion in long view of the tendon. 1.0 to 2.0 cm depth is all that is needed to visualize areas of the insertion of the Achilles paying particular attention to capturing the entire proximal to distal length of any enthesophyte. Interventions are performed dynamically, with the aid of real-time grey-scale and color Doppler imaging.

2.1.3. Needle Insertion and Injection. A 2 mL mixture of 1 mL of 1% lidocaine and 1 mL of 50% dextrose is placed in a syringe. A 25-gauge 1.5 inch standard needle is guided under real-time ultrasound guidance to the insertion of the calcaneal tendon and specifically underneath/anterior to any identified enthesophyte and in very close proximity to calcification. Injections are generally approached from the medial or lateral side in short axis with preference given to shortest injection distance. When the needle tip is clearly visualized at the desired location, 1-2 mL of the solution is slowly injected depending on size of enthesophytic area with 15–20 fenestrations as area becomes anesthetized. Successful targeting of the desired location is confirmed by spread of anechoic fluid within and around the calcaneal tendon just deep/anterior to the enthesophyte (Figure 1, Table 1).

3. Results

21 patients with clinically diagnosed insertional Achilles tendinosis were referred to the Sports Medicine Department. Of this group, 10 patients were found to have enthesopathy on ultrasound evaluation. This group included 7 males and 3 females with a mean age of 47 years (range 29–57 years). Achilles pain had been present for a mean of 25 months (range 3–120 months) without significant symptomatic improvement. Ultrasound-guided prolotherapy injection was performed on 5 of the 10 patients.

None of the treated patients had previously received any type of injection therapy. Patients primary pain complaint was with push off. Initially these five patients had an average pain level of 5/10 by visual analog scale (VAS) at rest and 8/10 with sport activity such as running. The Victorian

TABLE 1: Ultrasound-guided prolotherapy injection of insertional Achilles calcific tendinosis in the primary care setting.

Indications	Painful calcific tendinosis unresponsive to conservative therapy
Ultrasound-guided technique	A linear or small footprint high frequency (7–12 MHz) ultrasound probe is used to visualize any calcified area or enthesopathy and target the area just inferiorly for injection
Positioning	Patient is placed in prone position with a towel or pillow under the distal tibia while the foot hangs freely
Needle approach	In plane or out plane of plane approach with a 25-gauge 1.5 inch standard needle
Important anatomy	Achilles tendon, calcaneus, enthesophyte, and Plantaris tendon
Potential complications	Significant complications have not been reported. Possible complications that are typical of similar injections are pain, bleeding, infection, and local irritation

Institute of Sport Assessment-Achilles questionnaire (VISA-A), a previously validated questionnaire used for assessing the index of severity of Achilles tendinopathy, was also used as an objective measure to assess level of improvement. The VISA-A consists of eight questions that measure domains of pain, function in daily living, and sporting activity. Results range from 0 to 100, where 100 represents the perfect score [5]. The average VISA-A score for these patients before prolotherapy injections was 37.

All five patients reported drastic pain relief as well as a return to normal gait and sports activity within 8 weeks of receiving prolotherapy. At that time, the average pain level by VAS at rest was 1/10 with two patients reporting complete pain relief at rest. The average pain level by VAS with sport activity was reported as a 3/10. The average VISA-A score after prolotherapy injections was 84, indicating a sizeable clinical improvement in pain and function. Four patients received an isolated prolotherapy injection. One patient received a second injection 4 weeks after the initial injection. All patients denied recurrence of previous pain levels and symptoms.

4. Case Presentation #1

A 42-year-old healthy male presented to the Sports Medicine Department with complaint of left Achilles pain for 10 years. He complained of 5/10 sharp pain when walking and 10/10 with running. The pain significantly limited various activities of daily function. His VISA-A score at that time was 35. The patient had been doing physical therapy in conjunction with eccentric home exercises 5 days per week for the previous 8 weeks. He had also tried activity modification as well as nonsteroidal anti-inflammatory drugs with minimal relief. Plain films of the heel were unremarkable but MRI revealed a longitudinal partial tear of the central fibers of the distal Achilles tendon with chronic inflammatory changes. Ultrasound evaluation in the clinic showed a prominent enthesophyte along with insertional mixed echogenicity of

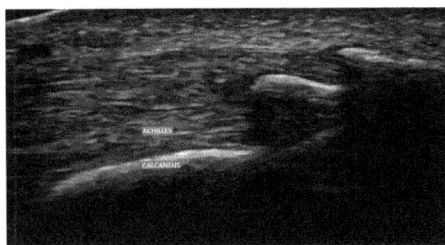

FIGURE 2: Long axis view ultrasound evaluation in a male with long-time chronic symptoms shows enthesophyte irregularity of the cortex of the calcaneus as well as intratendinous calcification at the Achilles tendon insertion.

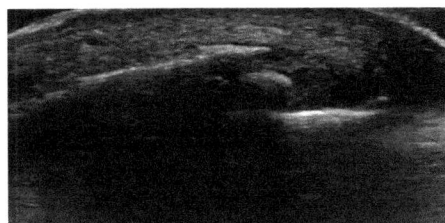

FIGURE 3: Axial view ultrasound evaluation in a patient with subacute symptoms also shows a large enthesophyte at the insertion of the Achilles tendon.

the Achilles tendon. The patient continued physical therapy after prolotherapy injection and within a few weeks the patient reported drastic improvement in pain levels. After two months, he reported near complete resolution of pain with levels decreased to 1/10 at rest and 3/10 with running. His follow-up postprolotherapy VISA-A score was 82 (Figure 2).

5. Case Presentation #2

A 49-year-old female presented to the Sports Medicine Department with the complaint of right Achilles pain for the past 5 months. The patient was an avid runner and reported running about 50 kilometers per week. She reported 4/10 sharp pain when walking and 7/10 with running. Her VISA-A score at that time was 42. She failed conservative therapy that included activity modification, physical therapy, and eccentric exercises, as well as nonsteroidal anti-inflammatory drugs without relief. Plain films of the heel were unremarkable. Ultrasound evaluation showed a prominent enthesophyte in proximity to the insertion of the Achilles tendon. Ultrasound also revealed heterogeneity throughout the Achilles tendon. Similar to the patient in case presentation #1, the patient continued physical therapy after injection and within a few weeks the patient reported drastic improvement. After a couple of months, she reported near complete resolution of pain, with no pain at rest and 1/10 with running. Her follow-up postprolotherapy VISA-A score was 95 (Figure 3).

6. Discussion

Prolotherapy is increasingly being used as treatment for a variety of musculoskeletal disorders such as lower back pain [6], knee instability secondary to anterior cruciate ligament injury [7], and osteoarthritis [8], as well as ankle sprains and meniscal injuries [9]. Specifically, in relation to our cases, dextrose prolotherapy seems to show significant clinical efficacy according to case series data for Achilles insertional tendinopathy [1]. Prolotherapy is understood to elicit a proliferant cellular response by inducing inflammation, subsequent growth factor production leading to increased fibroblast proliferation (either locally or systemic), and increased production of extracellular matrix materials [10]. A possible explanation for the success in our cases of enthesopathy is that over time the strongest portion of the tendon was able to "win out" over the bone while being under tensile strength. As the enthesophyte grew, the already weaker tendon insertion deep to the enthesophyte was subjected to a less nourishing environment and began terminal breakdown.

Limitation to procedure efficacy is the fact that sometimes prolotherapy is performed using palpation to guide needle placement. Without visualization, there is higher probability of nonoptimal placement of injectable fluid. Ultrasound guidance will not only aid in precise needle placement but also identify which patients are better candidates for injection as demonstrated by visual evidence of calcification.

Insertional Achilles tendinopathy will often show sonographic evidence of hypoechoicity, intratendinous tears, and increased tendon size. Some subsets of these patients will show calcification at the insertion and/or evidence of enthesopathy. The patients we have treated for this condition fall into this subset category and expand on positive outcomes reported previously [3]. The difference in these cases is that the patients had pain primarily with push off at the area of the enthesophyte and that care was taken to only and specifically inject the small area of tissue between the enthesophyte and the calcaneus. We see potential benefit in both subacute and chronic cases as evidenced by the two previous case presentations.

One limitation to our study given the small sample size is the question of how often prolotherapy injections are needed. Preliminarily, it seems plausible that one injection alone may be adequate given four of our patients only needed one injection. It is however conceivable that some patients with severe refractory cases maybe need additional injections. An additional limitation of our study is that follow-up ultrasound evaluation after clinical improvement was not performed. It would be interesting to see if there was any improvement or regression of calcified areas given the reported improvement in symptoms. It is a possible consideration that the clinical improvement observed is confounded by c-existing pathology of the Achilles tendon as opposed to enthesopathy alone. Previous studies have shown improved sonographic appearance of the tendon after prolotherapy to include neovascularization as well as reduction in tendon size and severity of hypoechoic regions. Regardless of exact etiology of insertional Achilles tendon pain, patients clinically improve with administration of prolotherapy, but more extensive studies and clinical trials are warranted to potentially isolate calcific causes and evaluate the efficacy of our technical approach aimed at injections specifically underneath the enthesopathy.

The numbers are small but the reported outcomes in these patients are encouraging. Ultrasound-guided prolotherapy injection seems to be most beneficial where conservative therapy has failed and there is evidence of enthesopathy or calcific findings and the technique is done as specified. Ultrasound guidance should be the technique of choice for prolotherapy injection for this condition as it provides the highest likelihood that the injectable fluid is placed in deep to the enthesophyte or calcified area.

Competing Interests

The authors declare that they have no competing interests.

References

[1] N. J. Maxwell, M. B. Ryan, J. E. Taunton, J. H. Gillies, and A. D. Wong, "Sonographically guided intratendinous injection of hyperosmolar dextrose to treat chronic tendinosis of the Achilles tendon: a pilot study," *American Journal of Roentgenology*, vol. 189, no. 4, pp. W215–W220, 2007.

[2] L. M. Sanderson and A. Bryant, "Effectiveness and safety of prolotherapy injections for management of lower limb tendinopathy and fasciopathy: a systematic review," *Journal of Foot and Ankle Research*, vol. 8, no. 1, article 57, 2015.

[3] M. Ryan, A. Wong, and J. Taunton, "Favorable outcomes after sonographically guided intratendinous injection of hyperosmolar dextrose for chronic insertional and midportion achilles tendinosis," *American Journal of Roentgenology*, vol. 194, no. 4, pp. 1047–1053, 2010.

[4] C. A. Q. Martins, R. T. Bertuzzi, R. A. Tisot et al., "Dextrose prolotherapy and corticosteroid injection into rat Achilles tendon," *Knee Surgery, Sports Traumatology, Arthroscopy*, vol. 20, no. 10, pp. 1895–1900, 2012.

[5] J. M. Robinson, J. L. Cook, C. Purdam et al., "The VISA-A questionnaire: a valid and reliable index of the clinical severity of Achilles tendinopathy," *British Journal of Sports Medicine*, vol. 35, no. 5, pp. 335–341, 2001.

[6] M. J. Yelland, P. P. Glasziou, N. Bogduk, P. J. Schluter, and M. McKernon, "Prolotherapy injections, saline injections, and exercises for chronic low-back pain: a randomized trial," *Spine*, vol. 29, no. 1, pp. 9–16, 2004.

[7] K. D. Reeves and K. M. Hassanein, "Long term effects of dextrose prolotherapy for anterior cruciate ligament laxity," *Alternative Therapies in Health and Medicine*, vol. 9, no. 3, pp. 58–62, 2003.

[8] K. D. Reeves and K. Hassanein, "Randomized, prospective, placebo-controlled double-blind study of dextrose prolotherapy for osteoarthritic thumb and finger (DIP, PIP, and trapeziometacarpal) joints: evidence of clinical efficacy," *Journal of Alternative and Complementary Medicine*, vol. 6, no. 4, pp. 311–320, 2000.

[9] B. D. Fullerton, "High-resolution ultrasound and magnetic resonance imaging to document tissue repair after prolotherapy: a report of 3 cases," *Archives of Physical Medicine and Rehabilitation*, vol. 89, no. 2, pp. 377–385, 2008.

[10] M. Cusi, J. Saunders, B. Hungerford, T. Wisbey-Roth, P. Lucas, and S. Wilson, "The use of prolotherapy in the sacroiliac joint," *British Journal of Sports Medicine*, vol. 44, no. 2, pp. 100–104, 2010.

15

Bilateral Diabetic Knee Neuroarthropathy in a Forty-Year-Old Patient

Patrick Goetti, Nicolas Gallusser, and Olivier Borens

Department of Orthopedics and Traumatology, Lausanne University Hospital, rue du Bugnon 46, 1011 Lausanne, Switzerland

Correspondence should be addressed to Patrick Goetti; patrick.goetti@chuv.ch

Academic Editor: Bayram Unver

Diabetic osteoarthropathy is a rare cause of neuropathic joint disease of the knee; bilateral involvement is even more exceptional. Diagnosis is often made late due to its unspecific symptoms and appropriate surgical management still needs to be defined, due to lack of evidence because of the disease's low incidence. We report the case of a forty-year-old woman with history of diabetes type I who developed bilateral destructive Charcot knee arthropathy. Bilateral total knee arthroplasty was performed in order to achieve maximal functional outcome. Follow-up was marked by bilateral tibial periprosthetic fractures treated by osteosynthesis with a satisfactory outcome. The diagnosis of Charcot arthropathy should always be in mind when dealing with atraumatic joint destruction in diabetic patients. Arthroplasty should be considered as an alternative to arthrodesis in bilateral involvement in young patients.

1. Introduction

The first anatomopathological description of neuropathic joint destruction was reported by Jean-Martin Charcot in 1868. While many disorders have been related to neuropathic joint arthropathy, diabetes mellitus is nowadays the primary etiology [1–4]. The prevalence of diabetic osteoarthropathy lies between 0.1 and 13% [5]. Bilateral Charcot arthropathy is a rare condition [6]. The diagnosis is often made late due to the unspecific early presentation of brutal inflammatory joint pain, which can also be misdiagnosed as common fracture, infectious, rheumatic arthritis, deep venous thrombosis, algoneurodystrophy, or erysipelas [7]. The diagnosis is made with standard X-rays and inflammatory parameters on blood tests. Due to its low incidence, the appropriate surgical treatment is still controversial with a trend going towards total knee arthroplasty (TKA).

2. Case Presentation

A forty-year-old woman with history of type I diabetes mellitus complicated with diabetic neuropathy and Charcot disease of her right foot is referred from her general practitioner with right knee pain without history of trauma.

The initial X-rays revealed a Schatzker type V tibial plateau fracture which was surgically treated by open reduction and lateral plate osteosynthesis using a locking compression plate (LCP) (Figures 1, 2, and 3). Progressive secondary fracture displacement on follow-up X-rays associated with necrosis of the medial tibial plateau and finally plate failure at three months postoperatively was observed (Figure 4). Varus pseudolaxity was present on clinical examination, a low-grade infection was suspected, and removal of hardware and wide debridement were performed. A postoperative CT-scan showed complete articular destruction of the medial and lateral tibial plateau (Figure 5). Sonication of the implant and standard microbiological exams remained negative. Due to the important destruction of the proximal tibia, a cemented rotating hinged knee prosthesis (RHK, Zimmer®) was implanted. Postoperatively the patient stayed for six weeks with partial weight bearing. Knee range of motion (ROM) was 105/0/0° (flexion/extension/hyperextension) at nine days postoperatively. Wound healing was uneventful in a satisfied patient with no complaints about her knee.

Eighteen months after initial management of the right knee, the patient presented at our outpatients' clinic with complaints of progressive invalidating contralateral knee pain. Performing the X-rays of the left knee, we were

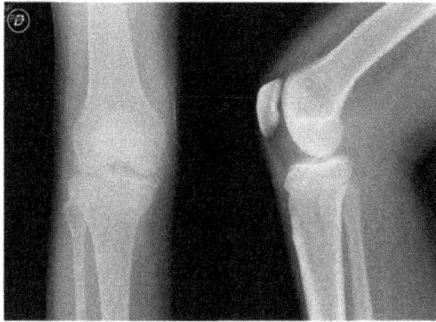

FIGURE 1: Initial X-rays of the right knee.

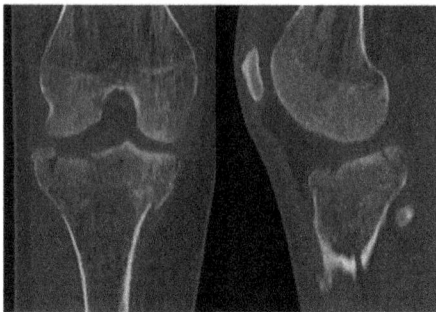

FIGURE 2: Initial CT-scan of the right knee.

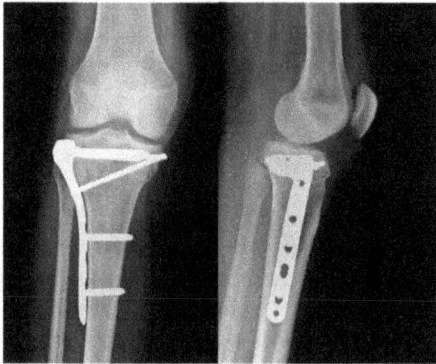

FIGURE 3: X-rays of the right knee after osteosynthesis.

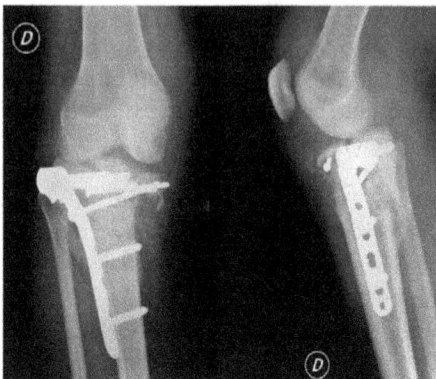

FIGURE 4: Follow-up X-rays at three months postoperatively of the right knee.

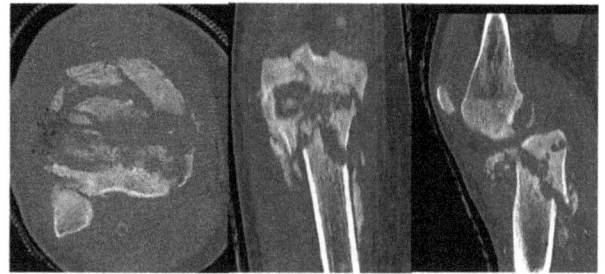

FIGURE 5: CT-scan after plate removal of the right knee.

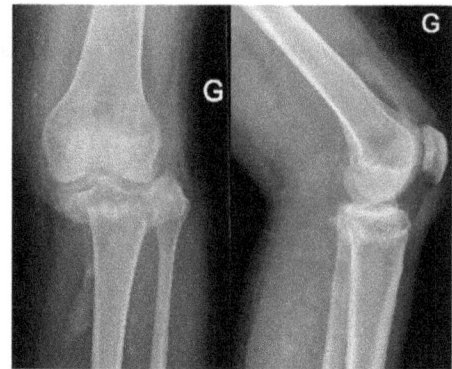

FIGURE 6: Initial X-rays of the left knee.

suspicious of a Charcot arthropathy (Figure 6). None-weight bearing immobilization of the left limb was initiated and one month later a cemented Zimmer® RHK prosthesis was implanted. Reeducation was performed with partial weight bearing of the left limb and knee ROM was 90/0/0° at seven days postoperatively. At one month postoperatively she started complaining of increasing left diaphyseal tibial pain without trauma. X-rays revealed a periprosthetic fracture around the tibial shaft. The patient was taken back to the operating room (OR) for revision surgery with replacement of the tibial stem and cerclage of the tibial shaft fracture. At three months postoperatively the patient still needed two crutches to walk. The scars were calm, and knee ROM was 100/0/3° on the left side and 120/0/5° on the right side (Figure 7).

At ten months postoperatively the patient was readdressed with left tibial pain. X-rays revealed a displaced fracture below the tip of the revision tibial stem, which had appeared at seven months postoperatively and had been initially treated with cast immobilization and none-weight bearing at an outside hospital. The patient was taken back to the OR and LCP plating of the distal left tibia and peroneus was performed.

At one year postoperatively the patient was addressed to emergency department with a periprosthetic fracture of the proximal right tibia without any trauma. Revision surgery with replacement of the tibial implant by a long stem bridging the fracture line was performed. At six weeks postoperatively the patient was able to walk with two crutches and presented good wound healing. Knee ROM was 95/0/0° on both sides.

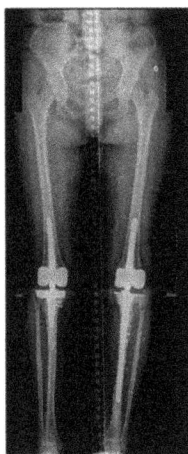

FIGURE 7: Follow-up X-rays, three months after osteosynthesis of the left tibial periprosthetic fracture.

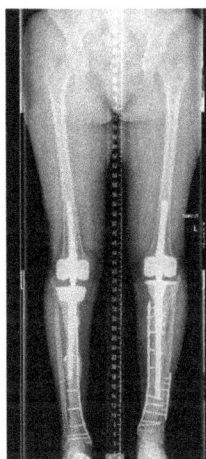

FIGURE 8: Follow-up X-rays, twelve months after osteosynthesis of the right tibial periprosthetic fracture.

She was finally seen again two months later after a fall down the stairs with a periprosthetic fracture of the distal tibia. The fracture was dealt with by LCP plating of the right distal tibia. After consultation of our Rheumatology Department, a six-month off-label prescription of teriparatide (Forsteo®) was introduced to promote bone healing and prevent further fractures. Follow-up was uneventful at one year postoperatively. She walked with two crutches and knee ROM was 95/0/0° on both sides (Figure 8).

3. Discussion

Neuropathic arthropathy is a rare complication of diabetes mellitus, which can occur in one or more joints. Knee involvement however is exceptional [5]. Standard treatment implies long term glycemic control to obtain disease stabilization and none-weight bearing cast immobilization [7]. Nevertheless, this treatment is difficult to apply to the knee especially in the case of a young and active patient.

Medical treatment with alendronate and calcitonin has been proposed, but there is at the moment not enough evidence in the literature to recommend their systematic clinical use [8]. In our case we introduced teriparatide at the end of the surgical management. To our knowledge, there is only one case report of a successful use of teriparatide in ankle Charcot arthropathy [9]; we think there is a need for further studies to confirm this indication. The gold standard for surgical treatment used to be arthrodesis due to the high complication rates of TKR [10, 11]. With recent improvement in long term survival of total knee replacement in neuropathic joint destruction with 85% survival at 8 years as reported by Parvizi [12, 13], TKR is nowadays a valid option with a higher functional outcome than arthrodesis by conserving knee joint function and with fewer issues on leg length discrepancy.

Neuropathic arthropathy can be classified in three stages using standard radiology (developmental, coalescence, and reconstructive) using the Eichenholtz classification. A better outcome is obtained if implantation occurs after the initial developmental phase [14]. In our case, total knee arthroplasty was performed rather early.

We chose a cemented fixation to achieve a good primary fixation and an RHK design was used because of the pre-existing deformity and associated ligamentous insufficiency. One described complication of early implantation is aseptic loosening due to the increased stress on the bone cement interface, which was not present in our case [15]. We were on the other hand confronted with a high complication rate with bilateral periprosthetic fractures. We refer them to the stress riser induced by the modulus mismatch between the stem and the patient's extremely narrow tibial diaphysis.

4. Conclusion

The diagnosis of Charcot arthropathy should always be in mind when dealing with atraumatic joint destruction in diabetic patients. There is still a lack of consensus regarding the optimal treatment when operative management is indicated. In our opinion total knee arthroplasty (TKA) should be preferred over arthrodesis in young patients. Nonetheless, TKA for neuropathic arthropathy is associated with high complication rates. It is technically very demanding and often needs operative techniques and implants otherwise reserved for complex revision arthroplasties.

Competing Interests

The authors declare that they have no competing interests.

References

[1] R. C. Cassidy and W. O. Shaffer, "Charcot arthropathy because of congenital insensitivity to pain in an adult," *Spine Journal*, vol. 8, no. 4, pp. 691–695, 2008.

[2] D. Biotti, R. Fuerea, G. Deschamps, and S. Durupt, "Neurogenic osteoarthropathy of the knee associated with spina bifida: a diagnosis not to be missed," *La Revue de Médecine Interne*, vol. 30, no. 11, pp. 985–987, 2009.

[3] D. S. Feldman, D. E. Ruchelsman, D. B. Spencer, J. J. Straight, M. E. Schweitzer, and F. B. Axelrod, "Peripheral arthropathy in hereditary sensory and autonomic neuropathy types III and IV," *Journal of Pediatric Orthopaedics*, vol. 29, no. 1, pp. 91–97, 2009.

[4] A. Sudanese, S. Paderni, E. Guerra, and F. Bertoni, "Neurogenic arthropathy of the knee due to chronic alcoholism: two case reports," *La Chirurgia Degli Organi di Movimento*, vol. 88, no. 4, pp. 427–434, 2003.

[5] R. G. Frykberg and R. Belczyk, "Epidemiology of the Charcot foot," *Clinics in Podiatric Medicine and Surgery*, vol. 25, no. 1, pp. 17–28, 2008.

[6] B. D. Fullerton and L. A. Browngoehl, "Total knee arthroplasty in a patient with bilateral Charcot knees," *Archives of Physical Medicine and Rehabilitation*, vol. 78, no. 7, pp. 780–782, 1997.

[7] D. L. Nielson and D. G. Armstrong, "The natural history of Charcot's neuroarthropathy," *Clinics in Podiatric Medicine and Surgery*, vol. 25, no. 1, pp. 53–62, 2008.

[8] A. Jostel and E. B. Jude, "Medical treatment of charcot neuroosteoarthropathy," *Clinics in Podiatric Medicine and Surgery*, vol. 25, no. 1, pp. 63–69, 2008.

[9] K. Tamai, K. Takamatsu, and K. Kazuki, "Successful treatment of nonunion with teriparatide after failed ankle arthrodesis for Charcot arthropathy," *Osteoporosis International*, vol. 24, no. 10, pp. 2729–2732, 2013.

[10] L. Marmor, "The marmor knee replacement," *Orthopedic Clinics of North America*, vol. 13, no. 1, pp. 55–64, 1982.

[11] C. S. Ranawat and J. J. Shine, "Duo condylar total knee arthroplasty," *Clinical Orthopaedics and Related Research*, vol. 94, pp. 185–195, 1973.

[12] J. Parvizi, J. Marrs, and B. F. Morrey, "Total knee arthroplasty for neuropathic (Charcot) joints," *Clinical Orthopaedics and Related Research*, vol. 416, pp. 145–150, 2003.

[13] D. K. Bae, S. J. Song, K. H. Yoon, and J. H. Noh, "Long-term outcome of total knee arthroplasty in charcot joint: a 10- to 22-year follow-up," *Journal of Arthroplasty*, vol. 24, no. 8, pp. 1152–1156, 2009.

[14] S. Yoshino, J. Fujimori, A. Kajino, M. Kiowa, and S. Uchida, "Total knee arthroplasty in Charcot's joint," *Journal of Arthroplasty*, vol. 8, no. 3, pp. 335–340, 1993.

[15] J. M. Hartford, S. B. Goodman, D. J. Schurman, and G. Knoblick, "Complex primary and revision total knee arthroplasty using the condylar constrained prosthesis: an average 5-year follow-up," *Journal of Arthroplasty*, vol. 13, no. 4, pp. 380–387, 1998.

16

Avulsion Fracture of the Coracoid Process at the Coracoclavicular Ligament Insertion: A Report of Three Cases

Takeshi Morioka,[1] **Kiyohisa Ogawa,**[1] **and Masaaki Takahashi**[2]

[1]*Department of Orthopedic Surgery, Eiju General Hospital, 2-23-16 Higashi-Ueno, Taito-ku, Tokyo 110-8645, Japan*
[2]*Department of Orthopedic Surgery, National Hospital Organization Tokyo Medical Center, 2-5-1 Higashigaoka, Meguro-ku, Tokyo 152-8902, Japan*

Correspondence should be addressed to Kiyohisa Ogawa; ogawa51@jcom.home.ne.jp

Academic Editor: Pedro Carpintero

Avulsion fracture at the site of attachment of the coracoid process of the coracoclavicular ligament (CCL) is extremely rare. We presented three adult cases of this unusual avulsion fracture associated with other injuries. Case 1 was a 25-year-old right-handed male with a left distal clavicular fracture with an avulsion fracture of the coracoid attachment of the CCL; this case was treated surgically and achieved an excellent outcome. Case 2 was a 39-year-old right-handed male with dislocation of the left acromioclavicular joint with two avulsion fractures: one at the posteromedial surface of the coracoid process at the attachment of the conoid ligament and one at the inferior surface of the clavicle at the attachment site of the trapezoid ligament; this case was treated conservatively, and unfavorable symptoms such as dull pain at rest and sharp pain during some daily activities remained. Case 3 was a 41-year-old right-handed female with a right distal clavicular fracture with an avulsion fracture of the coracoid attachment of the conoid ligament; this case was treated conservatively, and the distal clavicular fracture became typical nonunion. These three cases corresponded to type I fractures according to Ogawa's classification as the firm scapuloclavicular connection was destroyed and also to double disruption of the superior shoulder suspensory complex. We recommend surgical intervention when treating patients with this type of acute or subacute injury, especially in those engaging in heavy lifting or overhead work.

1. Introduction

The coracoid process can fracture at various sites [1, 2]. However, avulsion fracture at the site where the coracoclavicular ligament (CCL) attaches to the coracoid process is very rare; an extensive literature search found only six such cases [3–8]. Four of these cases were adolescents in whom avulsion fracture of the coracoid apophysis attached by the CCL occurred [5–7]. Fracture of three adolescent cases was associated with complete acromioclavicular separation [5, 6]. Presented here are three cases of adults with similar unusual avulsion fractures associated with other injuries including acromioclavicular joint (ACJ) dislocation and distal clavicular fracture. These three patients were provided with a written explanation of the importance of the publication of their cases and gave their consent.

2. Case Presentation

2.1. Case 1. A 25-year-old right-handed male office worker became inebriated with a friend at a social function and they fell together, with his friend landing on top of his left shoulder. The patient experienced severe left shoulder pain soon after the fall, visited a local orthopedic clinic on the day of the injury, and was referred to our hospital the next day.

Examination showed swelling around the left distal clavicle and shoulder pain that increased with elevation of the shoulder. Past medical and family histories were noncontributory. Radiography demonstrated a left distal clavicular fracture (type 2b according to Craig's classification and type 3B1 according to Robinson's classification) with an avulsion fracture of the coracoid attachment of the CCL [9] (Figure 1(a)).

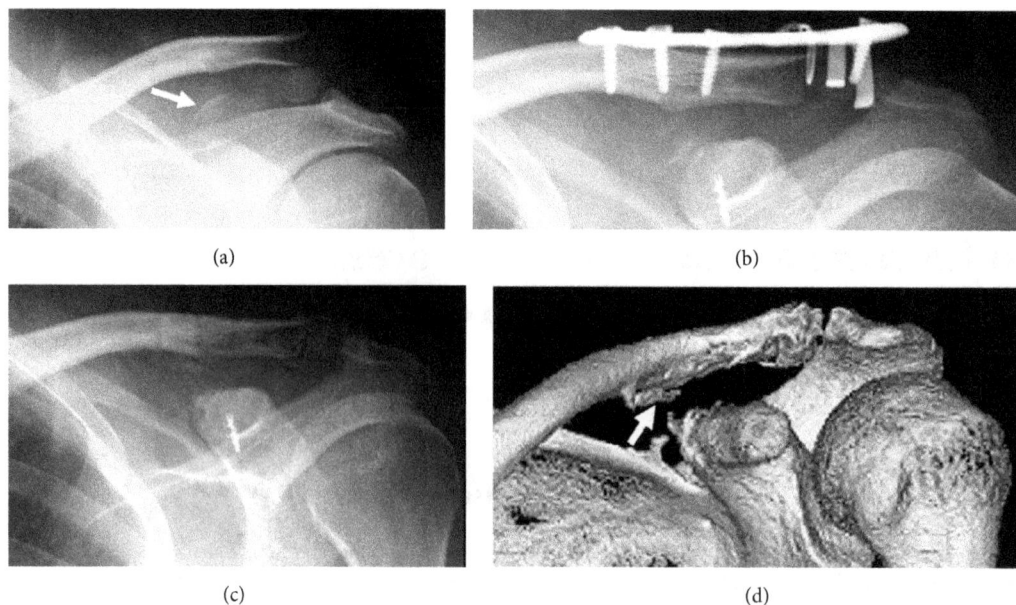

(a)   (b)

(c)   (d)

FIGURE 1: Imaging of Case 1. (a) Radiogram taken at the first visit showing distal clavicular fracture and avulsion fracture of the upper side of the coracoid process (arrow). (b) Postoperative radiogram revealing the well-reduced clavicular fracture and the fractured coracoid fragment. (c) Roentgenogram taken 1 year postoperatively indicating firm bony union of the distal clavicular and coracoid process fractures. (d) Three-dimensional computed tomography performed 1 year postoperatively demonstrating thin new bone formation at the conoid tubercle (arrow).

Surgery was performed on the third day after the injury via a horizontal incision just above the distal clavicle. The conoid ligament had been avulsed from the coracoid with a bone fragment of approximately 15 mm × 10 mm. A small part of the trapezoid ligament had also been avulsed with another small bone fragment; however, most of the trapezoid ligament was anatomically intact. A Scorpion® plate (Aimedic MMT, Tokyo, Japan) was used to secure the fractured distal clavicle. The conoid ligament with avulsed bone fragment was fixed to the fracture bed of the coracoid with a Ti Screw Suture Anchor with EasySlide™ Surface Treatment (Biomet, Warsaw, Indiana, USA) (Figure 1(b)).

After 3 days of immobilization in a sling, passive range of motion exercise of the shoulder was started. Active range of motion exercise was initiated at postoperative week 6. The Scorpion plate was removed at 8 months postoperatively. The fractured bones had achieved a firm union 1 year postoperatively (Figures 1(c) and 1(d)). The Constant score ratio to the normal side was 100% at 2 years postoperatively [10].

2.2. Case 2.

A 39-year-old right-handed male journal editor was hit by a car while walking. He was taken by ambulance to the emergency room of our hospital, where a physician diagnosed traumatic subarachnoid hemorrhage and anterior cruciate ligament injury of the right knee. The patient required hospitalization, during which he complained of persistent left shoulder pain. He was referred to us 3 weeks after the initial injury.

Examination revealed tenderness and swelling surrounding the ACJ. The left shoulder was painful on active movement, although its active and passive ranges of motion were not limited. Past medical and family histories were noncontributory. Radiographs showed dislocation of the left ACJ (type III according to Rockwood's classification) with fractures of the posteromedial surface of the coracoid process and of the inferior surface of the clavicle [11] (Figures 2(a) and 2(b)). The attachment site of the trapezoid ligament to the clavicle and that of the conoid ligament to the coracoid (compatible with the posteromedial side of the coracoid angle) appeared to be avulsed; hence, we assumed that the CCL function was lost. As 3 weeks had already elapsed since the injury, we initiated conservative therapy with a sling for 3 weeks.

Although bony union of the avulsion fractures was confirmed on the radiograms taken 1 year and 6 months after the injury, the coracoclavicular interval and ACJ space remained wide (Figure 2(c)). At 3 years and 6 months after the injury, physical examination showed mild posterior instability and superior protrusion of the distal end of the clavicle. The stress test for the ACJ was negative. The patient complained of dull pain at rest and sharp pain when downward traction was placed upon the arm or when he engaged in overhead work. The Constant score ratio was 88% [10].

2.3. Case 3.

A 41-year-old right-handed woman without occupation who suffered from osteoporosis due to anorexia nervosa fell on her right shoulder. She experienced severe right shoulder pain soon after the fall and presented at our orthopedic clinic on the day of the injury. She had undergone left femoral prosthetic replacement due to traumatic femoral neck fracture 3.5 months previously.

Examination revealed swelling around the left distal clavicle and shoulder pain that increased with shoulder

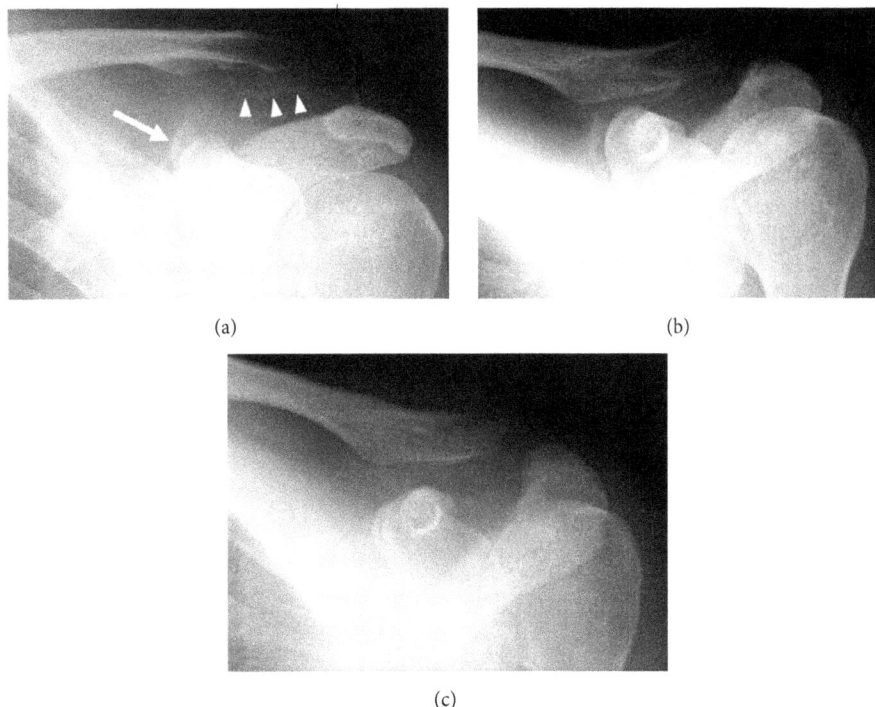

(a)

(b)

(c)

FIGURE 2: Imaging of Case 2. (a) Radiogram taken at the first visit showing the acromioclavicular dislocation and avulsion fracture of the superomedial side of the coracoid process (arrow) and the inferior side of the clavicle (arrow heads). (b) Angle up view taken at the first visit showing avulsion fracture of the coracoid located on the posteromedial side of the coracoid angle (compatible with the attaching site of the conoid ligament). (c) Radiogram taken 1 year and 6 months after the injury demonstrating firm union of the avulsed coracoid fragment.

movement. Radiography showed a right distal clavicular fracture (type 2b according to Craig's classification [9]) with an avulsion fracture of the coracoid attachment of the conoid ligament (Figure 3(a)). We recommended surgical treatment because of the probability that the CCL function was lost; however, the patient refused surgery.

After 3-month immobilization using a figure-of-eight splint and passive range of motion exercise of the shoulder was started. One month later, active shoulder ROM was begun, with some dull pain during movement. Five months after the initial shoulder injury, the patient was in a traffic accident that caused subdural hematoma with resultant right hemiplegia and aphasia. Hence, functional evaluation was impossible 1 year after the shoulder injury. Although bony union of the avulsion fracture of the coracoid was confirmed by computed tomography (CT), the distal clavicular fracture showed typical nonunion (Figures 3(b) and 3(c)).

3. Discussion

Fracture of the coracoid process occurs more frequently than previously thought and is well known to occur in various anatomical sites [1, 2]. Although coracoid fractures in adults have been classified into four or five types based on their anatomical position, Ogawa et al. [12] classified coracoid fractures into two types from a functional point of view according to the relationship between the fracture site and the CCL; type I fractures occurring proximal to this ligament attachment destroy the scapuloclavicular connection, whereas type II

fractures distal to this attachment basically preserve this connection. The cases presented above corresponded to type I fractures, as the scapuloclavicular connection had been destroyed. According to the characteristic fracture site, they should be considered as a subtype of type I fractures.

Nearly all type I fractures are complex injuries and are consistent with the double disruption of the superior shoulder suspensory complex (SSSC) proposed by Goss [13, 14]. There is no consensus regarding the typical mechanism of injury that produces type I fracture [14]. However, a number of reported cases had a common mechanism of injury that was clearly caused by force exerted on the lateral aspect of the shoulder [1, 2, 12–17]. This mechanism is consistent with the concept of lateral impaction injuries, in which a powerful impaction force exerted on the lateral aspect of the shoulder is transmitted via the humeral head to the scapula and clavicle to cause a range of injuries [18]. The mechanism of injury in our cases seems to match this concept. The immediate cause of type I fractures in the majority of cases, however, is unquestionably traction caused by the CCL associated with concurrent injuries, particularly ACJ dislocation, and distal clavicular or acromial fractures [14]. When the traction force is applied to the CCL, breakdown may occur in four different locations and forms: avulsion fracture of the CCL attachment to the clavicle, tear of the CCL itself, avulsion fracture of the CCL attachment to the coracoid process, and/or type I coracoid fracture. The site of the damage is determined by the relative mechanical strength of the bone and ligament, as well as the amount and direction of the applied force. The exact

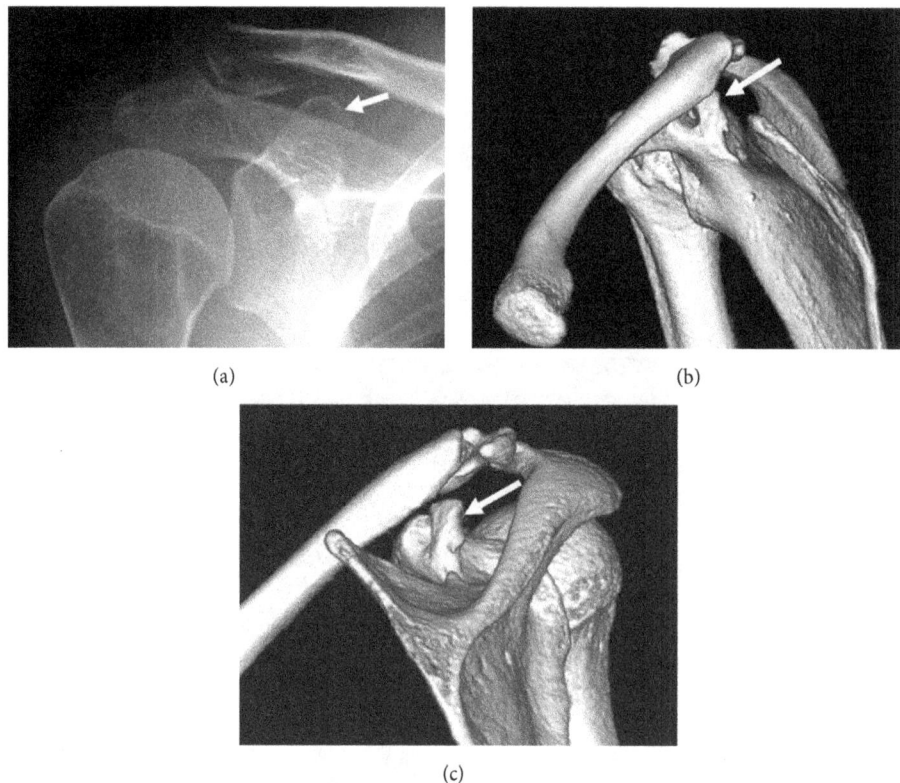

(a)

(b)

(c)

FIGURE 3: Imaging of Case 3. (a) Radiogram taken at the first visit revealing distal clavicular fracture (type 2b according to Craig's classification) and avulsion fracture of the posterior side of the coracoid process (arrow). (b and c) Three-dimensional computed tomography taken 1 year after the injury demonstrating nonunion of the lateral clavicular fracture and the malunited coracoid fragment migrating posterosuperiorly (arrow).

mechanism of injury producing avulsion fracture of the CCL attachment to the coracoid process remains unknown.

Our three cases correspond to double disruption of the SSSC, in which surgical treatment is indicated in acute cases [13]. The first case was treated surgically and had an excellent outcome. The second and third cases were treated conservatively, and the outcomes were not favorable. The second case still had unfavorable symptoms such as dull pain at rest and sharp pain while applying downward traction or engaging in overhead work 3 years and 6 months after the injury. The third case could not be functionally evaluated 1 year postoperatively, but CT showed nonunion of the distal clavicular fracture. A previously reported case of an adolescent treated conservatively also resulted in some aching during activity [5]. We therefore believe that surgical intervention, including precise repositioning of the fractured fragment and appropriate stabilization of associated injuries, should be considered when treating patients with this type of acute injury, especially for those engaging in heavy lifting or overhead work.

Competing Interests

The authors declare that there are no competing interests regarding the publication of this paper.

References

[1] K. Ogawa, Y. Toyama, S. Ishige, and K. Matsui, "Fracture of the coracoid process. Its classification and pathomechanism," *Journal of the Japanese Orthopaedic Association*, vol. 64, no. 10, pp. 909–919, 1990 (Japanese).

[2] K. S. Eyres, A. Brooks, and D. Stanley, "Fractures of the coracoid process," *The Journal of Bone & Joint Surgery—British Volume*, vol. 77, no. 3, pp. 425–428, 1995.

[3] G. A. Landoff, "Eine bisher nicht beschriebene Schädigung am Processus coracoideus," *Acta Chirurgica Scandinavica*, vol. 89, pp. 401–406, 1943 (German).

[4] H. G. Schaefer, "Clinical aspect of coracoid fractures," *Der Chirurg*, vol. 22, no. 4, pp. 172–173, 1951 (German).

[5] S. P. Montgomery and R. D. Loyd, "Avulsion fracture of the coracoid epiphysis with acromioclavicular separation. Report of two cases in adolescents and review of the literature," *The Journal of Bone & Joint Surgery—American Volume*, vol. 59, no. 7, pp. 963–965, 1977.

[6] Y. Nakagawa, H. Okumoto, and Y. Sakamoto, "Fractures of the coracoid process of the scapula—complex injury of the shoulder girdle," *Katakansetsu*, vol. 31, pp. 323–327, 2007 (Japanese).

[7] M. Leijnen, P. Steenvoorde, A. Da Costa, and S. Adhin, "Isolated apophyseal avulsion of the coracoid process: case report and review of literature," *Acta Orthopaedica Belgica*, vol. 75, no. 2, pp. 262–264, 2009.

[8] Y. Onada, T. Umemoto, K. Fukuda, and T. Kajino, "Coracoid process avulsion fracture at the coracoclavicular ligament attachment site in an osteoporotic patient with acromioclavicular joint dislocation," *Case Reports in Orthopedics*, vol. 2016, Article ID 9580485, 3 pages, 2016.

[9] M. D. McKee, "Clavicle fractures," in *Rockwood and Green's Fractures in Adults*, C. M. Court-Brown, J. D. Heckman, M. M. McQueen, W. M. Ricci, and P. Tornetta, Eds., pp. 1427–1473, Lippincott Williams & Wilkins, Philadelphia, Pa, USA, 8th edition, 2015.

[10] C. R. Constant and A. H. G. Murley, "A clinical method of functional assessment of the shoulder," *Clinical Orthopaedics and Related Research*, vol. 214, pp. 160–164, 1987.

[11] L. M. Galats, R. F. Hollis Jr., and G. R. Williams Jr., "Acromioclavicular joint injuries," in *Rockwood and Green's Fractures in Adults*, R. W. Bucholz, J. D. Heckman, C. M. Court-Brown, and P. Tornetta III, Eds., pp. 1210–1242, Lippincott Williams & Wilkins, Philadelphia, Pa, USA, 7th edition, 2010.

[12] K. Ogawa, A. Yoshida, and M. Takahashi, "Fracture of the coracoid process," *The Journal of Bone & Joint Surgery—British Volume*, vol. 79, pp. 17–19, 1997.

[13] T. P. Goss, "Double disruptions of the superior shoulder suspensory complex," *Journal of Orthopaedic Trauma*, vol. 7, no. 2, pp. 99–106, 1993.

[14] K. Ogawa, N. Matsumura, and H. Ikegami, "Coracoid fractures. Therapeutic strategy and surgical outcomes," *Journal of Trauma and Acute Care Surgery*, vol. 72, no. 2, pp. E20–E26, 2012.

[15] K. M. Wilson and J. C. Colwill, "Combined acromioclavicular dislocation with coracoclavicular ligament disruption and coracoid process fracture," *The American Journal of Sports Medicine*, vol. 17, no. 5, pp. 697–698, 1989.

[16] T. Martín-Herrero, C. Rodríguez-Merchán, and L. Munuera-Martínez, "Fractures of the coracoid process. Presentation of seven cases and review of the literature," *Journal of Trauma*, vol. 30, no. 12, pp. 1597–1599, 1990.

[17] M. DiPaola and P. Marchetto, "Coracoid process fracture with acromioclavicular joint separation in an American football player. A case report and literature review," *American Journal of Orthopedics*, vol. 38, no. 1, pp. 37–39, 2009.

[18] M. M. Scarlat, C. Cuny, B. A. Goldberg, D. T. Harryman II, and F. A. Matsen, "The lateral impaction of the shoulder," *International Orthopaedics*, vol. 23, no. 5, pp. 302–307, 1999.

17

Synovial Lipomatosis of the Glenohumeral Joint

Shaul Beyth and Ori Safran

Orthopedic Surgery Department, Hadassah Medical Center, 91120 Jerusalem, Israel

Correspondence should be addressed to Shaul Beyth; sbeyth@hadassah.org.il

Academic Editor: Kiyohisa Ogawa

Synovial lipomatosis (also known as lipoma arborescens) is a rare and benign lesion affecting synovium-lined cavities. It is characterized by hyperplasia of mature fat tissue in the subsynovial layer. Although the most commonly affected site is the knee joint, rarely additional locations such as tendon sheath and other joints are involved. We present a case of synovial lipomatosis of the glenohumeral joint in a 44-year-old man. The clinical data radiological studies and histopathologic results are described, as well as a review of the current literature.

1. Introduction

Synovial lipomatosis is a rare and benign lesion affecting synovium-lined cavities [1]. It most commonly affects the knee, but in rare cases also the hip, elbow, wrist, ankle, tendon sheath, and shoulder. This intra-articular condition of unknown etiology is marked by villous synovial proliferation with replacement of the subsynovial tissue by adipose tissue and mature fat cells [2]. Synovial lipomatosis may present itself as an inflammatory condition of the joint with or without systemic manifestations. Several cases with shoulder involvement were reported; only three of them related to the glenohumeral joint while the others involved the subacromial space. In two of these cases bone involvement was reported [2, 3]. We present a rare case of late posttraumatic synovial lipomatosis of the glenohumeral joint in a 44-year-old chef. Diagnosis was established on the basis of clinical data, imaging studies, and histopathology. A pertinent literature review is provided.

2. Case Presentation

A 44-year-old right hand dominant chef referred to the clinic complaining of recurrent episodes of right shoulder pain with prolonged asymptomatic periods between them. He described an episode that occurred four years earlier in which he was hospitalized for suspected glenohumeral joint infection. The suspected diagnosis was then based on a combination of severe shoulder pain, globally limited range of motion, fever of 38°C, and elevated ESR and CRP values (50 mm/hour and 12 mg%, resp.). At that time an ultrasound examination revealed a large amount of fluid in the glenohumeral joint and the bicipital tendon sheath. A synovial fluid sample was aspirated and a Gram stain showed only a few white blood cells but was negative for the presence of bacteria. The cultures were also negative. The patient's condition improved under nonsteroidal anti-inflammatory treatment and he was discharged. Three years later he had a similar episode for which he was treated as before.

He came to our outpatient clinic a few weeks later. His physical examination at that point was unremarkable. There was normal active range of motion as well as normal cuff strength and no signs of instability or impingement. Tests for subacromial and bicep irritation were negative.

Plain radiographs as well as a CT scan which were performed a few years earlier demonstrated a medium size Hill-Sachs lesion, without blunting of the anterior inferior glenoid (Figure 1). Only when confronted with the findings did the patient recall sustaining an indirect trauma to the shoulder some 20 years earlier for which he was unable to provide any documentation.

An MRI examination revealed large joint effusion and heterogeneous signal intensity within the periphery of the joint, suggestive of synovial hyperplasia (Figure 2).

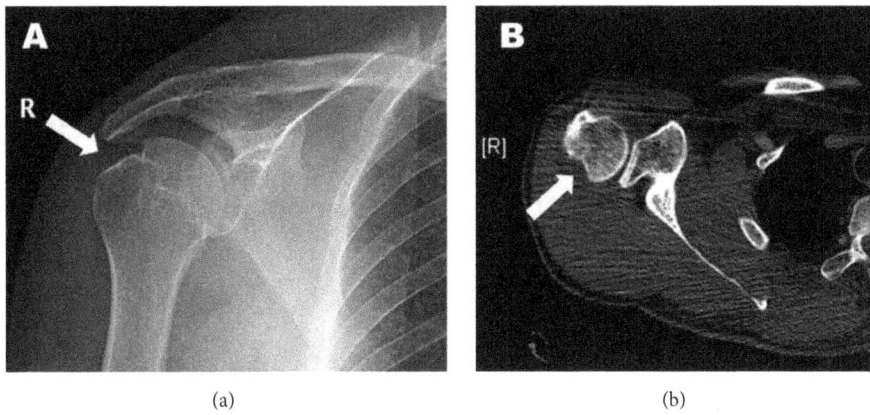

(a)

(b)

FIGURE 1: Preoperative imaging of the right shoulder. A medium size Hill-Sachs lesion is demonstrated in the posterosuperior aspect of the humeral head (arrow) in a plain AP radiograph of the shoulder (a) and in an axial plain image of a CT scan (b), suggesting previous anterior dislocation of the glenohumeral joint.

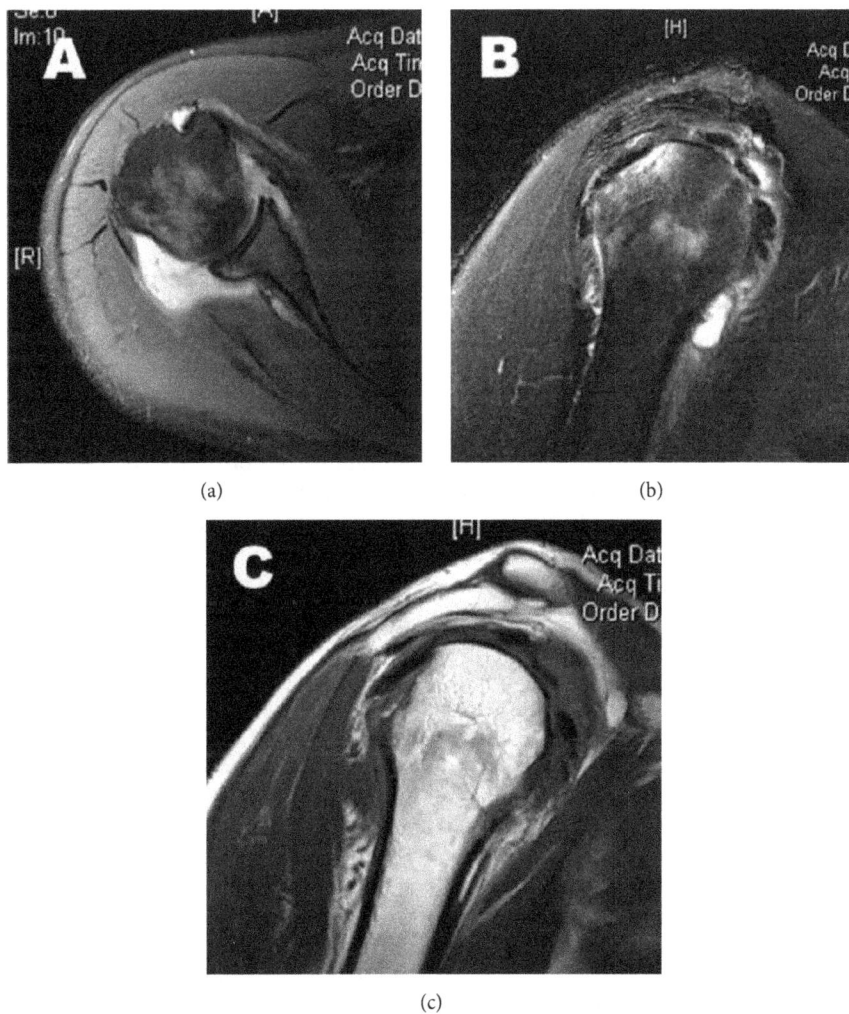

(a)

(b)

(c)

FIGURE 2: MRI of the right shoulder. (a) Axial proton density fat suppressed weighted image showing regions of low signal intensity within the joint effusion. (b) Sagittal proton density fat suppressed weighted image showing suppression of the signal intensity of the lesions, similar to subcutaneous fat. Bone erosion is present at the superior aspect of humeral head representing a Hill-Sachs fracture. (c) Sagittal T1-weighted image showing a large joint effusion and heterogeneous signal intensity within the periphery of the joint, suggestive of synovial hyperplasia.

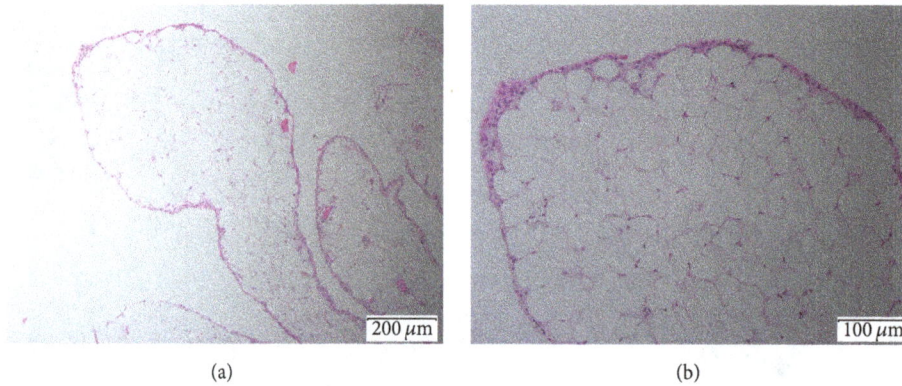

(a)

(b)

FIGURE 3: Histopathological photomicrographs. Hematoxylin and eosin stained sections of samples obtained from the glenohumeral joint during arthroscopy showing synovial lined villous proliferation which is diffusely infiltrated by mature fat cells while the periphery is lined by hypertrophic synovial cells and infiltrated by chronic inflammatory cells (bar size at lower right corner of images indicates 200 μm panel (a) and 100 μm panel (b)).

Due to the persistence of the symptoms the patient underwent arthroscopy of his right shoulder which demonstrated abundant yellowish villous synovial tissue in the glenohumeral region. The rotator cuff tendons as well as the articular cartilage were intact. The subacromial space was not involved. After samples were obtained, arthroscopic synovectomy was performed.

Histopathological examination of the retrieved tissue showed fragments of synovial villi with no acute inflammation or infection, with evidence of lipomatous metaplasia (Figure 3).

The patient's postoperative course was uneventful. Twelve months after surgery his pain has diminished with no recurrence of inflammatory episodes to date.

3. Discussion

Synovial lipomatosis is a rare benign lesion affecting synovium-lined cavities. It most commonly affects the knee [2] but rarely affects the hip [4, 5], elbow [6, 7], wrist [8], ankle [1, 9], tendon sheath [2, 6], and shoulder [3, 10, 11]. Although synovial lipomatosis is most commonly a monoarticular condition, several cases of multifocal disease have been reported [12, 13].

Since it was first described by Hoffa [14] in 1904, only several cases of synovial lipomatosis of the shoulder were reported, of which only three were related to the glenohumeral joint [3, 10, 11] and the others were describing subacromial space lesions [15–17]. Interestingly, although synovial lipomatosis is primarily a soft tissue condition, in two of these cases, bone erosion in young healthy patients was also present [3, 11]. The third reported patient was a 90-year-old woman, and therefore joint erosion may be assumed, although it was not reported [3].

In 1995 Laorr et al. published the first description of synovial lipomatosis of the shoulder in a 90-year-old patient. The diagnosis was based on clinical findings and imaging, and the patient was treated nonoperatively [3]. In et al. reported in 2008 a case of glenohumeral synovial lipomatosis diagnosed by arthroscopy in a 22-year-old male patient. The authors noticed bone erosion and arthritic changes of the joint and assumed a causative relation by which the synovial metaplasia induces degenerative joint disease [11]. One year later Chae et al. reported a similar case involving a 36-year-old male patient in whom the affected shoulder was also deranged [10]. In their report they emphasize the seven-year delay in diagnosis that may be attributed to the insidious nature of the disease.

Synovial lipomatosis may equally affect males and females, between the second and the ninth decades of life. It has been suggested that adolescent patients present an idiopathic primary form of the disease, whereas older individuals, young and older adults, exhibit a secondary process. Less than a handful of multifocal cases were described in young patients. The etiology was suggested to be linked to systemic conditions in some reports, specifically to fat metabolism due to coexisting short bowel syndrome in one case [18] and to chronic inflammatory diseases such as rheumatoid arthritis in another [12]. This may follow traumatic or degenerative injury to the joint with resultant chronic irritation of the synovium [9, 19]. This is somewhat contrary to the theory raised by In et al. and Chae et al., who considered the synovial lipomatosis to be the primary lesion and the bony involvement only secondary. Synovial lipomatosis as a reactive process has been further supported by observations made by Ikushima et al. who noticed decreased osteogenic activity and increased adipogenic activity of marrow cells in this condition [20]. The authors suggested that synovial chondromatosis is yet another form of the synovial reaction and supported their theory by the coincidence of the two conditions in two cases, as well as the similar age distribution of the two conditions. They concluded that the spectrum of late synovial reaction to injury may include several forms. In our case we found clear evidence of prior anterior shoulder dislocation that took place well before the onset of symptoms, consistent with this paradigm.

Clinically, synovial lipomatosis usually presents an inflammatory condition of the joint. Manifestations include painless swelling of the involved joint due to accumulation of synovial fluid. In addition, this condition of unknown etiology is marked by villous proliferation consisting of replacement of the subsynovial tissue by adipose tissue with mature fat cells [2]. Lack of pain and systemic manifestations in most cases may explain the long period that usually elapses until diagnosis. Indeed, our case is unique due to the documented significant pain accompanied by fever and systemic inflammatory response. Unfortunately, at that time clinicians were misled by the acute presentation and assumed joint infection, whereas accurate diagnosis was made only at a later stage.

Diagnosis of synovial lipomatosis is confirmed by histology. Although plain radiography and CT scan may not be very helpful, magnetic resonance imaging criteria have been published as an aid to diagnosis. These may include high signal intensity villous or nodular foci on both T1- and T2-weighted images that are suppressed on short tau inversion recovery (STIR) or fat saturation sequences, while the remaining nonfatty component of the hypertrophied synovium displays heterogeneous high signal intensity on T2 or STIR sequences and intermediate-to-low signal intensity on T1-weighted sequences. Degenerative or posttraumatic changes may be seen in the secondary (but not the primary) type of synovial lipomatosis. The subsynovial fatty proliferation usually presents in the diffuse villous form or in the focal nodular frond-like form. A mixed form of the two patterns may also be seen [3, 6, 10, 19, 21].

In 2003 Vilanova et al. reported a series of 33 cases of synovial lipomatosis in 32 knees and one shoulder in which the lesion was located in the subacromial bursa. Only 12 lesions were confirmed by histology, diagnosis of the remaining 21 joints based on MRI findings only [19]. These findings included joint effusion in all cases and other unspecified degenerative findings in all but two knees, whereas other intra-articular lesions were less common. A cuff tear identified by MRI was assumed to be related to the synovial lipomatosis of the shoulder case, as suggested before [15, 17].

Differential diagnosis of synovial lipomatosis of the shoulder should include pigmented villonodular synovitis, rheumatoid arthritis, tuberculous arthritis gouty arthropathy and synovial osteochondromatosis. Although clinically these may be indistinguishable from synovial lipomatosis, correct diagnosis can be made based on detailed history, laboratory tests of blood, and synovial fluid as well as imaging, particularly by magnetic resonance.

Asymptomatic and therefore undiagnosed cases of synovial lipomatosis should be assumed to exist. When symptomatic, synovial lipomatosis is commonly treated nonoperatively by physical therapy and anti-inflammatory medications aimed at controlling the reactive episode. Failure of these modalities may indicate the need for invasive measures.

Treatment of synovial lipomatosis by radionuclide therapy in one case yielded significant reduction of lesion volume at six months [22]. No clinical benefit was confirmed. An additional case treated by radionuclide therapy was described by Erselcan et al. Here a 36-year-old woman was treated with intra-articular administration of yttrium-90 in conjunction with 40 mg methylprednisolone acetate. The authors described the clinical benefit at one-year follow-up, supported by MRI findings [23]. Although radionuclide therapy was reported for these two cases, the treatment of choice for synovial lipomatosis is arthroscopic radical synovectomy. This minimally invasive procedure facilitates early postoperative recovery. Recurrence of synovial lipomatosis after synovectomy is uncommon.

4. Conclusions

Synovial lipomatosis (lipoma arborescens) is an uncommon intra-articular condition of unknown etiology, with less than a handful of cases reported in the glenohumeral joint. The etiology is unclear, but synovial lipomatosis was suggested to represent a late reaction of the synovium to injury in young and older adults. Although it commonly presents insidiously with local soft tissue swelling and joint effusion, on rare occasions it may manifest with an acute local and systemic inflammatory response that is difficult to differentiate from septic shoulder. Clinical and radiological evaluation may facilitate diagnosis. Arthroscopic synovectomy may result in prolonged remission of symptoms.

Competing Interests

The authors declare that they have no competing interests.

Acknowledgments

The authors thank Dr. Alexander Mali for the histopathological evaluation, description, and images.

References

[1] S. A. Babar, A. Sandison, and A. W. Mitchell, "Synovial and tenosynovial lipoma arborescens of the ankle in an adult: a case report," *Skeletal Radiology*, vol. 37, no. 1, pp. 75–77, 2008.

[2] T. Hallel, S. Lew, and M. Bansal, "Villous lipomatous proliferation of the synovial membrane (lipoma arborescens)," *The Journal of Bone & Joint Surgery—American Volume*, vol. 70, no. 2, pp. 264–270, 1988.

[3] A. Laorr, C. G. Peterfy, P. F. J. Tirman, and A. E. Rabassa, "Lipoma arborescens of the shoulder: magnetic resonance imaging findings," *Canadian Association of Radiologists Journal*, vol. 46, no. 4, pp. 311–313, 1995.

[4] E. R. Noel, J. G. Tebib, C. Dumontet et al., "Synovial lipoma arborescens of the hip," *Clinical Rheumatology*, vol. 6, no. 1, pp. 92–96, 1987.

[5] R. S. Wolf, G. N. Zoys, V. A. Saldivar, and R. P. Williams, "Lipoma arborescens of the hip," *The American Journal of Orthopedics*, vol. 31, no. 5, pp. 276–279, 2002.

[6] A. J. Doyle, M. V. Miller, and J. G. French, "Lipoma arborescens in the bicipital bursa of the elbow: MRI findings in two cases," *Skeletal Radiology*, vol. 31, no. 11, pp. 656–660, 2002.

[7] M. Levadoux, J. Gadea, P. Flandrin, E. Carlos, R. Aswad, and M. Panuel, "Lipoma arborescens of the elbow: a case report," *Journal of Hand Surgery*, vol. 25, no. 3, pp. 580–584, 2000.

[8] A. Napolitano, "Lipoma arborescens of the synovial fluid; clinical contribution to a case located at the synovia of the wrist," *Progresso Medico*, vol. 13, no. 4, pp. 109–118, 1957.

[9] G.-S. Huang, H.-S. Lee, Y.-C. Hsu, H.-W. Kao, H.-H. Lee, and C.-Y. Chen, "Tenosynovial lipoma arborescens of the ankle in a child," *Skeletal Radiology*, vol. 35, no. 4, pp. 244–247, 2006.

[10] E. Y. Chae, H. W. Chung, M. J. Shin, and S. H. Lee, "Lipoma arborescens of the glenohumeral joint causing bone erosion: MRI features with gadolinium enhancement," *Skeletal Radiology*, vol. 38, no. 8, pp. 815–818, 2009.

[11] Y. In, K.-A. Chun, E.-D. Chang, and S.-M. Lee, "Lipoma arborescens of the glenohumeral joint: a possible cause of osteoarthritis," *Knee Surgery, Sports Traumatology, Arthroscopy*, vol. 16, no. 8, pp. 794–796, 2008.

[12] I. Bejia, M. Younes, A. Moussa, M. Said, M. Touzi, and N. Bergaoui, "Lipoma arborescens affecting multiple joints," *Skeletal Radiology*, vol. 34, no. 9, pp. 536–538, 2005.

[13] L. Silva, G. Terroso, L. Sampaio et al., "Polyarticular lipoma arborescens—a clinical and aesthetical case," *Rheumatology International*, vol. 33, no. 6, pp. 1601–1604, 2013.

[14] A. Hoffa, "The influence of the adipose tissue with regard to the pathology of the knee joint," *JAMA*, vol. 43, no. 12, pp. 795–796, 1904.

[15] J. S. Dawson, F. Dowling, B. J. Preston, and L. Neumann, "Case report: lipoma arborescens of the sub-deltoid bursa," *British Journal of Radiology*, vol. 68, no. 806, pp. 197–199, 1995.

[16] R. Kim, Y. Kim, J. Choi, S. Shin, Y. Kim, and L. Kim, "Lipoma arborescens associated with osseous/chondroid differentiation in subdeltoid bursa," *International Journal of Shoulder Surgery*, vol. 7, no. 3, pp. 116–119, 2013.

[17] J.-F. Nisolle, E. Blouard, V. Baudrez, Y. Boutsen, P. De Cloedt, and W. Esselinckx, "Subacromial-subdeltoid lipoma arborescens associated with a rotator cuff tear," *Skeletal Radiology*, vol. 28, no. 5, pp. 283–285, 1999.

[18] C. Siva, R. Brasington, W. Totty, A. Sotelo, and J. Atkinson, "Synovial lipomatosis (lipoma arborescens) affecting multiple joints in a patient with congenital short bowel syndrome," *Journal of Rheumatology*, vol. 29, no. 5, pp. 1088–1092, 2002.

[19] J. C. Vilanova, J. Barceló, M. Villalón, J. Aldomà, E. Delgado, and I. Zapater, "MR imaging of lipoma arborescens and the associated lesions," *Skeletal Radiology*, vol. 32, no. 9, pp. 504–509, 2003.

[20] K. Ikushima, T. Ueda, I. Kudawara, and H. Yoshikawa, "Lipoma arborescens of the knee as a possible cause of osteoarthrosis," *Orthopedics*, vol. 24, no. 6, pp. 603–605, 2001.

[21] S. K. Sanamandra and K. O. Ong, "Lipoma arborescens," *Singapore Medical Journal*, vol. 55, no. 1, pp. 5–11, 2014.

[22] J. O'Doherty, R. Clauss, J. Scuffham, and A. Khan, "Lipoma arborescens successfully treated with (90)Y synovectomy," *Clinical Nuclear Medicine*, vol. 39, no. 2, pp. e187–e189, 2014.

[23] T. Erselcan, O. Bulut, S. Bulut et al., "Lipoma arborescens; successfully treated by yttrium-90 radiosynovectomy," *Annals of Nuclear Medicine*, vol. 17, no. 7, pp. 593–596, 2003.

18

Lumbar Scoliosis Combined Lumbar Spinal Stenosis and Herniation Diagnosed Patient Was Treated with "U" Route Transforaminal Percutaneous Endoscopic Lumbar Discectomy

Binbin Wu,[1] Shaobo Zhang,[2] Qingquan Lian,[1] Haibo Yan,[3] Xianfa Lin,[4] and Gonghao Zhan[1]

[1]*Department of Anesthesiology and Pain Medicine, The Second Affiliated Hospital and Yuying Children's Hospital of Wenzhou Medical University, Wenzhou 325027, China*
[2]*Department of Anesthesiology and Pain Medicine, The Hospital of Integrated Traditional and Western Medicine, Taizhou 317500, China*
[3]*Department of Orthopaedics, The First People's Hospital of Wenling, Taizhou 317500, China*
[4]*Department of Anesthesiology and Pain Medicine, The First People's Hospital of Wenling, Taizhou 317500, China*

Correspondence should be addressed to Binbin Wu; wbb19880117@163.com and Gonghao Zhan; wenzhoumz@163.com

Academic Editor: Hitesh N. Modi

The objective was to report a case of a 63-year-old man with a history of low back pain (LBP) and left leg pain for 2 years, and the symptom became more serious in the past 5 months. The patient was diagnosed with lumbar scoliosis combined with lumbar spinal stenosis (LSS) and lumbar disc herniation (LDH) at the level of L4-5 that was confirmed using Computerized Topography and Magnetic Resonance Imaging. The surgical team preformed a novel technique, "U" route transforaminal percutaneous endoscopic lumbar discectomy (PELD), which led to substantial, long-term success in reduction of pain intensity and disability. After removing the osteophyte mass posterior to the thecal sac at L4-5, the working channel direction was changed to the gap between posterior longitudinal ligament and thecal sac, and we also removed the herniation and osteophyte at L3-4 with "U" route PELD. The patient's symptoms were improved immediately after the surgical intervention; low back pain intensity decreased from preoperative 9 to postoperative 2 on a visual analog scale (VAS) recorded at 1 month postoperatively. The success of the intervention suggests that "U" route PELD may be a feasible alternative to treat lumbar scoliosis with LSS and LDH patients.

1. Introduction

Lumbar spinal stenosis (LSS) is the most common spinal degenerative condition and usually related to the occurrence of low back pain (LBP), functional limitations, and disability [1]. The causes can be intervertebral joint hypertrophy, osteophytes, and lumbar disc herniation (LDH) [2]. It has been reported that almost 9% of general population and about 47% of people older than 60 years are diagnosed with LSS and their 2-year cost of treatment is 4 billion dollars in the United States alone. LSS is one of the most common spinal pathologies affecting patients that are older than 65 years [3, 4]. In addition, approximately 80% of Chinese adults with LSS experience low back or leg pain or both during their lifetime [5]. Majority of patients have significant pain alleviation through massage and physical therapies, but approximately 20% suffer from intractable pain and suffer greatly [6].

Open discectomy (OD) has been regarded as the standard surgical procedure for LSS during the last decades [7]; however, OD needs to extensively resect the lamina in the regions of facets, causing iatrogenic instability and more postoperative morbidity [8], such that the outcome is not satisfying [9]. Recent advancements in minimal invasive discectomy operations include the transforaminal percutaneous endoscopic lumbar discectomy (PELD) approach that has many advantages compared to older techniques in terms of protecting the lamina, muscles, ligaments, and spinal canal, as well as long-term success by minimizing postoperative

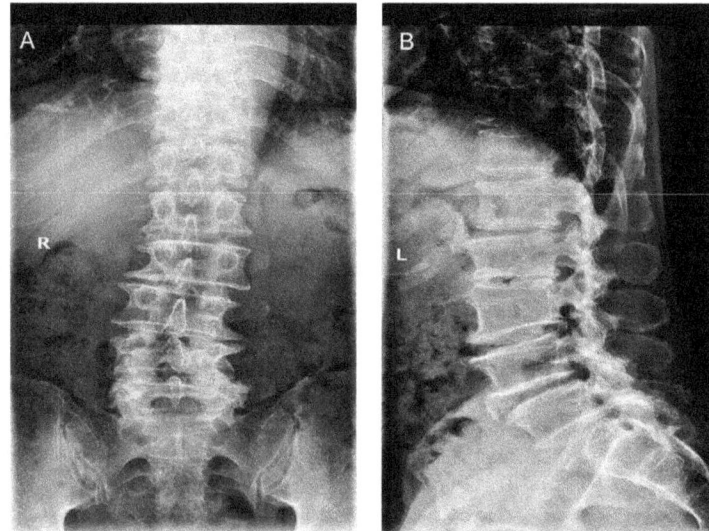

FIGURE 1: The preoperative anteroposterior (A) and left lateral (B) X-ray images of the patient, showing lumbar scoliosis, lumbar degeneration, and vertebral instability.

pain, epidural scarring, segment instability, and slippage [7, 8, 10]. Despite the advantages, the applications of "U" route PELD are limited due to controversy regarding its therapeutic efficacy and indication to treat LSS and LDH [11].

The objective of the case report was to describe the "U" route PELD technique, which could effectively treat lumbar scoliosis combined with lumbar stenosis, caused by herniation and/or osteophyte on L3-4 and L4-5 discs, with the aim of enriching the knowledge and further applications of "U" route PELD.

2. Case Presentation

2.1. History and Examination. A 63-year-old man presented with LBP and left leg pain for 2 years with symptoms worsening in the recent 5 months. The patient consulted our department for treatment, and the neurological examination revealed lumbar scoliosis, limited lumbar spine flexibility, L3-4 interspinous tenderness, and marked tenderness on the left side of L5. In addition, the patient reports radiating pain on the left leg and weakened shallow feel on both lower limbs. The straight leg raising test on the two sides and pelvic compression test were negative, and no muscle weakness or reflex was found. The visual analog scale (VAS) pain ratings of LBP and left leg pain were both reported as 9 of 10.

The lumbar X-ray examination revealed lumbar scoliosis, lumbar degeneration, and L2 vertebral slip (Figure 1). The Computerized Topography (CT) indicated a L3-4 and L4-5 lumbar stenosis combined with intervertebral disc herniation and lumbar joint facets degeneration unexpected for his age (Figure 2). The Magnetic Resonance Imaging (MRI) confirmed results from the CT scan but also suggested lumbar stenosis at L3-4 and L4-5; thecal sacs at the both levels were compressed by herniation (Figure 3). After completion of preoperative tests and examinations, we estimated that the existing lumbar stenosis at L3-4 and L4-5 was due to spinal osteoarthritis and herniation and that of L4-5 was more

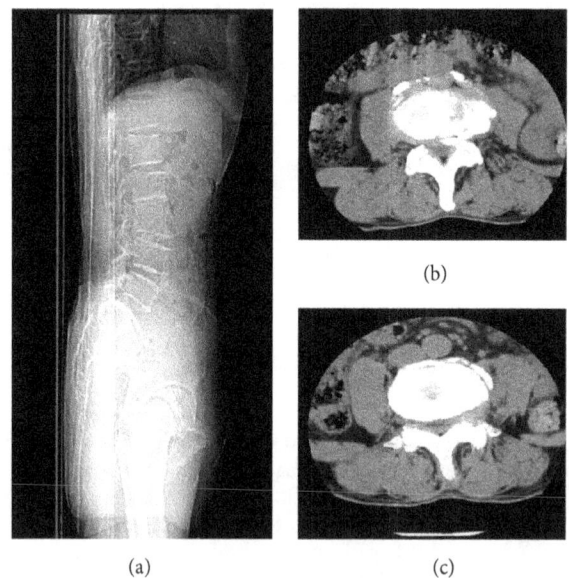

FIGURE 2: The sagittal (a) and coronal CT images of L3-4 (b) and L4-5 (c) revealed lumbar stenosis combined with intervertebral disc herniation at both levels and combined lumbar facet joint degenerative changes.

serious. Meanwhile, based on the patient's clinical history, we concluded that conservative physical treatments might be ineffective and a spine surgery would be a better choice. After the patient was informed of the disadvantages and advantages of both OD and "U" route PELD, he chose "U" route PELD surgery.

2.2. Intervention. All procedures were performed following the standard transforaminal endoscopic discectomy technique after local anesthesia was administered [12]. The patient lay prone on an operating table on the contralateral side,

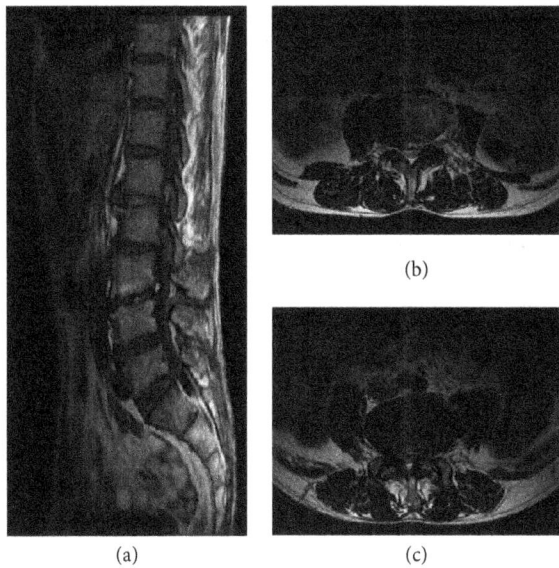

FIGURE 3: Both the T1 sagittal (a) and coronal MRI images of L3-4 (b) and L4-5 (c) suggested that the herniation and lumbar stenosis compressed the thecal sac at both levels, and lumbar degenerative changes were also reported.

and C-arm fluoroscopy technique was used to determine the affected discs and pedicles. Thus, the surgeons drew lines from the mid-pedicular annulus of L3-4 and L4-5 to the facet lateral margin and extended them to the body surface, and the skin entry point was about 10 cm from the midline. After a routine disinfection procedure, subcutaneous tissue and trajectory tract were infiltrated with 1.0–1.5 mL of 1% lidocaine at the L4-5 level. Following this, an 18-gauge needle was inserted to reach the facet of L5 superior articular process under a fluoroscopic guidance, and with a puncture angle of about 15°. Then, we retreated the stylet followed by injecting another 20 mL 1% lidocaine for further anesthesia and inserted a guide wire as the direction of the needle. After that, the needle was retreated and a 0.8 cm incision was made at the position of guide wire firstly; secondly, a serial dilation and working channel were inserted as the direction of guide wire; thirdly, we retreated the guide wire and dilation and inserted the guide bar into the working channel. To prevent the occurrence of postoperative spinal instability, the guide bar was passed over the facet of L5 superior articular process without damaging any bone tissue. However, at that moment, the patient complained radiating pain on his left leg when the surgeon planned to insert the guide bar into his spinal canal. We estimated that the pain resulted from nerve root compression as we repeatedly adjusted the position of the guide bar. However, all adjustments could not avoid touching nerve root and the pain was persistent. Therefore, we changed the puncture path to the superior and interior articular process facets at the level of L4-5 and resected the facets partly for decompression. After the guide bar being inserted into the posterior of thecal sac (Figure 4), the working channel was rotated around the direction of the guide bar, and the endoscope was introduced. Besides, a continuous irrigation

system for a clear endoscopic view was used. Then, we removed the osteophyte and reshaped the ligamentum flavum firstly. Following that, the working channel was adjusted to remove the herniation mass in the gap between posterior longitudinal ligament and thecal sac, just like a "U" route. At the end, the operative field was copiously irrigated and meticulous hemostasis was obtained, and suture was placed at the incision after the channel was removed.

The spinal stenosis was also observed at the L3-4 level; for further treatment, we inserted the guide bar to reach the location of L4 superior articular process facet after the determination of landmarks and skin window as described above. After local anesthesia, the working channel reached the location of herniation and osteophyte at L3-4 as the guidance of the guide bar, and the mass between thecal sac and posterior longitudinal ligament was removed under endoscope successfully. At the end of the operation, the patient reported the low back pain was alleviated, the VAS pain rating was about 2 of 10, and the leg pain absolutely disappeared. All of the resected mass was collected on a plate (Figure 5), and the irrigation, meticulous hemostasis, and suture were done as described above. Thus, treating the LSS mainly caused by LDH and osteophyte combined lumbar scoliosis with PELD was performed. An MRI scan was done 1 month postoperatively; in addition, the patient reported his LBP 1 of 10 on a VAS scale and 0 of 10 on a VAS scale of leg pain. MRI imaging 1 month postoperatively suggested disc edema at L3-4 and L4-5; herniation and stenosis were alleviated compared with preoperative images (Figure 6).

3. Discussion

It has been demonstrated that PELD is a relatively safe, minimally invasive procedure for LSS and LDH compared with OD, with merits such as less tissue trauma and blood loss, shorter mean disability period, and recovery time. The procedure requires a small incision of 0.6–0.8 cm and 3 days of in-patient stay [7, 13, 14]. Despite the above advantages and inspiring clinical results, PELD is not universally adopted because of some disadvantages, such as difficulty in anatomical delineation during the endoscopic approach and the learning curve to disassociate the neural structure from the instruments or to develop skillset and experience to safely perform the surgery. In order to circumvent iatrogenic persistence of neuropathic postoperative pain, many new techniques have been developed, and the PELD is also being advanced [15–20]. Several years ago, PELD was not a recommended therapy for patients with highly migrated herniation and lumbar stenosis, but a recently developed "U" route PELD becomes an available treatment for these pathologies regardless of laterality or herniation [8, 21]. And we can reach the operation area with the working channel bypassing the vertebral facets without destroying any anatomical structure of the spine. But for this case, because of inducing radiating pain when we rotated in guide bar, we resected the articular process facets at L4-5 for decompression for this patient. Lumbar scoliosis leads to mispositioning during the surgery, and we circumvented this

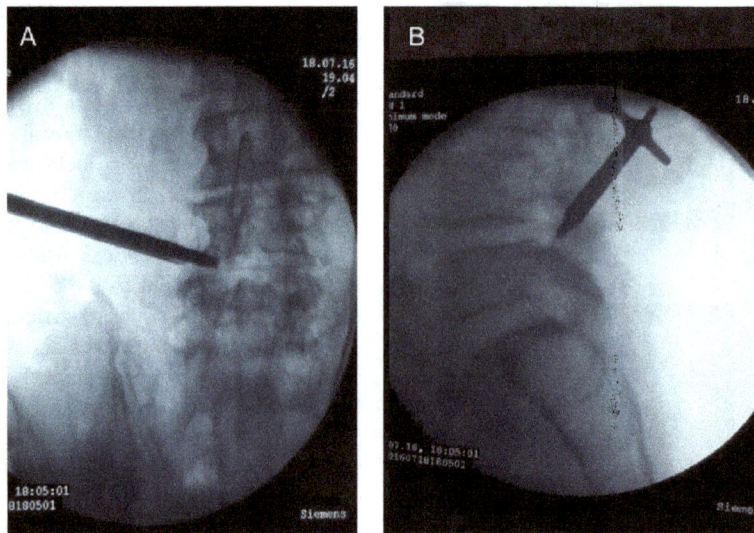

FIGURE 4: The location pictures after successfully reaching the operation area at L4-5 with a guide bar.

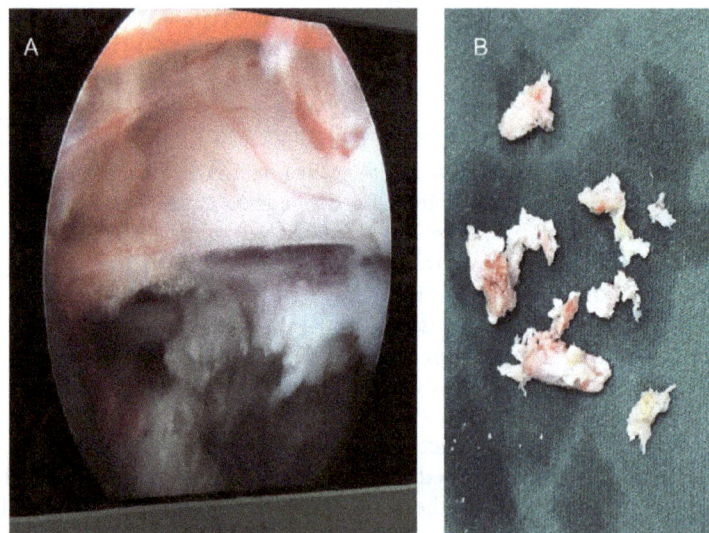

FIGURE 5: The sight under the endoscope at L4-5 (A); the herniation mass and bone hyperplasia were collected at the plate (B).

potential issue by adjusting the direction and orientation of the needle repeatedly, although the needed may be stopped several times due to anatomical channel abnormalities in the process. As a result, an osteophyte formation with majority developing near the ligamentum flavum was treated, and then we changed the direction of working channel to the gap between posterior longitudinal ligament and thecal sac; this is just like a "U" route, a newly developed approach of PELD, and is heatedly discussed; however, there are not many studies published about it. And during a 3-month follow-up, no spine instability was observed as a result from the surgery. Moreover, many studies have suggested endoscopic disc surgery by experienced and well-trained surgeons can achieve more favorable and sustainable clinical results equivalent to the standard microsurgical technique [20, 22]. Therefore, the clinical outcome of PELD is closely

related to the proficiency of surgeons. The surgeon of the operation in this study has carried out more than 2,000 cases of LBP with PELD, including LSS and LDH patients, in China alone.

The patient's VAS pain rating decreased to 2 after the surgery and was 1 when he was discharged, no pain on his leg. And we cannot absolutely exclude the possibility that the slight pain at back may be related to minor injury of the paraspinal muscles during the operation, although the postoperative 1-month MRI indicated disc edema of both levels of L3-4 and L4-5. In addition, both the follow-up results at 1 month and 3 months after surgery suggested that no complications happened to the patient, despite the fact that there are no images for postoperative 3 months here. All these indicated the success of the surgery. With this case, we might demonstrate that the "U" route PELD could be an alternative

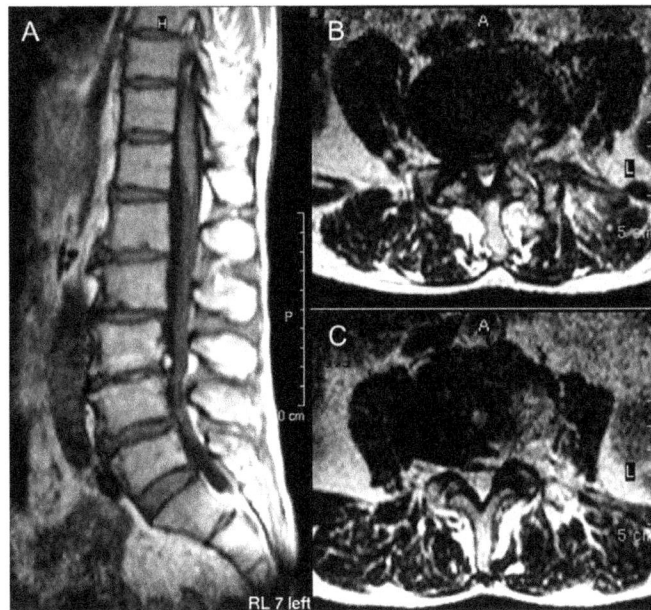

FIGURE 6: Both the T1 sagittal (A) and coronal MRI images of L3-4 (B) and L4-5 (C) at 1-month postoperatively, indicating that the herniation and stenosis at both levels were alleviated compared with the preoperative results, despite edema being observed.

treatment for patients diagnosed by lumbar scoliosis with LSS and LDH, but we also need a larger-sample study with long-term follow-up in this area.

Competing Interests

The authors declare that there is no conflict of interests.

Acknowledgments

The study was supported by the funding of Zhejiang Medical Association (2015ZYC-A28) and Wenzhou Science and Technology Project (Y20160392). The authors thank Taha Abdullah, M.S., department of Physiology, Northwestern University Feinberg School of Medicine, for language help.

References

[1] C. Ammendolia, K. Stuber, C. Tomkins-Lane et al., "What interventions improve walking ability in neurogenic claudication with lumbar spinal stenosis? A systematic review," *European Spine Journal*, vol. 23, no. 6, pp. 1282–1301, 2014.

[2] P. Campbell, G. Wynne-Jones, S. Muller, and K. M. Dunn, "The influence of employment social support for risk and prognosis in nonspecific back pain: a systematic review and critical synthesis," *International Archives of Occupational and Environmental Health*, vol. 86, no. 2, pp. 119–137, 2013.

[3] S. L. Parker, S. S. Godil, S. K. Mendenhall, S. L. Zuckerman, D. N. Shau, and M. J. Mcgirt, "Two-year comprehensive medical management of degenerative lumbar spine disease (lumbar spondylolisthesis, stenosis, or disc herniation): a value analysis of cost, pain, disability, and quality of life: clinical article," *Journal of Neurosurgery: Spine*, vol. 21, no. 2, pp. 143–149, 2014.

[4] L. Kalichman, R. Cole, D. H. Kim et al., "Spinal stenosis prevalence and association with symptoms: the Framingham Study," *Spine Journal*, vol. 9, no. 7, pp. 545–550, 2009.

[5] R. Chen, J. Xiong, Z. Chi, and B. Zhang, "Heat-sensitive moxibustion for lumbar disc herniation: a meta-analysis of randomized controlled trials," *Journal of Traditional Chinese Medicine*, vol. 32, no. 3, pp. 322–328, 2012.

[6] O. P. Gautschi, D. Cadosch, and G. Hildebrandt, "Acute low back pain—assessment and management," *Praxis*, vol. 97, no. 2, pp. 58–68, 2008.

[7] X. Li, Y. Han, Z. Di et al., "Percutaneous endoscopic lumbar discectomy for lumbar disc herniation," *Journal of Clinical Neuroscience*, vol. 33, pp. 19–27, 2016.

[8] X. Wu, G. Fan, X. Guan et al., "Percutaneous endoscopic lumbar discectomy for far-migrated disc herniation through two working channels," *Pain Physician*, vol. 19, no. 4, pp. E675–E680, 2016.

[9] T. Aizawa, H. Ozawa, T. Kusakabe et al., "Reoperation for recurrent lumbar disc herniation: a study over a 20-year period in a Japanese population," *Journal of Orthopaedic Science*, vol. 17, no. 2, pp. 107–113, 2012.

[10] Y. Ahn, S.-H. Lee, W.-M. Park, and H.-Y. Lee, "Posterolateral percutaneous endoscopic lumbar foraminotomy for L5-S1 foraminal or lateral exit zone stenosis. Technical note," *Journal of neurosurgery*, vol. 99, no. 3, pp. 320–323, 2003.

[11] R. Kim, R. H. Kim, C. H. Kim et al., "The incidence and risk factors for lumbar or sciatic scoliosis in lumbar disc herniation and the outcomes after percutaneous endoscopic discectomy," *Pain Physician*, vol. 18, no. 6, pp. 555–564, 2015.

[12] A. T. Yeung and P. M. Tsou, "Posterolateral endoscopic excision for lumbar disc herniation: surgical technique, outcome, and complications in 307 consecutive cases," *Spine*, vol. 27, no. 7, pp. 722–731, 2002.

[13] Y. Tamaki, T. Sakai, R. Miyagi et al., "Intradural lumbar disc herniation after percutaneous endoscopic lumbar discectomy: case report," *Journal of Neurosurgery: Spine*, vol. 23, no. 3, pp. 336–339, 2015.

[14] J. Mizuno, Y. Hirano, and Y. Nishimura, "Establishment of endoscopic spinal neurosurgery and its current status," *No shinkei geka. Neurological surgery*, vol. 44, no. 3, pp. 203–209, 2016.

[15] G. Choi, S.-H. Lee, P. Lokhande et al., "Percutaneous endoscopic approach for highly migrated intracanal disc herniations by foraminoplastic technique using rigid working channel endoscope," *Spine*, vol. 33, no. 15, pp. E508–E515, 2008.

[16] No Author Listed, "Endoscopic laser foraminoplasty," *Clinical Privilege White Paper*, no. 60, pp. 1–13, 2012.

[17] M. T. N. Knight, D. R. Ellison, A. Goswami, and V. F. Hillier, "Review of safety in endoscopic laser foraminoplasty for the management of back pain," *Journal of Clinical Laser Medicine and Surgery*, vol. 19, no. 3, pp. 147–157, 2001.

[18] C.-W. Lee, K.-J. Yoon, S.-S. Ha, and J.-K. Kang, "Foraminoplastic superior vertebral notch approach with reamers in percutaneous endoscopic lumbar discectomy: technical note and clinical outcome in limited indications of percutaneous endoscopic lumbar discectomy," *Journal of Korean Neurosurgical Society*, vol. 59, no. 2, pp. 172–181, 2016.

[19] H. C. Ki, I. J. Chang, M. L. Seung, W. K. Byoung, Y. K. Saeng, and S. K. Hyeun, "Strategies for noncontained lumbar disc herniation by an endoscopic approach: transforaminal suprapedicular approach, semi-rigid flexible curved probe, and 3-dimensional reconstruction CT with discogram," *Journal of Korean Neurosurgical Society*, vol. 46, no. 4, pp. 312–316, 2009.

[20] S. Ruetten, M. Komp, H. Merk, and G. Godolias, "Use of newly developed instruments and endoscopes: full-endoscopic resection of lumbar disc herniations via the interlaminar and lateral transforaminal approach," *Journal of Neurosurgery: Spine*, vol. 6, no. 6, pp. 521–530, 2007.

[21] Z.-Z. Li, S.-X. Hou, W.-L. Shang, Z. Cao, and H.-L. Zhao, "Percutaneous lumbar foraminoplasty and percutaneous endoscopic lumbar decompression for lateral recess stenosis through transforaminal approach: technique notes and 2 years follow-up," *Clinical Neurology and Neurosurgery*, vol. 143, pp. 90–94, 2016.

[22] C. Birkenmaier, M. Komp, H. F. Leu, B. Wegener, and S. Ruetten, "The current state of endoscopic disc surgery: review of controlled studies comparing full-endoscopic procedures for disc herniations to standard procedures," *Pain Physician*, vol. 16, no. 4, pp. 335–344, 2013.

19

Successful Closed Reduction of a Lateral Elbow Dislocation

Kenya Watanabe, Takuma Fukuzawa, and Katsuhiro Mitsui

Department of Orthopedics, Nagano Prefectural Suzaka Hospital, Suzaka, Nagano, Japan

Correspondence should be addressed to Kenya Watanabe; watanabekenya@hotmail.com

Academic Editor: Johannes Mayr

In this report, we present a case of lateral elbow dislocation treated with closed reduction. Lateral elbow dislocation is rare, and a closed reduction is reported with even less frequency. The reduction can be hindered by swelling and soft tissue interposition, and we describe the use of a nonoperative reduction technique performed under mild sedation with early physiotherapy to avoid joint stiffness. No additional complication was observed, and the normal range of elbow movement and function was obtained by early physiotherapy.

1. Introduction

Elbow dislocation is a common injury, and posterior dislocation, specifically, is a frequent form. Simple lateral elbow dislocation is rare and often associated with neurovascular issues with difficulty in performing closed reduction [1]. Reduction can be hindered by swelling and soft tissue interposition. In this rare case of lateral dislocation treated with closed reduction under mild sedation, we describe the use of a nonoperative reduction technique and early physiotherapy to avoid joint stiffness.

2. Case Report

A 68-year-old woman fell on her right side with her right elbow flexed while carrying her luggage. After the trauma, she found her elbow in a valgus position and repositioned the joint herself through flexed and internal rotation. She was admitted to the emergency center of our hospital because of right elbow pain and deformity. She presented with a flexed elbow and the hand placed on her abdomen. The neurologic examination revealed mild numbness in her 4-5th digits only. The radial pulse was palpable. Anteroposterior and lateral radiographs of the elbow showed lateral convergent displacement of the radius and ulna relative to the humerus without fracture signs (Figure 1).

Upon diagnosis of lateral elbow dislocation, we attempted closed reduction under sedation with 15 mg pentazocine hydrochloride and 25 mg hydroxyzine hydrochloride i.m. as well as local anesthesia with 10 mg lidocaine.

The reduction maneuver was performed in the image intensifier room with the patient in the supine position. Initially, we attempted gentle longitudinal traction on the axis in the flexed position with an assistant holding the axilla as a countertraction while simultaneously checking lateral images of the elbow. After the first try was unsuccessful, we applied longitudinal traction on the axis in the stretched position while checking anteroposterior images of the elbow. The operator distracted her wrist distally and moved the dislocated proximal forearm medially. After this maneuver, we felt a click; however, the image intensifier revealed that the elbow joint was not reduced fully, and we suspected that only the ulnohumeral joint was reduced on the trochlea of the humerus (Figure 2). The operator gently pushed the radial head with the elbow flexed and we heard a click to indicate full reduction. Postreduction radiographs were obtained without signs of fracture (Figure 3). Though obvious varus and valgus instability of the joint was observed, redislocation was not observed in the range of motion from 30° to 90° (Figure 4). Elbow arthrography revealed a completely torn medial collateral ligament (MCL) and a suspected partial tear of the lateral collateral ligament (LCL, Figure 5). CT scan and MRI revealed no sign of fracture and additional information.

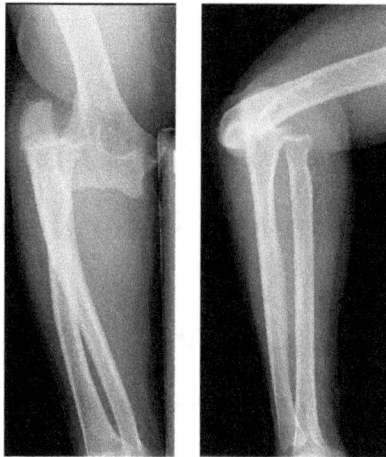

FIGURE 1: Anteroposterior and lateral radiographs of the elbow revealed lateral convergent displacement of the radius and ulna relative to the humerus without fracture signs.

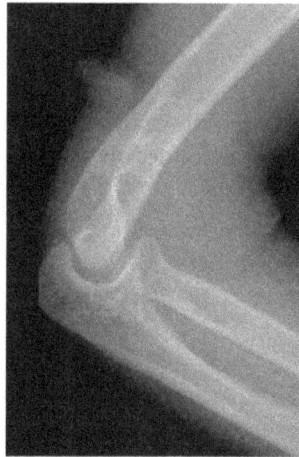

FIGURE 2: During reduction maneuver, the image intensifier revealed that only the ulnohumeral joint was reduced.

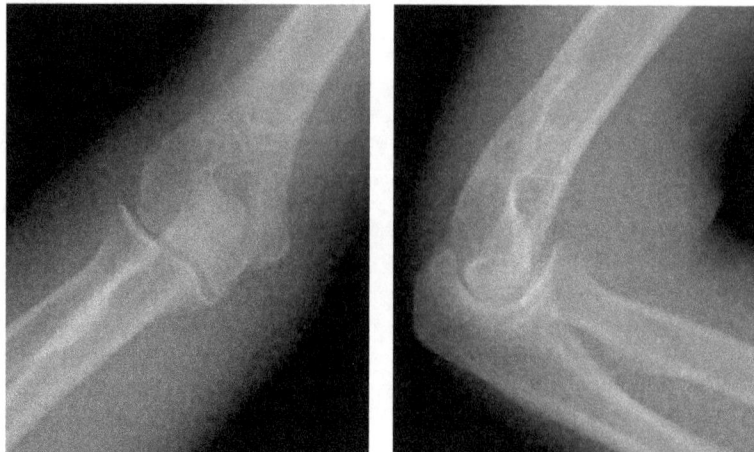

FIGURE 3: Postreduction radiographs revealed no fractures.

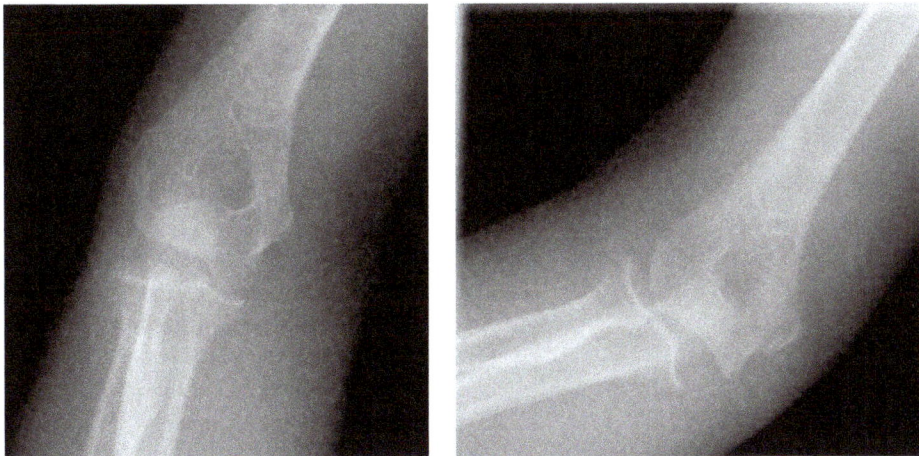

FIGURE 4: Postreduction radiographs revealed obvious varus and valgus instability of the joint. However, redislocation was not observed in the range of motion from 30° to 90°.

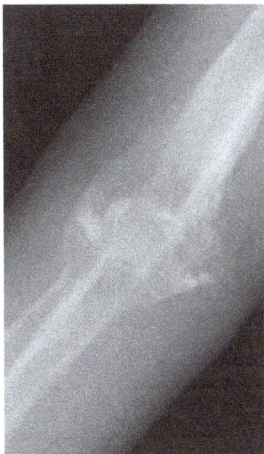

FIGURE 5: The elbow arthrography revealed a complete tear of the medial collateral ligament and a suspected partial tear of the lateral collateral ligament.

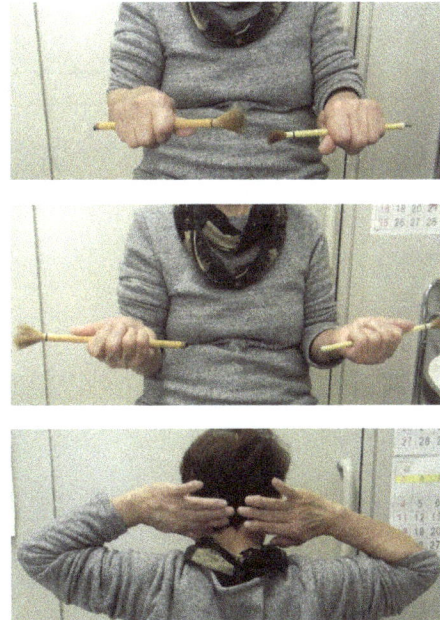

FIGURE 6: After 8 weeks, the elbow range of motion was from 0° to 125°, supination to 90°, and pronation to 90°.

A motor nerve conduction velocity study of the ulnar nerve revealed decreased velocity and prolonged latency.

The elbow joint was immobilized at 90° of flexion with the forearm in supination in a posterior plaster cast for 3 weeks. Mild physiotherapy started at 2 weeks after the trauma and the elbow was examined weekly. The plaster was removed 3 weeks after the trauma. After 8 weeks, the elbow range of motion was from 0° to 125°, supination to 90°, and pronation to 90° (Figure 6). Radiographs revealed mild calcification around the anterior articular capsule, MCL, and LCL; however, the patient did not complain of elbow pain (Figure 7). The decreased velocity and prolonged latency of the ulnar nerve improved steadily (Figure 8). Medical examination 20 weeks after trauma measured her grip strength at 17 (right)/19 (left) kg, and she had not experienced any trouble in daily living. At 6 months, she had no sensory disturbance distributed by the ulnar nerve, and her score of the DASH - JSSH: Japanese Society for Surgery of the Hand version of the

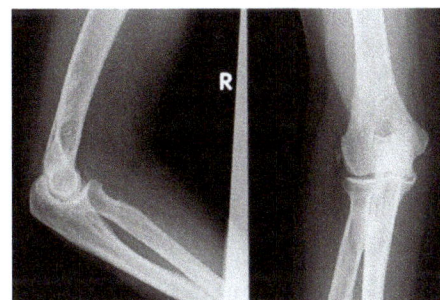

FIGURE 7: Eight weeks after the trauma, radiographs revealed mild calcification around the anterior articular capsule, medial collateral ligament, and lateral collateral ligament.

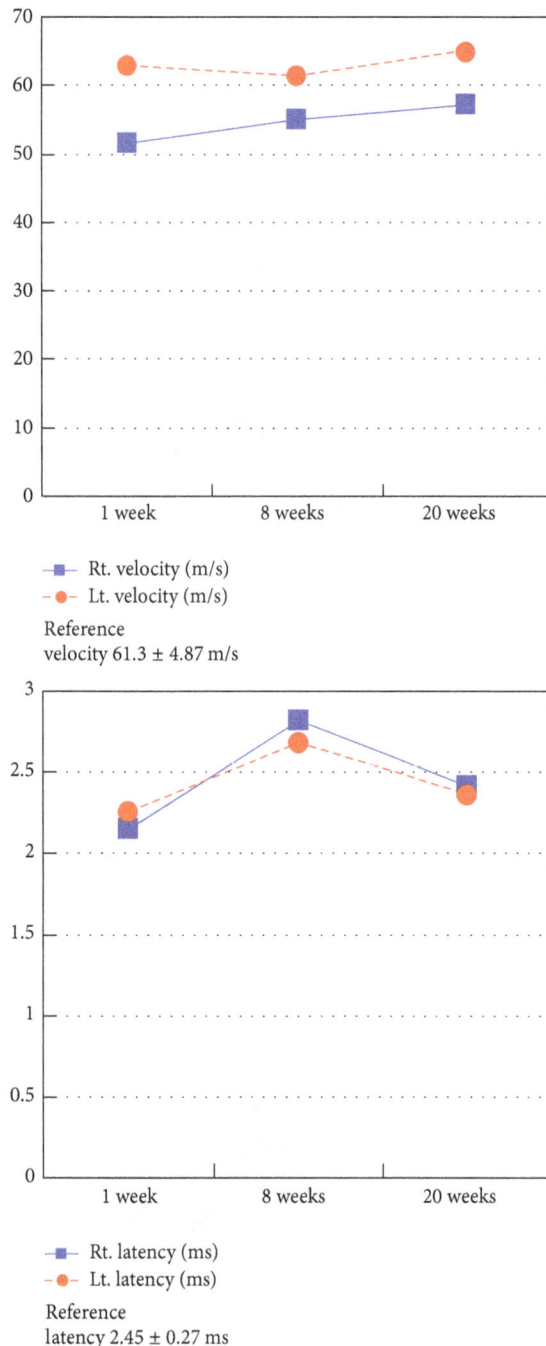

FIGURE 8: Decreased velocity and prolonged latency of the ulnar nerve improved steadily.

Disability of Arm, Shoulder, and Hand questionnaire [1] was 0.86.

3. Discussion

In a systematic review of the literature, three cases of lateral dislocation were reported in 342 patients with dislocated elbows, and one case of anterolateral dislocation was reported [2]. Ulnar nerve involvement after lateral dislocation is typically reported [3] as observed in our case. The reduction of pure lateral elbow dislocation is known to be difficult owing to high risk of incarceration such as swelling, soft tissue interposition such as anconeus muscle, brachialis muscle, ulnar nerve, or associated fractures [4, 5].

Several reduction maneuvers for pure lateral traumatic dislocation of the elbow have been reported. Modification of the gravity-aided "hanging arm" technique originally described for shoulder dislocations by Stimson (modified Stimson's technique [3]) and longitudinal traction on the axis in the semiflexed position, without forcing the elbow in extension [6], is reported as a reducing maneuver. In this case, reduction verified by the image intensifier suggests that this is a reliable method.

Even if obvious varus or valgus instability of the joint was observed, redislocation was not observed in flexion and extension indicating that simple lateral dislocation of the elbow joint can be treated without surgical treatment [3, 4, 6]. Physiotherapy started 2-3 weeks after trauma allowing patients to regain the normal range of elbow movements. Prolonged immobilization of the elbow joint after elbow dislocation is not recommended, as immobilization for more than 14 days may be associated with stiffness [2].

4. Conclusion

Lateral dislocation of the elbow joint is rare and its closed reduction is even rarer. Testing the stability is important for early physiotherapy to avoid joint stiffness. Excellent functional outcomes can be achieved even if followed by nonoperative therapy.

Consent

Written informed consent was obtained from the patient for the publication of this case report and the accompanying images.

Competing Interests

The authors declare there is no conflict of interests.

References

[1] T. Imaeda, S. Toh, Y. Nakao et al., "Validation of the japanese society for surgery of the handversion of the disability of the arm, shoulder, and hand questionnaire," *Journal of Orthopaedic Science*, vol. 10, no. 4, pp. 353–359, 2005.

[2] J. de Haan, N. W. L. Schep, W. E. Tuinebreijer, P. Patka, and D. den Hartog, "Simple elbow dislocations: a systematic review of the literature," *Archives of Orthopaedic and Trauma Surgery*, vol. 130, no. 2, pp. 241–249, 2010.

[3] S. K. Khan, R. Chopra, and D. Chakravarty, "Successful closed manipulation of a pure lateral traumatic dislocation of the elbow joint using a modified Stimson's technique: a case report," *Journal of Medical Case Reports*, vol. 2, article no. 170, 2008.

[4] E. J. Exarchou, "Lateral dislocation of the elbow," *Acta Orthopaedica*, vol. 48, no. 2, pp. 161–163, 1977.

[5] M. Chhaparwal, A. Aroojis, M. Divekar, S. Kulkarni, and S. V. Vaidya, "Irreducible lateral dislocation of the elbow," *Journal of Postgraduate Medicine*, vol. 43, no. 1, pp. 19–20, 1997.

[6] B. Gokcen, S. Ozyurek, A. Atik, A. K. Sivrioglu, E. Kaya, and K. Keklikci, "Successful closed manipulation of simple lateral dislocation of the elbow joint: a case report," *Oman Medical Journal*, vol. 28, no. 6, 2013.

20

Leg Lengthening as a Means of Improving Ambulation Following an Internal Hemipelvectomy

Wakyo Sato,[1] Hiroshi Okazaki,[2] and Takahiro Goto[3]

[1]*Department of Rehabilitation Medicine, Tokyo Metropolitan Tama Medical Center, 2-8-29 Musashidai, Fuchu-Shi, Tokyo 183-8524, Japan*

[2]*Department of Orthopedic Surgery, Japan Labour Health and Welfare Organization, Kanto Rosai Hospital, 1-1 Kizukisumiyoshi-cho, Nakahara-ku, Kawasaki City, Kanagawa 211-8510, Japan*

[3]*Department of Musculoskeletal Oncology, Tokyo Metropolitan Cancer and Infectious Diseases Center Komagome Hospital, 3-18-22 Honkomagome, Bunkyo-ku, Tokyo 113-8677, Japan*

Correspondence should be addressed to Wakyo Sato; wakyo_sato@tmhp.jp

Academic Editor: Elke R. Ahlmann

Reconstructive surgery following an internal hemipelvectomy for a malignant pelvic tumor is difficult due to the structural complexity of the pelvis and the massive extension of the tumor. While high complication rates have been encountered in various types of reconstructive surgery, resection without reconstruction reportedly involved fewer complications. However, this method often results in limb shortening with resultant instability during walking. We reported herein leg lengthening performed to correct lower limb shortening after an internal hemipelvectomy, which improved ambulatory stability and overall QOL. An 18-year-old male patient came to our hospital to correct a lower limb discrepancy resulting from a left internal hemipelvectomy. His left pelvis and proximal femur had been resected, and the femur remained without an acetabular roof. His left lower limb was about 8 centimeters shorter. The left tibia was lengthened 8 centimeters with an external fixator. After the lengthening, the patient was able to walk without support and his gait remarkably improved. Additionally he no longer required placing a wallet in his back pocket as a pad as a means of raising the left side of his torso while sitting. Leg lengthening was a useful method of improving ambulation after an internal hemipelvectomy.

1. Introduction

The treatment of pelvic tumors involving the acetabulum in particular is difficult due to the anatomical complexity of the pelvis and the massive extension of the tumor [1]. Ablation of the affected lower limb was a standard procedure in the past, but, as medicine advanced, limb-sparing procedures such as the internal hemipelvectomy have become popular [2]. Reconstructing the pelvis after an internal hemipelvectomy has nonetheless remained difficult. Prosthetic implantation [3, 4], bone graft, bone cement reconstruction, arthrodesis, hip transposition, or a combination of some of these methods has been employed [4, 5]. Although reconstructive surgery is preferable to amputation, a complication rate as high as 50–60% has been cited in connection with this method [3, 6–10].

Resection without reconstruction, that is, the "flail hip," is an alternative form of pelvic tumor treatment [11, 12] but the result was reportedly poor in terms of restoration of function [6, 13]. Other, more recent reports, on the other hand, demonstrated a lower complication rate and higher functional score for this procedure [8, 12] in which the shortening of the lower limb resulted in a gait abnormality. Rectifying the discrepancy in length has reportedly improved lower extremity stability and ambulation [12, 14].

The purpose of this paper is to assess bone lengthening as a method of correcting leg length discrepancy and improving ambulation following an internal hemipelvectomy, especially

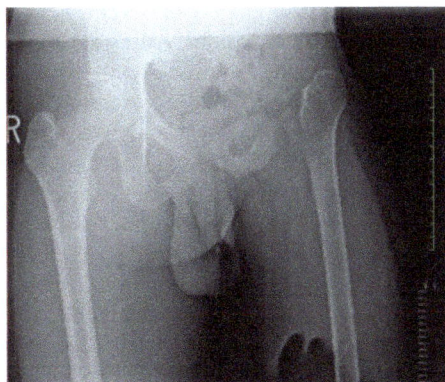

FIGURE 1: Radiograph of the hip joints at first visit.

in cases involving a nearly complete resection of the half pelvis and the ipsilateral proximal femur.

2. Case Presentation

A 13-year-old boy received the diagnosis of clear cell chondrosarcoma in his left ilium and underwent a left internal hemipelvectomy. The whole left ilium, most of the left ischium, part of superior pubis ramus, and the left femoral head and neck were resected. The total iliacus and the psoas major muscle were resected while the tendon of the psoas muscle was left intact. About half of the left gluteus maximus and medius muscles were left and resutured to the abdomen or back muscles after bone resection, preserving the extension and abduction functions of the left hip joint. The left adductor muscles were left intact.

At 18 years old, the patient came to our hospital to correct the discrepancy in the length of his legs. A hip radiograph showed evidence of surgical resection of the left pelvis, femoral head, and neck (Figure 1). A radiograph of the entire lower limb revealed that the tip of the residual left femur moved upward about 4 centimeters on the left leg compared with the right leg in the standing position (Figure 2). The patient walked with a limp and required a crutch. The umbilicus-medial malleolus distance (UMD) was 87 cm/82 cm (right/left) when in the standing position on the right leg and 87 cm/77 cm when on the left leg.

Before the operation to lengthen the limb, we gauged the desired effect using a shoe-lift to simulate changes in limb length. After several trials, an 8-centimeter shoe-lift raised the pelvis sufficiently to achieve evenness in the height and position of the hips. Then, the left tibia was lengthened using an unilateral external fixator (Hifixator®, Nagano Keiki Co. Ltd., Ueda, Japan). The osteotomy was performed at the proximal tibia, and three half pins 6 mm in diameter were inserted above and below the osteotomy site (Figure 3). The patient began walking with crutches on the day after the operation. Weight-bearing was strongly encouraged. Lengthening began at one week after the operation at an average rate of 0.5 mm/day. The total increase in length was 8 cm, and the duration of fixator mount use was 17.5 months.

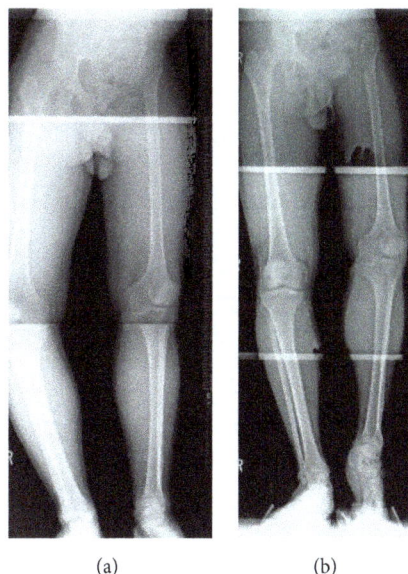

(a)   (b)

FIGURE 2: Radiographs of entire lower limbs before leg lengthening showed tip of the residual left femur had moved upward about 4 cm in standing position (a) compared with the right leg (b).

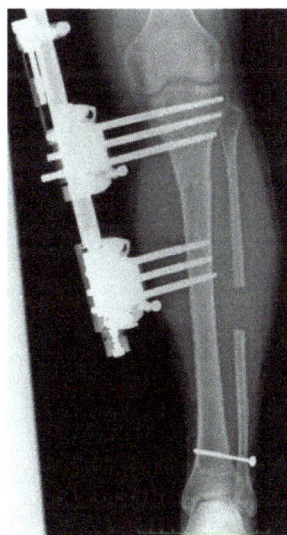

FIGURE 3: Radiograph of the left tibia after lengthening operation.

A below-the-knee cylinder brace was worn when walking for 9 months after fixator removal.

The patient was able to walk short distances without a crutch after fixator removal. One year later, he was able to walk without any assistance. Five years after fixator removal, he was able to walk 4-5 kilometers continuously without any apparent gait abnormality and could stand on the left leg steadily (Figure 4). The radiograph of the entire lower limbs in the standing position showed the tip of the left femur in the same position as when the 8 cm shoe-lift was used (Figure 5). Furthermore, after lengthening, the patient no longer required placing a wallet in his back pocket to adjust his height in the seated position. The patient expressed great

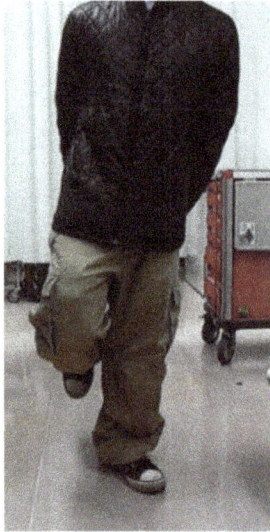

FIGURE 4: Photograph showed he stood on the left leg steadily without any support.

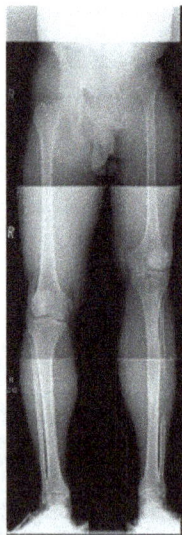

FIGURE 5: Radiograph of entire lower limbs at 5 years after leg lengthening.

satisfaction with the results. The Musculoskeletal Tumor Society Score (MSTS) [15] was 26 (87%).

3. Discussion

The annual incidence of bone malignancies is about 4–7 cases/million children under 15 years of age [16, 17]. Nearly two-thirds of the malignancies occur in the pelvis [18].

While nonreconstruction following an hemipelvectomy can prevent complications such as those that occur when reconstruction is performed, some gait impairment will result from the discrepancy in limb length and the resultant instability of the lower limb.

As a solution to this problem, Eilber et al. [14] reported that a shoe-lift or compensatory pelvic tilt was effective in

rectifying an average discrepancy of 3.5 cm. Schwartz et al. [12] reported that a shoe-lift compensating for approximately 50% of the total discrepancy improved stability and ambulation. Catagani and Ottaviani [19] reported favorable results with an increase of 6.4 cm in leg length using an Ilizarov apparatus.

In the present case, the discrepancy was approximately 8 centimeters although some variation resulted from the difference in loading on the affected and healthy limb. The 8 cm shoe-lift was effective, but in addition to being uncomfortably heavy, this height also made the patient prone to tripping over and too heavy to walk. Nonetheless the surgical lengthening was generally very favorable, allowing the patient not only to walk without any ambulatory aids but also to sit on a chair without using a wallet to bolster his torso.

Another concern following the procedure was the possibility of the tip of the residual femur penetrating overlying soft tissue by loading during ambulation. In a study of the course of 98 untreated cases of congenital hip dislocation (CHD) among patients aged 17–65 involving a total of 132 hips, Kono [20] reported that 68 patients suffered complete dislocation of the hip. In 64 of these cases, the femoral head was situated in the gluteus muscle without the acetabulum but was able to maintain stability and mobility during the patients' lifetime. The features of our case resembled those of a complete CHD with an unstable lower limb. Although our patient suffered from a gait abnormality like that of the CHD patients, surgical intervention restored lower limb stability and enabled him to walk without any ambulatory aids.

To assess the functional efficacy of flail hips, Takami et al. [21] reviewed 5 cases with MSTS scores between 53% and 93%. Schwartz et al. [12] reported 8 nonreconstruction cases with MSTS scores at 53.3–80.0% of normal values. These reports demonstrated that nonreconstruction methods are capable of producing acceptable outcomes. Our case also demonstrated a favorable result with a MSTS score of 87%.

The present report features only one case of surgical intervention to treat the shortening of a lower limb due to an hemipelvectomy. The result was nonetheless very favorable from both the clinical perspective and patient satisfaction. We consider this method as a viable option for the treatment of impaired ambulation due to an hemipelvectomy.

4. Conclusion

Lengthening the shortened limb was a useful method of improving ambulation following an internal hemipelvectomy.

Competing Interests

The authors declare that there is no conflict of interests regarding the publication of this paper.

References

[1] R. P. H. Veth, R. van Hoesel, M. Pruszczynski, J. Hoogenhout, B. Schreuder, and T. Wobbes, "Limb salvage in musculoskeletal oncology," *The Lancet Oncology*, vol. 4, no. 6, pp. 343–350, 2003.

[2] R. Nagarajan, J. P. Neglia, D. R. Clohisy, and L. L. Robison, "Limb salvage and amputation in survivors of pediatric lower-extremity bone tumors: what are the long-term implications?" *Journal of Clinical Oncology*, vol. 20, no. 22, pp. 4493–4501, 2002.

[3] A. Abudu, R. J. Grimer, S. R. Cannon, S. R. Carter, and R. S. Sneath, "Reconstruction of the hemipelvis after the excision of malignant tumours," *The Journal of Bone and Joint Surgery—British Volume*, vol. 79, no. 5, pp. 773–779, 1997.

[4] R. L. Satcher Jr., R. J. O'Donnell, and J. O. Johnston, "Reconstruction of the pelvis after resection of tumors about the acetabulum," *Clinical Orthopaedics and Related Research*, no. 409, pp. 209–217, 2003.

[5] E. Schwameis, M. Dominkus, P. Krepler et al., "Reconstruction of the pelvis after tumor resection in children and adolescents," *Clinical Orthopaedics and Related Research*, no. 402, pp. 220–235, 2002.

[6] R. Windhager, J. Karner, H.-P. Kutschera, P. Polterauer, M. Salzer-Kuntschik, and R. Kotz, "Limb salvage in periacetabular sarcomas: review of 21 consecutive cases," *Clinical Orthopaedics and Related Research*, no. 331, pp. 265–276, 1996.

[7] A. J. S. Renard, R. P. H. Veth, H. W. B. Schreuder et al., "The saddle prosthesis in pelvic primary and secondary musculoskeletal tumors: functional results at several postoperative intervals," *Archives of Orthopaedic and Trauma Surgery*, vol. 120, no. 3-4, pp. 188–194, 2000.

[8] A. Hillmann, C. Hoffman, G. Gosheger, R. Rödl, W. Winkelmann, and T. Ozaki, "Tumors of the pelvis: complications after reconstruction," *Archives of Orthopaedic and Trauma Surgery*, vol. 123, no. 7, pp. 340–344, 2003.

[9] L. R. Menendez, E. R. Ahlmann, Y. Falkinstein, and D. C. Allison, "Periacetabular reconstruction with a new endoprosthesis," *Clinical Orthopaedics and Related Research*, vol. 467, no. 11, pp. 2831–2837, 2009.

[10] U. Aydinli, C. Ozturk, U. Yalcinkaya, O. Tirelioglu, and S. Ersozlu, "Limb-sparing surgery for primary malignant tumours of the pelvis," *Acta Orthopaedica Belgica*, vol. 70, no. 5, pp. 417–422, 2004.

[11] H. H. Steel, "Partial or complete resection of the hemipelvis. An alternative to hindquarter amputation for periacetabular chondrosarcoma of the pelvis," *The Journal of Bone and Joint Surgery—American Volume*, vol. 60, no. 6, pp. 719–730, 1978.

[12] A. J. Schwartz, P. Kiatisevi, F. C. Eilber, F. R. Eilber, and J. J. Eckardt, "The friedman-eilber resection arthroplasty of the pelvis," *Clinical Orthopaedics and Related Research*, vol. 467, no. 11, pp. 2825–2830, 2009.

[13] M. I. O'Connor, "Malignant pelvic tumors: limb-sparing resection and reconstruction," *Seminars in Surgical Oncology*, vol. 13, no. 1, pp. 49–54, 1997.

[14] F. R. Eilber, T. T. Grant, D. Sakai, and D. L. Morton, "Internal hemipelvectomy—excision of the hemipelvis with limb preservation. An alternative to hemipelvectomy," *Cancer*, vol. 43, no. 3, pp. 806–809, 1979.

[15] W. F. Enneking, W. Dunham, M. C. Gebhardt, M. Malawar, and D. J. Pritchard, "A system for the functional evaluation of reconstructive procedures after surgical treatment of tumors of the musculoskeletal system," *Clinical Orthopaedics and Related Research*, no. 286, pp. 241–246, 1993.

[16] C. A. Arndt and W. M. Crist, "Common musculoskeletal tumors of childhood and adolescence," *The New England Journal of Medicine*, vol. 341, no. 5, pp. 342–352, 1999.

[17] T. Marugame, K. Katanoda, T. Matsuda et al., "The Japan cancer surveillance report: incidence of childhood, bone, penis and testis cancers," *Japanese Journal of Clinical Oncology*, vol. 37, no. 4, pp. 319–323, 2007.

[18] R. Nagarajan, D. R. Clohisy, J. P. Neglia et al., "Function and quality-of-life of survivors of pelvic and lower extremity osteosarcoma and Ewing's sarcoma: the Childhood Cancer Survivor Study," *British Journal of Cancer*, vol. 91, no. 11, pp. 1858–1865, 2004.

[19] M. A. Catagani and G. Ottaviani, "Ilizarov method to correct limb length discrepancy after limb-sparing hemipelvectomy," *Journal of Pediatric Orthopaedics Part B*, vol. 17, no. 6, pp. 293–298, 2008.

[20] S. Kono, "Untreated severe congenital hip dislocations," *Journal of the Japanese Orthopaedic Association*, vol. 41, no. 5, pp. 473–478, 1967.

[21] M. Takami, M. Ieguchi, K. Takamatsu et al., "Functional evaluation of flail hip joint after periacetabular resection of the pelvis," *Osaka City Medical Journal*, vol. 43, no. 2, pp. 173–183, 1997.

A Case of Penicillin-Resistant *Veillonella* Prosthetic Joint Infection of the Knee

Claudia R. Libertin,[1,2,3] **Joy H. Peterson,**[2] **Mark P. Brodersen,**[4,5] **and Tamara Huff**[4,5]

[1]*Division of Infectious Diseases, Mayo Clinic Health System (MCHS-W), Waycross, GA, USA*
[2]*Departments of Pathology and Laboratory Medicine, Mayo Clinic Health System-Waycross, Waycross, GA, USA*
[3]*Division of Infectious Diseases, Mayo Clinic, Jacksonville, FL, USA*
[4]*Department of Orthopedics, Mayo Clinic Health System-Waycross, Waycross, GA, USA*
[5]*Department of Orthopedic Surgery, Mayo Clinic, Jacksonville, FL, USA*

Correspondence should be addressed to Claudia R. Libertin; libertin.claudia@mayo.edu

Academic Editor: Koichi Sairyo

Veillonella sp. and *V. dispar* are emerging pathogens. This is the third case of a monomicrobial *Veillonella* sp. prosthetic joint infection (PJI) among knees and hips; this is the second prosthetic knee infection described. The infection was treated with a 2-stage procedural approach combined with 6 weeks of ceftriaxone with excellent clinical response. There was no relapse in 2 years of follow-up care. This case exemplifies the importance of incubating anaerobic cultures for at least 7 days to grow some anaerobic pathogens.

1. Introduction

Diagnosing prosthetic joint infections takes a disciplined approach by orthopedic surgeons to make a bacterial diagnosis [1]. Prosthetic joint infections due to *Veillonella* sp. as the sole pathogen remain rarely reported. *Veillonella* sp. are small, strictly anaerobic gram-negative cocci that are found in the oral, respiratory, genitourinary, and intestinal tracts [2]. Infections such as bacteremia [3], meningitis [4], endocarditis [5], osteomyelitis [6, 7], and prosthetic joint infections (PJI) [8, 9] have been described. This is only the second prosthetic knee infection [9] reported due solely to *Veillonella* sp. and only the third prosthetic joint infection [8] including hips. In addition to supporting that *Veillonella* acts as a pathogen, this case exemplifies the need for microbiology laboratories to follow standard microbiologic practices such as incubating anaerobic cultures for a minimum of 7 days.

Informed consent was obtained from the patient to report this case.

2. Case Report

A 61-year-old man with well-controlled, noninsulin-dependent diabetes and a history of an uncomplicated left total knee arthroplasty implanted 2 years before presented with a 2-month history of acute knee pain with progressive swelling, erythema, and an inability to ambulate. He had no fevers, chills, or night sweats. He received no empiric antibiotics. Besides a swollen and warm left knee, he had extensive caries and gingivitis on examination. His X-rays revealed a well fixed total knee arthroplasty (Figure 1).

Two aspirates of the knee done in a clinic at Mayo Clinic Health System-Waycross (MCHS-W; formerly Satilla Regional Medical Center) revealed brown, purulent-appearing fluid (Table 1). White blood cell count from the initial aspiration was 72,696 cell/uL with 88% polys. Gram stain showed white blood cells, but no organisms were seen. Only cultures were requested on the second knee aspirate done in the clinic. The clinic aspirate samples were submitted to a national commercial microbiology laboratory and not MCHS-W hospital's microbiology laboratory. Cultures were reported to have no growth on two separate occasions (Table 1). Because of persistent pain, the orthopedic surgeon admitted the patient to MCHS-W hospital to remove the prosthesis, place a static antibiotic spacer, and submit 4 operative tissue specimens to the Department of Laboratory Medicine and Pathology. His white blood cell count was

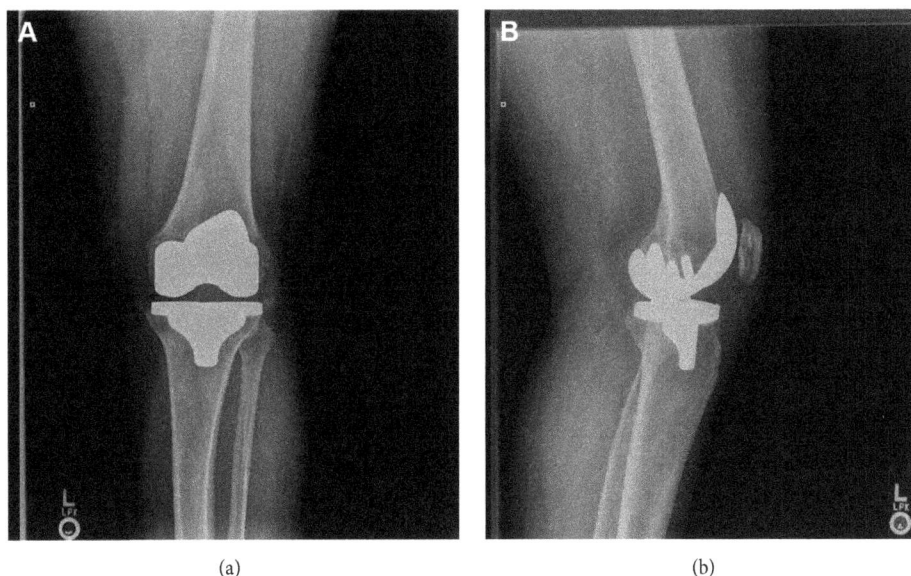

FIGURE 1: Anterior-posterior (a) and lateral (b) radiographs of left primary total knee arthroplasty from initial clinic presentation.

TABLE 1: Impact of anaerobic incubation time on growth detection.

Knee sample	Fluid appearance	Culture Orders	Laboratory	Duration of incubation	Microbiologic results
Arthrocentesis #1	Brown, purulent	Aerobic & anaerobic cultures	National commercial lab	48 hours	No growth
Arthrocentesis #2	Brown, purulent	Aerobic culture hold for 7 days	National commercial lab	72 hours	No growth
Synovial operative tissue ×4	No description	Aerobic & anaerobic cultures	MCHS-Waycross	10 days	Veillonella sp.

MCHS: Mayo Clinic Health System.

$15.8 \times 10^5/\mu L$, erythrocyte sedimentation rate was 100 mm/hour, and C-reactive protein was 138 mg/L. The patient was started on parenteral vancomycin and ciprofloxacin empirically for a presumed diagnosis of culture-negative PJI (CN PJI) by the orthopedic team. While hospitalized, an infectious disease consultation was obtained. Prior negative aerobic cultures and inadequate incubation times for anaerobic cultures raised suspicion that an anaerobic organism is the pathogen. The consultant confirmed with the microbiology laboratory that an anaerobic culture had indeed been submitted and requested that the anaerobic cultures be held for 10 days. It was discovered that the MCHS-W hospital laboratory, which is a rural community microbiology laboratory, only held anaerobic cultures for 2 days unless otherwise requested.

All operative samples were plated on Remel media (Remel, Lenexa, KS). Blood agar (BAP) and chocolate agar were incubated at 35°C in 5% CO_2; MacConkey agar and thioglycolate broth were incubated at 35°C in ambient air. BAP and phenyl ethyl alcohol agar were incubated anaerobically with the Anoxomat System (Advanced Instruments, INC; MART Microbiology, BV, Drachten, Netherlands). Bactec Pediatric Plus/F bottles (Becton Dickinson, Sparks, MD)

were not inoculated. All original aerobic and anaerobic plates showed no growth at 2 days. On day 4, a gram stain performed directly from the thioglycolate broth of all 4 specimens revealed small gram-negative cocci. All 4 thioglycolate broths were plated to BAP CO_2 and BAP anaerobic. All BAP CO_2 subcultures were no growth. All BAP anaerobic subcultures grew small round translucent colonies that stained as gram-negative cocci. The Remel RapID ANA II System identified the organism as Veillonella sp. Because Veillonella sp. yield a negative biochemical profile except for the production of catalase and nitrate reduction, the bacterial isolate was sent to Mayo Medical Laboratories (MML, Rochester, MN) for confirmation. The Bruker Biotyper was used to identify the pathogen by MALDI-TOF (Matrix Assisted Laser Desorption Ionization-Time of Flight) methodology. Bruker MALDI-TOF identified the isolate as Veillonella parvula to an acceptable level of 2.173 (an acceptable identification to the genus level with a confidence level is as low as 1.70). The isolate was further speciated by real time polymerase chain reaction (PCR) on the microbial identification kit from Applied Bio systems. The master-mix of primers/probes is made in-house; all components are purchased individually. Primers and

TABLE 2: *Veillonella* isolate.

Antibiotic	MIC (mcg/mL)	CLSI guidelines		Interpretation
		Susceptible	Resistant	
Penicillin	8	≤0.5	>1	Resistant
Clindamycin	≤0.5	≤2	>4	Susceptible
Metronidazole	1	≤8	>16	Susceptible
Ceftriaxone	8	≤16	>32	Susceptible
Ciprofloxacin	0.12	No interpretive criteria given		No interpretation

CLSI: Clinical Laboratory Standards Institute; MIC: minimal inhibitory concentration tested by Etest methodology performed by Mayo Medical Laboratory.

TABLE 3: Monomicrobial *Veillonella* prosthetic joint infections.

Case report	Year	PJI site	Symptoms	X-ray	Organism	E test sensitivities	Surgical	Medical treatment	Follow-up evaluation
Marchandin et al. [9]	2001	Knee	Pain & swelling functional incapacity	Prosthetic loosening	*Veillonella dispar*	Penicillin (S) Amoxicillin/clavulanate (S) clindamycin (S)	2-stage procedure	Amoxicillin + rifampicin × 6 months	6 months
Zaninetti-Schaerer et al. [8]	2004	Hip	Pain & functional incapacity	Prosthetic loosening	*Veillonella* sp.	Not reported	Retained prosthesis	Ceftriaxone 3 wks, then ampicillin, followed by imipenem, for a total of 3 months; lifelong po clindamycin	Not reported
Current	2016	Knee	Pain & swelling functional incapacity	No prosthetic loosening	*Veillonella* sp.	Penicillin (R)	2-stage procedure	Ceftriaxone 2 gm qd × 6 wks	2 years

PJI: prosthetic joint infection, R: resistant, and S: sensitive.

probes are purchased from Integrated DNA Technologies, INC (IDT, Coralville, Iowa). MML performs dual PCR with Applied Biosystems and then performs 16S rRNA sequencing with IDT primers and probes. 16S rRNA sequencing was done at Mayo Medical Laboratory. After performing 16S rRNA sequencing on the *Veillonella* isolate differentiation among 3 possible species: *V. parvula*, *V. dispar*, and *V. rodentium* could not be determined. All three comparison strains were ATCC reference strains. The percentages of similarity were 99.54, 99.49, and 99.25, respectively.

Susceptibilities were performed by Etest methodology (bioMerieux, Durham, NC) on *Brucella*-based agar at MML and are reported in Table 2.

The patient received 6 weeks of parenteral ceftriaxone in the community following the removal of the prosthesis. During antibiotic therapy, extensive dental work and extractions were performed since his dental caries, dental abscesses, and gingivitis could have been a potential source of the infection. After completion of the therapy and an antibiotic holiday, interventional radiology attempted unsuccessfully to aspirate the knee. At reimplantation, frozen bone sections were negative for bacteria and acute inflammation. Figure 2 shows the reimplanted knee arthroplasty. The patient's recovery

from reimplantation was uneventful. Two years later, he has not had a relapse of PJI in that knee.

3. Discussion

Marchandin et al. [9] described the first report of a monomicrobial prosthetic joint infection caused by *Veillonella dispar* in a prosthetic knee in 2001. All *Veillonella* sp. reported to cause monomicrobial PJI are listed and compared in Table 3. The two PKIs of the knees had similar clinical presentations of joint swelling associated with pain and functional incapacity. Our patient did not have evidence of prosthesis loosening radiographically (Figure 1), as the other cases did. Our patient's isolate was identified by MALTI-TOF methodology followed by real-time PCR and by 16S rRNA sequencing with IDT primer/probes to confirm the pathogen, but determination of the species was not made. Our patient received 6 weeks of ceftriaxone therapy after removal of the prosthesis. Two years later, there were no manifestations of a relapse of infection. Zaninetti-Schaerer et al. [8] described a monomicrobial *Veillonella* sp. prosthetic hip infection which was associated with bacteremia. That infection was treated with 3 weeks of ceftriaxone followed by amoxicillin and

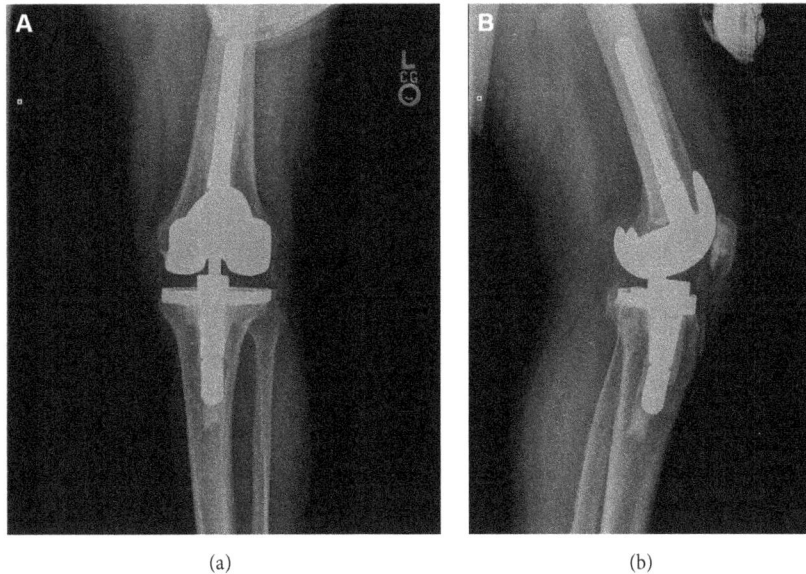

FIGURE 2: Anterior-posterior (a) and lateral (b) radiographs after second stage of reimplantation of cemented revision left total knee arthroplasty.

imipenem for a total of 3 months. Lifelong oral clindamycin without prosthesis was prescribed. Ongoing monitoring of the patient post treatment was not documented. Of these three monomicrobial prosthetic joint infections, our patient did well with a standard 6 weeks of ceftriaxone therapy after prosthesis removal. In all three PJIs from *Veillonella* sp., dental sources were suspected but never definitively proven.

The susceptibility profile of our isolate is typical of those reported in recent literature [10–12]; most strains of *Veillonella* sp. are now penicillin resistant (Table 2). Resistance to vancomycin is an innate resistance. Manchandin et al. isolate was penicillin susceptible [9]. Susceptibilities on the isolate from the total hip arthroplasty (THA) *Veillonella* sp. infection were not reported [8].

Unfortunately, our patient was initially falsely diagnosed as a CN PJI based on the fact that the orthopedic surgeon had ordered anaerobic cultures when the patient was seen in the clinic. Two knee aspirates were performed but sent to a commercial laboratory from our clinic instead of the hospital microbiology laboratory. Cultures revealed no growth (Table 1). CN PJI can result from sampling practices by surgeons, failure to order anaerobic cultures, methodologies used in the microbiology laboratory, and most commonly prior use of antimicrobial therapy within the 3 months before cultures are obtained [13]. The inappropriate empiric initiation of vancomycin and ciprofloxacin occurred initially because the surgeon had ordered anaerobic cultures and even had requested from the national commercial laboratory that they be held for 7 days with the cultures reported as negative. The inadequate incubation times for anaerobic organism detection resulted in the reporting of false negative results. The requesting of anaerobic cultures, submitting 4 tissue specimens, and incubating anaerobic cultures for a minimum of 7 days are vital in making a bacteriologic diagnosis [1, 14]. It is critical to confirm with the microbiology laboratories

used to process and identify patients' organisms that the incubation standards for isolating anaerobic cultures are followed. Even if the anaerobic incubation time had not been extended by the infectious disease physician at MCHS-W, the organism would have been recovered from aerobic cultures in that the organism was growing in thioglycolate broth on day 4. This case reveals the importance of clinicians being diligent in confirming that each step in the process of identifying a bacterial isolate is done according to the standard of practice in that discipline.

In summary, we report the second case of monomicrobial *Veillonella* sp. prosthetic knee infection successfully treated with a 2-stage orthopedic approach and 6 weeks of ceftriaxone therapy. This case supports *Veillonella* sp. as an emerging pathogen causing monomicrobial PJIs. It also exemplifies the importance of all microbiology laboratories to analyze an anaerobic sample properly utilizing adequate microbiological practices as advised by national standards and for clinicians to confirm that the standards are done.

Competing Interests

The authors declare that they have no competing interests.

Acknowledgments

The 16S rRNA sequencing was done by Brian Connelly, Technical Specialist, at Mayo Medical Laboratory, Rochester, MN.

References

[1] American Academy of Orthopaedic Surgeons: the diagnosis of periprosthetic joint infections of the hip and knee: guideline and evidence report, 2010, http://www.aaos.org/Research/guidelines/PJIguideline.pdf.

[2] E. A. Delwiche, J. J. Pestka, and M. L. Tortorello, "The Veil-lonellae: gram-negative cocci with a unique physiology," *Annual Review of Microbiology*, vol. 39, pp. 175–193, 1985.

[3] J. W. Liu, J. J. Wu, L. R. Wang, L. J. Teng, and T. C. Huang, "Two fatal cases of *Veillonella* bacteremia," *European Journal of Clinical Microbiology & Infectious Diseases*, vol. 17, no. 1, pp. 62–64, 1998.

[4] M. A. Bhatti and M. O. Frank, "Veillonella parvula meningitis: case report and review of Veillonella infections," *Clinical Infectious Diseases*, vol. 31, no. 3, pp. 839–840, 2000.

[5] T. W. Boo, B. Cryan, A. O'Donnell, and G. Fahy, "Prosthetic valve endocarditis caused by Veillonella parvula," *The Journal of Infection*, vol. 50, no. 1, pp. 81–83, 2005.

[6] R. A. Barnhart, M. R. Weitekamp, and R. C. Aber, "Osteomyelitis caused by Veillonella," *The American Journal of Medicine*, vol. 74, no. 5, pp. 902–904, 1983.

[7] K. A. Borchardt, M. Baker, and R. Gelber, "*Veillonella parvula* septicemia and osteomyelitis," *Annals of Internal Medicine*, vol. 86, no. 1, pp. 63–64, 1977.

[8] A. Zaninetti-Schaerer, C. Van Delden, S. Genevay, and C. Gabay, "Total hip prosthetic joint infection due to Veillonella species," *Joint Bone Spine*, vol. 71, no. 2, pp. 161–163, 2004.

[9] H. Marchandin, H. Jean-Pierre, C. Carrière, F. Canovas, H. Darbas, and E. Jumas-Bilak, "Prosthetic joint infection due to Veillonella dispar," *European Journal of Clinical Microbiology and Infectious Diseases*, vol. 20, no. 5, pp. 340–342, 2001.

[10] V. L. Sutter and S. M. Finegold, "Susceptibility of anaerobic bacteria to 23 antimicrobial agents," *Antimicrobial Agents and Chemotherapy*, vol. 10, no. 4, pp. 736–752, 1976.

[11] M. Litterio, M. Matteo, G. Fiorilli, and E. Rubeglio, "Susceptibility of *Veillonella* spp. to ten different antibiotics," *Anaerobe*, vol. 5, no. 3-4, pp. 477–478, 1999.

[12] D. Ready, R. Bedi, P. Mullany, and M. Wilson, "Penicillin and amoxicillin resistance in oral Veillonella spp," *International Journal of Antimicrobial Agents*, vol. 40, no. 2, pp. 188–189, 2012.

[13] E. F. Berbari, C. Marculescu, I. Sia et al., "Culture-negative prosthetic joint infection," *Clinical Infectious Diseases*, vol. 45, no. 9, pp. 1113–1119, 2007.

[14] E. J. Baron, J. M. Miller, M. P. Weinstein et al., "A guide to utilization of the microbiology laboratory for diagnosis of infectious diseases: 2013 recommendations by the infectious diseases society of America (IDSA) and the American Society for Microbiology (ASM)," *Clinical Infectious Diseases*, vol. 57, no. 4, pp. e22–e121, 2013.

22

Fixation of a Proximal Humeral Fracture Using a Novel Intramedullary Cage Construct following a Failed Conservative Treatment

John Macy

Copley Hospital, Morrisville, VT 05661, USA

Correspondence should be addressed to John Macy; macemd@comcast.net

Academic Editor: George Mouzopoulos

A majority of proximal humeral fractures are preferably treated conservatively. However, surgical management may be beneficial in proximal humeral fractures with significant displacement or angulation. Unfortunately, the complication rates associated with current surgical procedures for fracture fixation, ORIF and IM devices, can be unacceptably high. A new technology, termed the PH Cage, addresses the technical limitations associated with current technologies available for fixation of proximal humeral fractures. It allows for intramedullary fixation of a PH fracture and provides direct load bearing support to the articular surface and buttresses the medial column during healing. We are presenting our first experience with the PH Cage for the fixation of a PH fracture, which had previously failed conservative management.

1. Introduction

Optimal management of proximal humeral (PH) fractures continues to be controversial. Since 71% of proximal humerus fractures occur in patients over sixty years in age, conservative management is currently preferred in a majority of these patients [1]. However, clinical studies have shown that nonoperative treatment of certain fracture types can significantly lower functional outcomes in some patients [2]. In spite of this evidence, surgical intervention may not be recommended because of potentially high complication rates associated with existing technologies for PH fracture fixation. However, as the degree of displacement and instability increases, conservative management of fractures results in suboptimal outcomes [3]. Surgical intervention may be preferred to optimally manage these significantly displaced two-, three- and four-part fractures.

Surgical techniques are constantly evolving to manage PH fractures either through reconstruction (with pins, plates, screws, and IM nails) or prosthetic replacement options (hemiarthroplasty and reverse shoulder arthroplasty). Of the current surgical treatments available, the evolution of locking plate technologies has increased the incidence of surgical interventions to fix PH fractures. Proximal humeral locking plates are indicated for the fixation of certain displaced two-, three-, and four-part PH fractures. Locking plates provide biomechanical strength and stability for restoring and fixing a fracture, especially for valgus impacted fractures. However, the overall clinical benefit of locking plates for PH fracture fixation is controversial, both in their ability to treat complex PH fractures and in the predictability of patient outcomes. When compared to conservative treatment in elderly patients, a recent randomized clinical trial showed better radiographic outcome with open reduction and internal fixation (ORIF) but statistically equivalent functional outcomes for patients with three-part fractures [4]. Additionally, complication rates associated with locking plate technologies can be unacceptably high.

Complication rates as high as 50% have been reported in literature for locking plates with associated revision rates at approximately 15% [5]. Complications include intra-articular screw penetration, hardware failure, subacromial impingement, varus collapse, and osteonecrosis [6]. To ensure optimal clinical outcomes, the current consensus is that the restoration of the medial calcar, metaphyseal buttressing, and anatomic reduction of the tuberosities are key [7]. The use of intramedullary fibular strut allografts has been reported to aid in reduction, as well as to provide buttress support to the medial column for patients with osteoporotic bone with good clinical outcomes [8]. However, there is a need for new technology that addresses the limitations of locking plates and IM devices for the fixation of proximal humeral fractures.

The PH Cage (Conventus Orthopaedics, Maple Grove MN, USA) is an intramedullary implant available for fixation of proximal humeral fractures. The PH Cage is made from nitinol and it expands once deployed below the articular surface, thus providing medial column buttress and head support on implantation. The PH Cage is indicated for the fixation of two-, three-, and four-part fractures similar to the locking plates. It can be surgically inserted in a retrograde or antegrade/intramedullary direction, percutaneously or through a traditional open approach. The intramedullary design of this implant enables medial column support, which is often required for PH fractures. Additionally, the PH Cage design also allows for unconstrained screw fixation of the tuberosities wherever it is needed (unlike current locking plates or IM devices that are directionally constrained). This report presents our first experience and outcome following the use of the PH Cage for treatment of a proximal humerus fracture malunion with severe varus angulation.

2. Case Report

A 70-year-old, right hand dominant, otherwise healthy and active, female presented to our clinic three (3) months after falling onto her left shoulder. She was initially treated elsewhere nonoperatively with sling immobilization and limited physical therapy. Upon presentation to us, she complained of persistent lateral shoulder pain and limited function in her left arm. Physical examination revealed her to be neurovascularly intact with no deltoid deficiency. She had limited active motion and painful passive motion associated with crepitation. Radiographs revealed a two-part, varus-angulated malunion with a large spike of bone protruding laterally, without evidence of AVN (Figure 1). The natural history, prognosis, treatment options, potential complications, and expected outcomes for both operative and nonoperative management were reviewed with the patient. Using a shared-decision making process, she elected to proceed with surgical management.

The patient was taken to the operating room for an ORIF procedure using the PH Cage. The patient was positioned in a modified beach chair setup using a shoulder specific table and articulated arm holder for the procedure. C-arm fluoroscopy was positioned "over the top" of the patient to allow for both AP and lateral views using internal/external rotation of the arm during the procedure. An extended deltopectoral incision was used to expose the fracture. The axillary nerve was identified inferiorly and laterally as it wrapped around the humerus close to the fracture site. Since the fracture was well healed, a surgical osteotomy was required for mobilization and reduction of the fracture. A reduction jig, which resembles the contours of a locking plate, was used for initial fracture fixation. The reduction jig comes attached with an optional plate, which may be

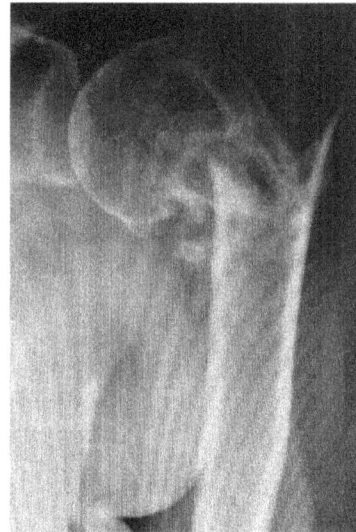

FIGURE 1: Preoperative radiograph depicting a two-part fracture of the proximal humerus. Note the varus malalignment of the head and lateral bone spike.

used per surgeons' discretion. Kirschner wires were used in conjunction with the reduction jig to obtain and maintain provisional reduction and fixation of the fracture. An 8 mm hole was drilled over a guide wire from the distal end of the reduction jig to approximately 5 mm below the articular surface of the head. The metaphyseal area below the head was then prepared using a tool specifically designed to break down the intramedullary cancellous bone without disrupting the subcortical bone. The PH Cage was then inserted in a retrograde manner, deployed, expanded, and then locked in position. The PH Cage is available in three different sizes: small, medium, and large. For this patient, a medium PH Cage was indicated.

The distal end of the PH Cage was locked to the plate using two 28 mm screws. At the proximal end, three screws were used to secure the fracture fragments to the PH Cage and the plate construct. One of these screws was a kickstand screw across the fracture line that was stabilized by the plate and the PH Cage on either side of the fracture. One additional screw was added outside of the plate to secure the greater tuberosity to the PH Cage construct. A titanium washer was added to that screw to buttress the screw head as well as to augment fixation of the rotator cuff. Intraop fluoroscopy confirmed adequate reduction and hardware position. The entire construct moved well as a unit under direct visualization and fluoroscopic control.

Postoperatively, the patient was immobilized in a sling for 6 weeks. She was started on pendulum/Codman exercises on POD1 and formal physical therapy involving gentle passive motion at week 1. The rehab protocol was advanced to active motion after 6 weeks and strengthening after 12 weeks. There were no intraoperative or postoperative complications. Her most recent follow-up X-rays obtained at 6 months after operation revealed a well healed fracture with anatomical alignment and no hardware complications or AVN (Figure 2). The PH Cage maintained the head and the screws in position,

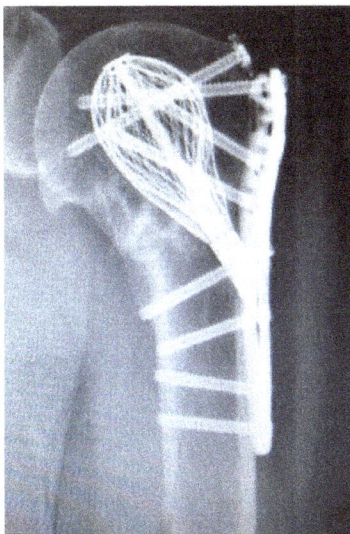

FIGURE 2: Radiograph at 6-month follow-up after fixation using a PH Cage and side plate construct.

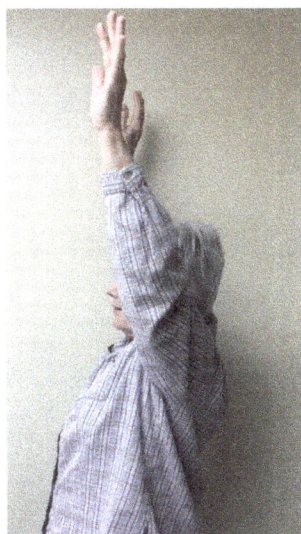

FIGURE 3: Patient exhibiting excellent range of motion at 6-month postop follow-up.

thus preventing varus collapse or intraarticular screw penetration. The patient exhibited excellent range of motion, strength, and function. She had no significant pain at last follow-up (Figure 3).

3. Discussion

Locking plate technologies are preferentially used for surgical fixation of proximal humeral fractures but the associated complication rates can be unacceptably high. Clinical studies have shown complication rates as high as 50% following PH fracture fixation using locking plates [5] and other IM devices. Many of these complications require reintervention to address either the soft tissue or implant-related issues. The primary implant-related complications reported for locking

plates are screw perforation of the humeral head and varus collapse of the fracture [6]. As locking plates have evolved, some of these complications have been addressed but there are inherent limitations in supporting varus fracture patterns using plates positioned on the lateral side of the humerus. Buttressing the medial column is key and it has been shown to be effective in providing biomechanical stability to a fracture, thus decreasing clinical complications associated with varus collapse [9]. As such the use of fibular strut allografts have been used as a potential solution to buttress the medial column, preventing varus collapse of the fracture [8]. Use of allograft struts, however, requires significant surgical dissection and potential disruption to important vascular support for fracture fragments and the inherent risks of graft failure, rejection, and disease transmission.

The PH Cage is a new technology that is able to fill the metaphyseal void created by the fracture, providing direct load bearing support below the articular surface of the humeral head. It also buttresses and supports the medial column, thus increasing the biomechanical stability of the fracture post fixation, without the need for allograft struts. The cage design also allows for unconstrained positioning of screws for tuberosity fixation. In this case, we used a standard deltopectoral surgical approach to reduce and fix the fracture using the PH Cage. The technique described is consistent with recent literature supporting the use of the PH Cage for fracture fixation [10]. The three-dimensional construct provides discretion in the number of and direction of screws used to fix the fracture fragments onto the PH Cage. In this particular case, the greater tuberosity screw was used outside the plate and the fragment was directly secured to the PH Cage construct. The design of the PH Cage locks the screw in place much like a locking plate would without limitations on the number and angle of screws.

This is a retrospective case review of one difficult proximal humerus fracture malunion that went on to anatomic healing and an excellent patient-reported outcome. The PH Cage has been used in multiple proximal humeral fracture types and settings. We are currently performing a prospective study evaluating the radiographic and clinical outcome of the PH Cage technology in comparison to existing technologies for the treatment of proximal humeral fractures.

Disclosure

The author is a paid consultant to Conventus Orthopaedics. However, no benefits have been or will be received for the subject of this article.

Competing Interests

The author declares that they have no competing interests.

References

[1] T. Lind, K. Krøner, and J. Jensen, "The epidemiology of fractures of the proximal humerus," Archives of Orthopaedic and Trauma Surgery, vol. 108, no. 5, pp. 285–287, 1989.

[2] B. Hanson, P. Neidenbach, P. de Boer, and D. Stengel, "Functional outcomes after nonoperative management of fractures of

the proximal humerus," *Journal of Shoulder and Elbow Surgery*, vol. 18, no. 4, pp. 612–621, 2009.

[3] S. Rasmussen, I. Hvass, J. Dalsgaard, B. S. Christensen, and E. Holstad, "Displaced proximal humeral fractures: results of conservative treatment," *Injury*, vol. 23, no. 1, pp. 41–43, 1992.

[4] P. Olerud, L. Ahrengart, S. Ponzer, J. Saving, and J. Tidermark, "Internal fixation versus nonoperative treatment of displaced 3-part proximal humeral fractures in elderly patients: a randomized controlled trial," *Journal of Shoulder and Elbow Surgery*, vol. 20, no. 5, pp. 747–755, 2011.

[5] R. C. Sproul, J. J. Iyengar, Z. Devcic, and B. T. Feeley, "A systematic review of locking plate fixation of proximal humerus fractures," *Injury*, vol. 42, no. 4, pp. 408–413, 2011.

[6] L. Vachtsevanos, L. Hayden, A. S. Desai, and A. Dramis, "Management of proximal humerus fractures in adults," *World Journal of Orthopaedics*, vol. 5, no. 5, pp. 685–693, 2014.

[7] R. Hertel, "Fractures of the proximal humerus in osteoporotic bone," *Osteoporosis International*, vol. 16, no. 2, pp. S65–S72, 2005.

[8] A. S. Neviaser, C. M. Hettrich, B. S. Beamer, J. S. Dines, and D. G. Lorich, "Endosteal strut augment reduces complications associated with proximal humeral locking plates," *Clinical Orthopaedics and Related Research*, vol. 469, no. 12, pp. 3300–3306, 2011.

[9] W.-B. Jung, E.-S. Moon, S.-K. Kim, D. Kovacevic, and M.-S. Kim, "Does medial support decrease major complications of unstable proximal humerus fractures treated with locking plate?" *BMC Musculoskeletal Disorders*, vol. 14, article 102, pp. 1–11, 2013.

[10] P. D. Paterson, E. W. Fulkerson, and A. K. Palmer, "Techniques for using a novel intramedullary cage technology for fixation of proximal humeral fractures," *Journal of Exercise, Sports & Orthopedics,*, vol. 3, no. 2, pp. 1–6, 2016.

23

A Delayed Postoperative C5 Palsy due to Spinal Cord Lesion: A Typical Clinical Presentation but Unusual Imaging Findings

Nobuaki Tadokoro, Yusuke Kasai, Katsuhito Kiyasu, Motohiro Kawasaki, Ryuichi Takemasa, and Masahiko Ikeuchi

Department of Orthopaedic Surgery, Kochi Medical School, Kochi University, Kochi, Japan

Correspondence should be addressed to Nobuaki Tadokoro; nobuaki.tadokoro@gmail.com

Academic Editor: Ali F. Ozer

Postoperative C5 palsy (C5 palsy) is a troublesome complication after cervical spine surgery and its etiology is still unclear. We experienced a case of C5 palsy after anterior decompression with fusion for cervical ossification of posterior longitudinal ligament with the typical clinical presentation of left deltoid and bicep weakness and left-arm pain without deterioration of myelopathy symptoms, albeit with the unusual imaging findings not shown preoperatively of a swelling in the spinal cord, and intramedullary high intensity change on T2-weighed MRI. The additional posterior surgery was carried out to decompress the swollen spinal cord. The abnormal findings disappear on MRI taken three weeks following the second surgery and the weakness improved fully within three months after the second surgery. This case report highlights the possibility of spinal cord lesion due to circulatory impairment as a cause of C5 palsy.

1. Introduction

Postoperative C5 palsy (C5 palsy) is defined as the deltoid/bicep muscle weakness without any deterioration of myelopathy symptoms after cervical spine surgery [1], which often appear several days after surgery. Although the nerve root tethering produced by spinal cord shifting after spinal cord decompressive surgery is now becoming a leading hypothesis [2–4], the cause of C5 palsy is still controversial and the spinal cord lesion is also hypothesized as the probable mechanism [5, 6].

We report a unilateral C5 palsy case, in which perioperative imaging studies provide evidence of spinal cord lesion.

2. Case Presentation

A 70-year-old female patient with cervical myelopathy presented at and was admitted to our hospital with aggravated quadriplegia due to ossification of posterior longitudinal ligament (OPLL). Her OPLL was mixed type from C2 vertebral body (VB) level down to C6 VB level, discontinuation at C3/4 with most cord compression, OPLL spinal canal occupancy ratio of 50%, and no C4/5 foraminal stenosis observed (Figure 1). Her clinical score, or cervical myelopathy Japanese Orthopaedic Association (JOA) score, was 9.5/17. There was no weakness of the deltoid and bicep muscles prior to surgery.

She underwent selective anterior cervical corpectomy of C4 and fusion with autoiliac bone grafting with plate fixation uneventfully. The intraoperative monitoring using transcranial electrical motor-evoked potentials with extremity muscle recordings including the deltoid and bicep muscles (MEP) and somatosensory-evoked potentials (SEP) showed no worsening of evoked potentials. Immediately after surgery, she experienced a favorable recovery of numbness in the extremities and no muscle weakness was observed.

The left deltoid and bicep weakness of manual muscle testing (MMT) 1~2 and left-arm pain occurred on the second postoperative day, though her symptoms such as walk disturbance, difficulty of hand dexterity, and numbness of extremities maintained postoperative improvement after the onset of left-arm symptoms. Imaging studies on the same day of left-arm symptoms onset demonstrated T2 high intramedullary signal change and spinal cord enlargement from C2 VB level

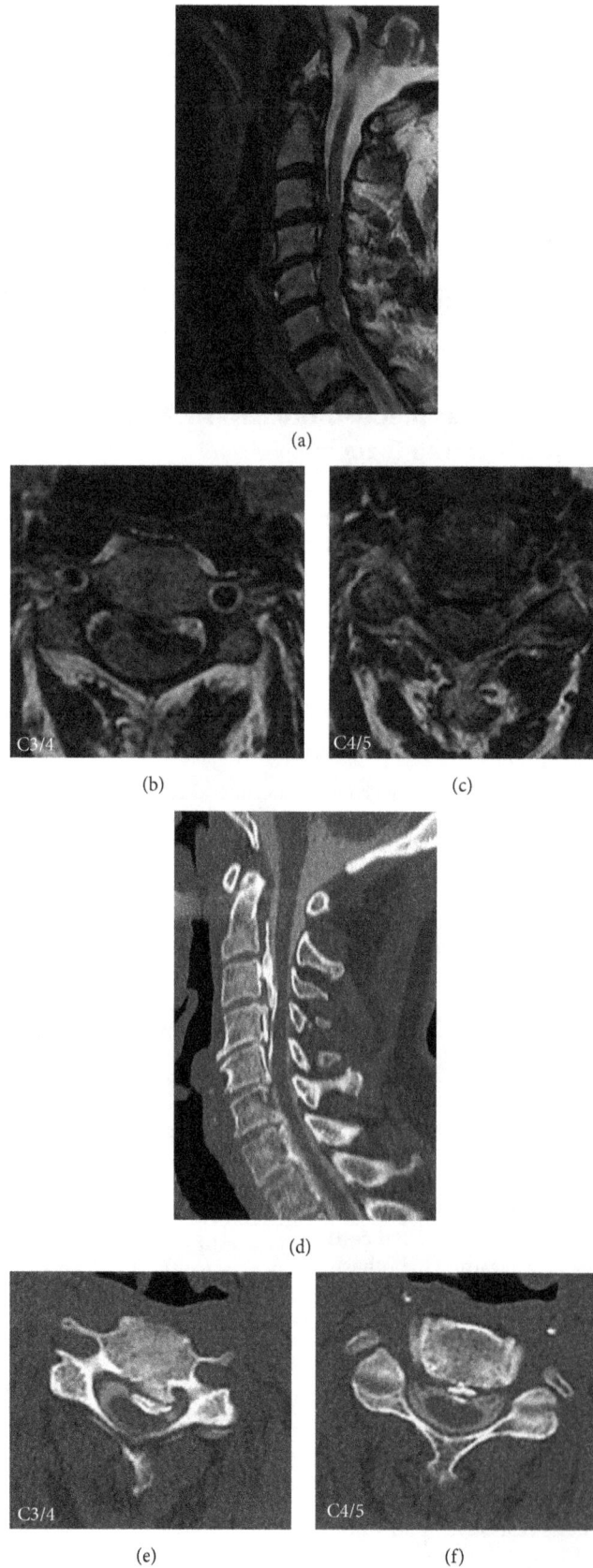

FIGURE 1: Preoperative images. Preoperative MRI (a, b, and c) and CT myelogram (d, e, and f) showed mixed-type OPLL compressing spinal cord, especially at C3-4 (OPLL canal occupying ratio: 50%). MRI showed no obvious cord signal change and cord enlargement (a, b, and c). The anterior-posterior diameters of right and left C4/5 foramen were 3.8 mm and 3.5 mm, respectively (f).

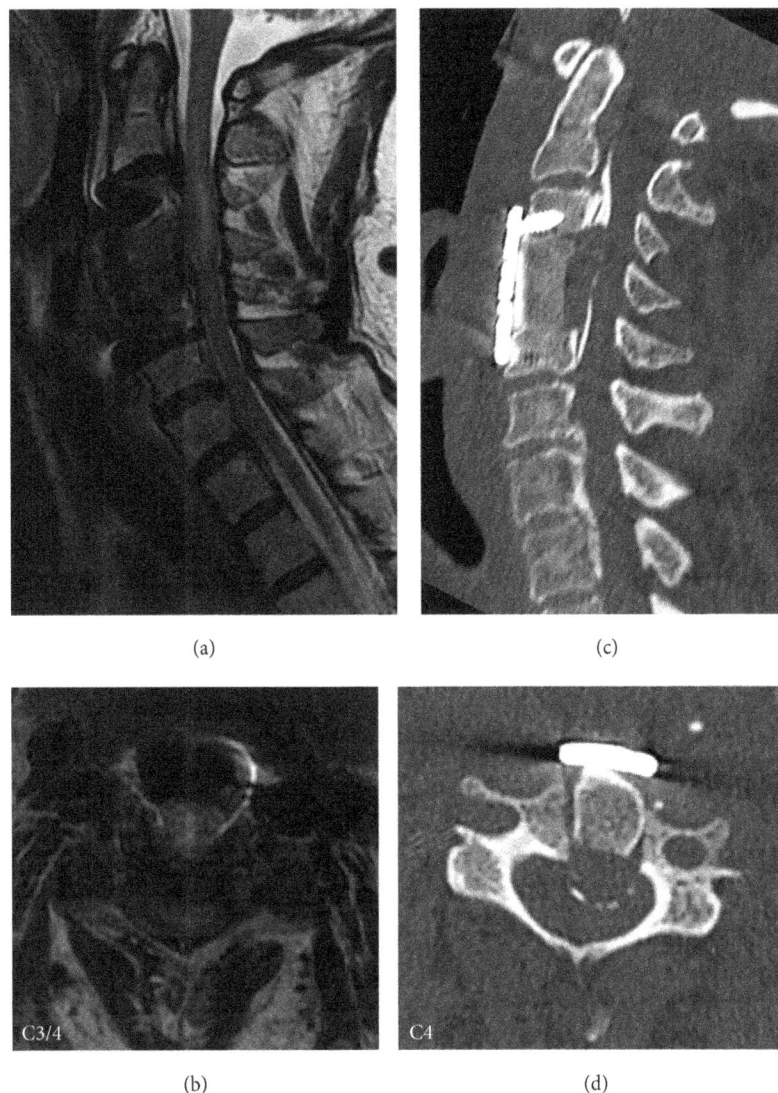

(a)   (c)

(b)   (d)

FIGURE 2: MRI and CT images taken at onset of C5 palsy. MRI (a, b) and CT imaging (c, d) obtained immediately after onset of C5 palsy showed the intramedullary T2 high signal change and spinal cord enlargement from C2 vertebral body level to C4 vertebral body level (a, b) without any graft dislodgement or implant malposition (c, d).

down to C4 VB level not evident prior to surgery on cervical MRI and no graft and implant malposition on CT images (Figure 2). Brain lesion was also ruled out by MRI and CT images. We diagnosed the patient with C5 palsy.

Although left-arm pain disappeared soon after administration of pregabalin, weakness of the deltoid and bicep muscles and T2 high intramedullary signal change and spinal cord enlargement remained unchanged. We recommended the additional C3–6 open-door laminoplasty with left C4/5 foraminotomy to this patient to decompress the spinal cord and left C5 root. She agreed to undergo a second round of surgery, which was performed ten days after the initial surgery. The C4/5 foraminal stenosis was not observed intraoperatively. The left deltoid and bicep muscles demonstrated reduced amplitude throughout the second round of surgery and the amplitude and latency of the rest of the muscles in MEP and SEP were the same compared with the first round of surgery in the intraoperative spinal cord monitoring

(Figure 3). T2 high intramedullary signal change disappeared on MRI taken three weeks after the second round of surgery (Figure 4). Her weakness started to recover after the second round of surgery and had recovered fully three months later. Her JOA score at the time of C5 palsy full recovery was 13.5/17 (recovery rate: 53.3%).

3. Discussion

Imaging studies after C5 palsy rarely demonstrate obvious spinal cord lesion or nerve root lesion; however, T2 high intramedullary signal change and spinal cord enlargement occurred after the onset of C5 palsy in this patient, which suggests spinal cord edema due to the impairment of circulation and is clear evidence of spinal cord lesion.

The fact that the spinal cord lesion caused only the selective unilateral C5 palsy was unclear; the longitudinal spinal cord lesion including the C5 motor segment after the first

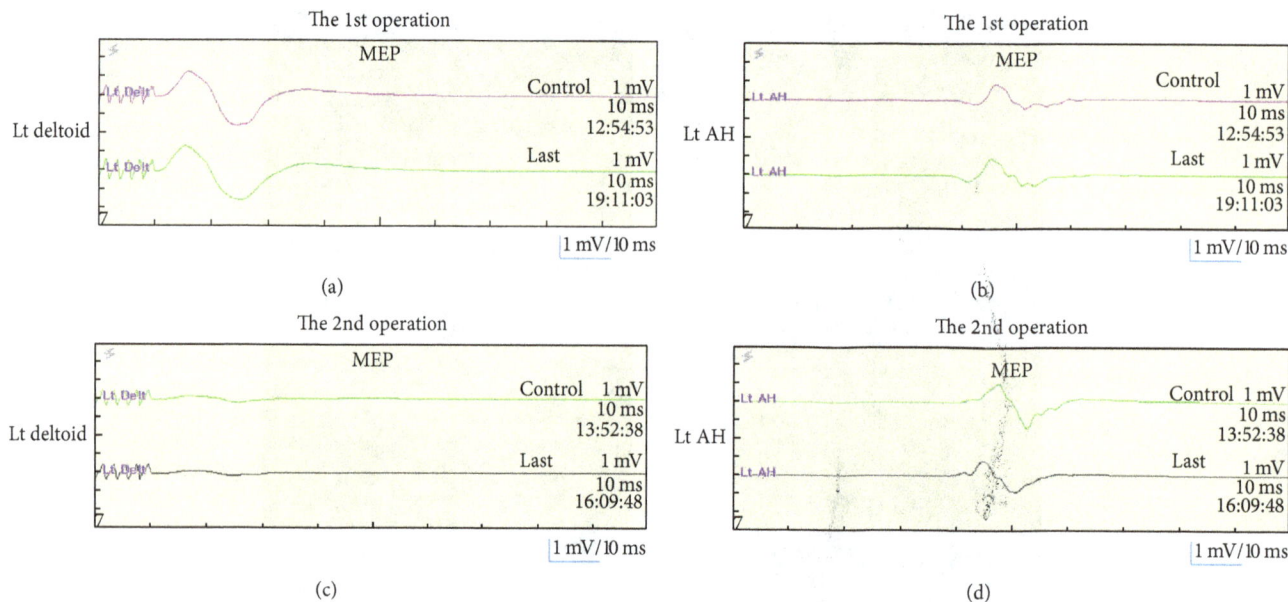

(a)

(b)

(c)

(d)

FIGURE 3: Intraoperative spinal cord monitoring. Although there was no worsening of left deltoid and left AH CMAPs during the 1st (a, b) and the 2nd (c, d), each operation was observed and low amplitude of left deltoid (c) and preserved amplitude of left AH CMAPs (d) in the 2nd operation compared to the 1st operation (a, b) were recorded, which means segmental C5 palsy occurred after the postoperative period of the 1st operation.

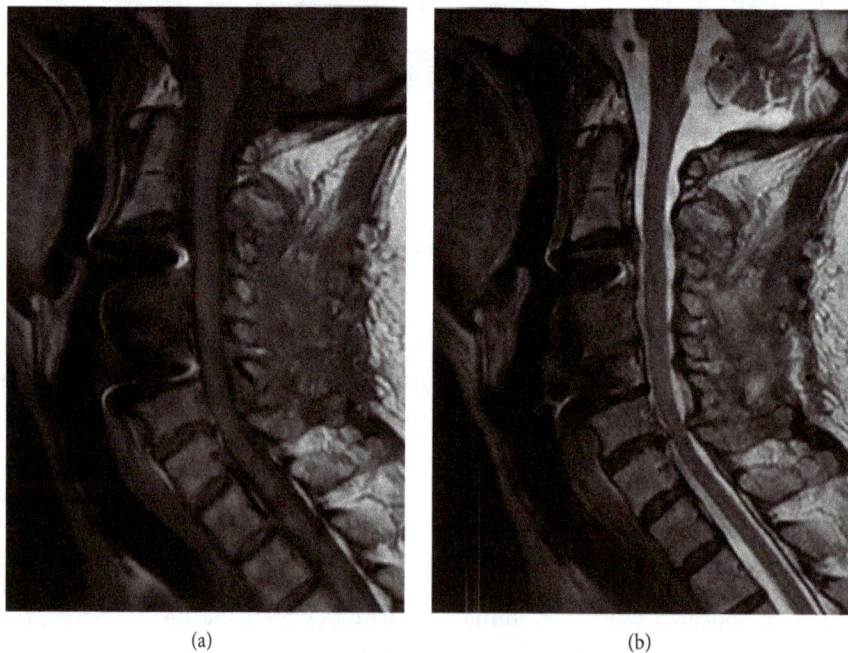

(a)

(b)

FIGURE 4: MRI taken three weeks after the second round of surgery. The spinal cord enlargement and intramedullary high intensity change disappear on T1 (a) and T2 (b) weighed MRI.

surgery and the left-oriented OPLL could partly explain that due to the ischemia-reperfusion injury [7]. Even though the reperfusion cord injury after spinal cord decompression might be excluded because of the residual cord compression induced by the cranial OPLL, the circulatory aspect of neural damage could be assumed by the intramedullary signal change and cord enlargement after C5 palsy onset and the early resolution after the second round of surgery.

In regard to the C4/5 foraminal stenosis, the mean diameters of C4/5 foramen with C5 palsy were reported below 2.7 mm [2–4]; however, that of this patient was 3.5 mm. No left C4/5 foraminal stenosis in the intraoperative findings also supports the spinal cord lesion responsible for C5 palsy.

The intraoperative spinal cord monitoring showed no worsening during the first round of surgery, which meant no intraoperative neurological damage. The deltoid and biceps muscle amplitude reduction, albeit the other MEP and SEP preservation, in the second round of surgery corresponds to the clinical picture of delayed-onset segmental C5 palsy without pyramidal and sensory tract injury.

The prognosis of C5 palsy with conservative treatment is generally good [8] but sometimes poor [9]. The possibility of symptom aggravation due to cord swelling could not excluded completely and the effect of this atypical imaging findings for the functional recovery was not clear. So, we performed the additional decompressive surgery for cord swelling and possible C5 root lesion, though not evident in imaging studies, which possibly affected her clinical course beneficially from the postoperative early resolution of cord abnormalities and good recovery of weakness.

4. Conclusion

We reported a case of a unilateral delayed segmental C5 palsy after anterior cervical decompression (corpectomy) with fusion. The clinical picture was typical for C5 palsy, but MRI showed clear evidence of spinal cord lesion possibly due to circulatory impairment. We recommend MRI investigation at the onset of postoperative neurological complications to examine the pathology in detail.

Competing Interests

The authors declare that there is no conflict of interests regarding the publication of this paper.

References

[1] H. Sakaura, N. Hosono, Y. Mukai, T. Ishii, and H. Yoshikawa, "C5 palsy after decompression surgery for cervical myelopathy: review of the literature," *Spine*, vol. 28, no. 21, pp. 2447–2451, 2003.

[2] S. Odate, J. Shikata, S. Yamamura, and T. Soeda, "Extremely wide and asymmetric anterior decompression causes postoperative C5 palsy: an analysis of 32 patients with postoperative C5 palsy after anterior cervical decompression and fusion," *Spine*, vol. 38, no. 25, pp. 2184–2189, 2013.

[3] K. Katsumi, A. Yamazaki, K. Watanabe, M. Ohashi, and H. Shoji, "Analysis of C5 palsy after cervical open-door laminoplasty: relationship between C5 palsy and foraminal stenosis," *Journal of Spinal Disorders & Techniques*, vol. 26, no. 4, pp. 177–182, 2013.

[4] S. Imagama, Y. Matsuyama, Y. Yukawa et al., "C5 palsy after cervical laminoplasty: a multicentre study," *The Journal of Bone and Joint Surgery B*, vol. 92, no. 3, pp. 393–400, 2010.

[5] K. Chiba, Y. Toyama, M. Matsumoto, H. Maruiwa, M. Watanabe, and K. Hirabayashi, "Segmental motor paralysis after expansive open-door laminoplasty," *Spine*, vol. 27, no. 19, pp. 2108–2115, 2002.

[6] K. Hasegawa, T. Homma, and Y. Chiba, "Upper extremity palsy following cervical decompression surgery results from a transient spinal cord lesion," *Spine*, vol. 32, no. 6, pp. E197–E202, 2007.

[7] S. K. Karadimas, A. M. Laliberte, L. Tetreault et al., "Riluzole blocks perioperative ischemia-reperfusion injury and enhances postdecompression outcomes in cervical spondylotic myelopathy," *Science Translational Medicine*, vol. 7, no. 316, article 6524, 2015.

[8] J. Z. Guzman, E. O. Baird, A. C. Fields et al., "C5 nerve root palsy following decompression of the cervical spine: a systematic evaluation of the literature," *The Bone & Joint Journal*, vol. 96, no. 7, pp. 950–955, 2014.

[9] C. Lim, S. Roh, S. Rhim, and S. Jeon, "Clinical analysis of C5 palsy after cervical decompression surgery: relationship between recovery duration and clinical and radiological factors," *European Spine Journal*, pp. 1–10, 2016.

24

Total Hip Arthroplasty for Implant Rupture after Surgery for Atypical Subtrochanteric Femoral Fracture

Yu Ozaki, Tomonori Baba, Hironori Ochi, Yasuhiro Homma, Taiji Watari, Mikio Matsumoto, and Kazuo Kaneko

Department of Orthopedic Surgery, Juntendo University School of Medicine, 2-1-1 Hongo, Bunkyo-ku, Tokyo, Japan

Correspondence should be addressed to Tomonori Baba; tobaba@juntendo.ac.jp

Academic Editor: Stamatios A. Papadakis

Treatment methods for delayed union and nonunion of atypical femoral fracture are still controversial. Moreover, no treatment method has been established for implant rupture caused by delayed union and nonunion. We encountered a 74-year-old female in whom nonunion-induced implant rupture occurred after treatment of atypical subtrochanteric femoral fracture with internal fixation using a long femoral nail. It was unlikely that sufficient fixation could be obtained by repeating osteosynthesis alone. Moreover, the patient was elderly and early weight-bearing activity was essential for early recovery of ADL. Based on these reasons, we selected one-stage surgery with total hip arthroplasty and osteosynthesis with inverted condylar locking plate as salvage procedures. Bone union was achieved at 6 months after surgery. This case illustrated that osteosynthesis-combined one-staged total hip arthroplasty could be considered as one of the options for nonunion-induced implant rupture of atypical femoral subtrochanteric fracture.

1. Introduction

Reportedly, delayed union and nonunion are likely to occur after treatment of atypical femoral fracture compared with those after normal fracture [1, 2]. However, treatment methods for delayed union and nonunion of atypical femoral fracture are still controversial. Moreover, no treatment method has been established for implant rupture caused by delayed union and nonunion [2, 3]. We encountered a patient in whom implant rupture occurred after treatment of atypical subtrochanteric femoral fracture with internal fixation using a long femoral nail. We treated this patient with invasive osteosynthesis-combined one-stage total hip arthroplasty.

2. Case Report

A 74-year-old female had a past medical history of Adult Still's disease and she had been treated with steroids for 23 years at the Department of Collagen Disease. Treatment of osteoporosis with bisphosphonates was initiated 4 years ago and the drug was switched to denosumab 1 year ago. She felt pain in the left femoral region 3 months before injury and underwent plain radiography. Breaking and a slightly radiolucent line were observed in the lateral subtrochanteric femoral cortex, and she was diagnosed with atypical incomplete subtrochanteric femoral fracture (Figure 1(a)). Then we measured bone turnover markers. Bone resorption and bone formation markers were suppressed (TRAP5b: 154 mU/dL, BAP: 11.2 μg/L, and PINP: 11.2 ng/mL), and serum levels of calcium (9.2 mg/dL) and phosphate (3.2 mg/dL) and the concentration of intact parathyroid hormone (65 pg/mL) were normal. Conservative treatment was planned, the drug was changed from denosumab to teriparatide, and she started walking with 2 crutches. There was a reduction in pain, but she fell and was unable to move her body, so she was transported to our hospital by ambulance. On plain radiography, transverse fracture accompanied by a spike was noted on the medial side. Atypical subtrochanteric femoral complete fracture was diagnosed (Figure 1(b)), and invasive osteosynthesis with a long femoral nail (Gamma3 long nail, Stryker) was performed (Figure 1(c)). Full weight-bearing exercise was applied as much as possible in treatment following surgery. Gait with a T-shape cane became stable and the patient was discharged 1 month after surgery. However, left thigh pain

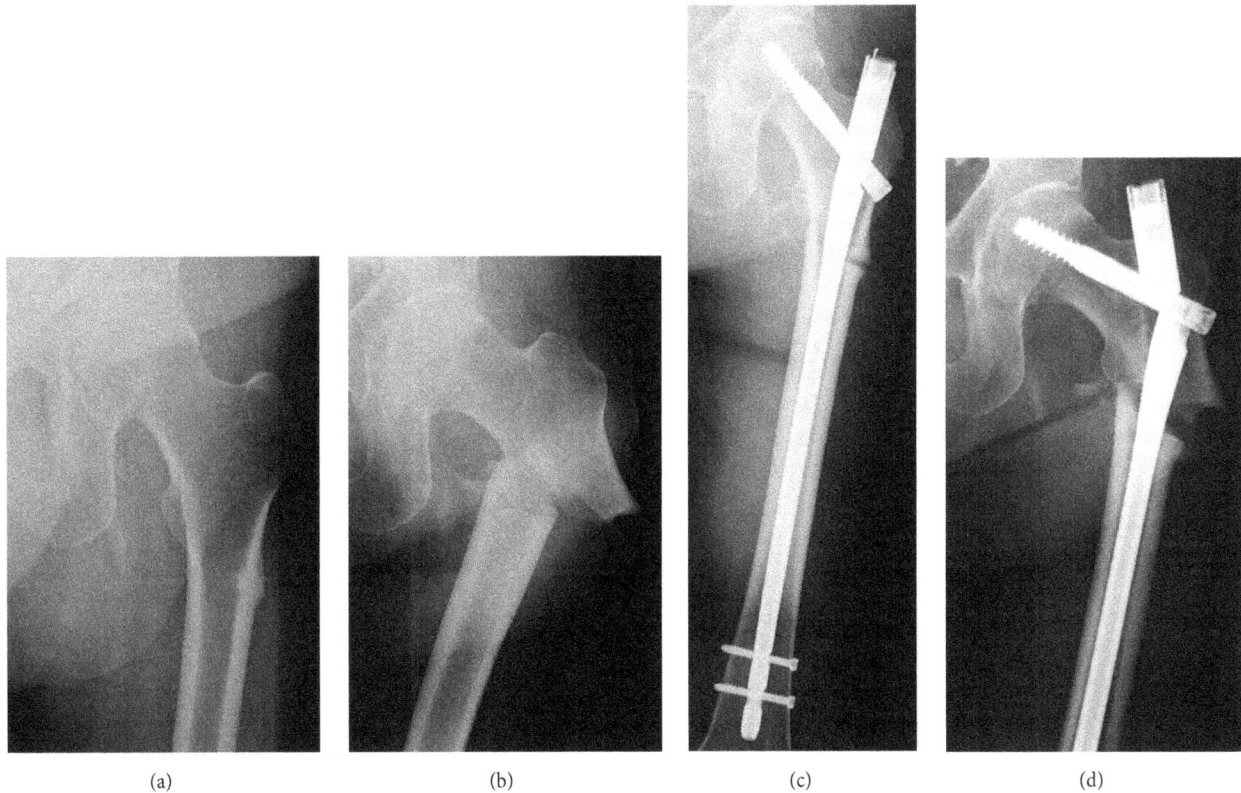

(a)   (b)   (c)   (d)

FIGURE 1: (a) An AP radiograph of the left femur shows a transverse fracture line and thickening of the lateral cortex at the subtrochanteric area. (b) A completely displaced fracture. (c) The internal fixation using a long femoral nail. (d) The nail breakage and opening of the fracture region.

appeared again 2 months after surgery, and nail breakage and opening of the fracture region due to delayed union were observed on plain radiography (Figure 1(d)). In reoperation, the implant was removed, and total hip arthroplasty through the posterior approach was performed. For the acetabular component, a dual mobility cup (MDM X3, Stryker) was used. For the femoral side, a distal fixation-type long stem (Restoration HA, Stryker) was used. As a modification of the surgery, varus of the proximal bone fragment was prevented using the Blocking Pin Technique (φ2.4 mm Kirschner wires) (Figures 2(a) and 2(b)) [4], and the stem was placed in the optimal position. The resected autologous femoral head was trimmed and transplanted into the bone defect formed between the screw insertion region and nonunion region. To fix the nonunion region, a condylar locking plate (LCP-DF, Synthes) for the opposite side was inverted and used, and osteosynthesis was also applied (Figure 2(c)). Low-Intensity Pulsed Ultrasound (LIPUS) treatment was initiated immediately after surgery. At the same time, administration of a PTH preparation was initiated. Weight-bearing exercise was initiated one week after surgery as treatment following surgery. She became able to walk with a cane 2 months after surgery and was discharged. Callus formation was observed 5 months after surgery and bone union was achieved at 6 months. Although radiolucent line at the lateral femoral cortex can still be seen, there was the callus formation in the three directions except for the lateral cortex (Figures 2(d) and 2(e)).

As of 2 years after surgery, there has been no problem with the implant (total hip arthroplasty and materials of osteosynthesis), and the patient's physical activity level returned to that before injury.

3. Discussion

In subtrochanteric femoral fracture, abduction, bending, and external rotation of the proximal bone fragment occur and adduction and shortening of the distal bone fragment occur due to strong muscles attaching to the region around the hip joint. Additionally, acquisition and retention of a favorable reduction position are difficult. Moreover, weight-bearing loads apply tension to the lateral bone cortex and pressure to the medial bone cortex in this region, resulting in a large load of stress concentration applied on the implant [5]. In addition to deterioration of bone quality, an influence of microdamage accumulation, due to remodeling failure, in atypical femoral fracture has been observed [6, 7]. When injury reaches complete fracture, many complications occur even if it is surgically treated, and the risk of delayed union/nonunion and accompanying implant rupture is high [1]. Atypical subtrochanteric femoral fracture is difficult to treat because it has properties of both subtrochanteric femoral fracture, which is biomechanically disadvantageous for bone union, and atypical femoral fracture, which is biologically disadvantageous.

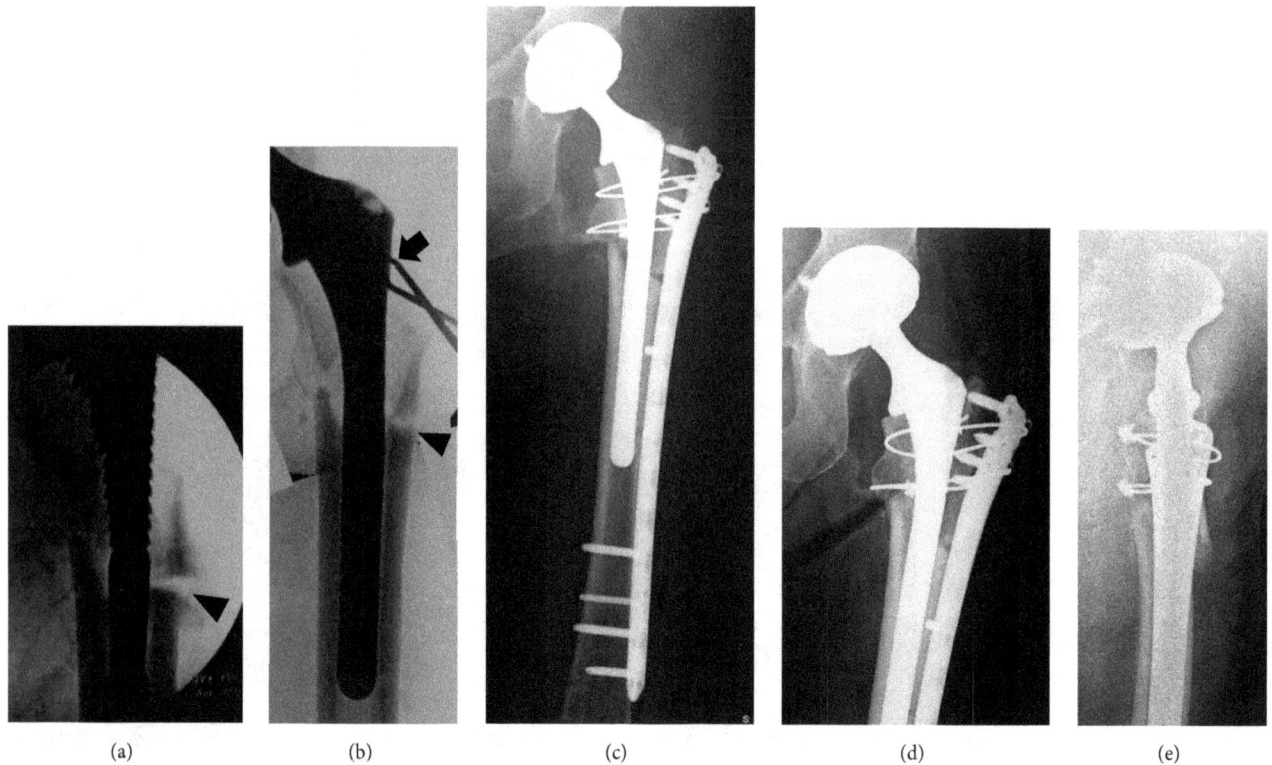

| | | | | |
| (a) | (b) | (c) | (d) | (e) |

FIGURE 2: (a) A trial broach with the optimum size was inserted, but reduction was not enough (arrowhead). (b) Varus of the proximal bone fragment was prevented using the Blocking Pin Technique (arrow), and the stem was placed in the optimal position (arrowhead). (c) The osteosynthesis-combined one-staged total hip arthroplasty. (d) AP and lateral views on radiograph obtained after second surgery six months show complete union of the fracture.

In this patient, conservative treatment was selected when incomplete atypical subtrochanteric femoral fracture was diagnosed, but poor prognosis of conservatively treated incomplete fracture has been occasionally reported [8, 9]. Considering the difficulty of surgery for complete atypical subtrochanteric femoral fracture, preventive internal fixation is recommended when incomplete fracture is diagnosed [8–10]. We recognized that surgery, not conservative treatment, should be indicated even though the fracture is incomplete when precursor pain is observed and a radiolucent line is observed in addition to breaking [6, 7, 11, 12].

There is room for discussion about whether osteosynthesis should be reapplied or an arthroplasty should be used for salvage procedures of nonunion-induced implant rupture. To our knowledge, no report recommended one-stage surgery with an arthroplasty. In the present patient, a radiolucent line extended widely from the nail breakage region to the lag screw insertion region, and exchange of the intramedullary nail was likely to be insufficient for initial fixation. In addition, poor outcomes of fixation of atypical femoral fracture with a plate alone have occasionally been reported [1, 13]. Thus, it was unlikely that sufficient fixation could be obtained by repeating osteosynthesis alone. Moreover, the patient was elderly and early weight-bearing activity was essential for early recovery of ADL. Based on these reasons, we selected the combination of total hip arthroplasty and osteosynthesis

as salvage procedures. The stem selected for the femoral side was a distal fixation-type long stem with an extensive porous coating so that a bypass is formed across the fracture region, aimed at early weight-bearing activity [14]. For the acetabular component, considering that the surgery was a reoperation in an elderly patient, the dual mobility cup was used to prevent dislocation [15]. To strongly fix the fracture region, condylar LCP was inverted and used for internal fixation because many screws can be inserted into the proximal bone fragment using this plate [16, 17]. Bone transplantation as salvage surgery for atypical fractures is reported to be effective, and we also collected cancellous bone from the excised femoral head and transplanted it to the bone defect region [2]. Promotion of fracture healing by PTH preparation alone or in combination with LIPUS in atypical femoral fracture has been reported, so we adopted it [18–20].

Ethical Approval

The study was carried out in accordance with the Declaration of Helsinki and the appropriate ethical framework

Consent

Written informed consent was obtained from the patient for publication of this case report and any accompanying images.

Competing Interests

The authors declare that they have no competing interests.

References

[1] M. L. Prasarn, J. Ahn, D. L. Helfet, J. M. Lane, and D. G. Lorich, "Bisphosphonate-associated femur fractures have high complication rates with operative fixation trauma," *Clinical Orthopaedics and Related Research*, vol. 470, no. 8, pp. 2295–2301, 2012.

[2] B. J. X. Teo, J. S. B. Koh, S. K. Goh, M. A. Png, D. T. C. Chua, and T. S. Howe, "Post-operative outcomes of atypical femoral subtrochanteric fracture in patients on bisphosphonate therapy," *The Bone & Joint Journal*, vol. 96, no. 5, pp. 658–664, 2014.

[3] B. J. O'Neill, S. O'hEireamhoin, D. I. Morrissey, and P. Keogh, "Implant failure caused by non-union of bisphosphonate-associated subtrochanteric femur fracture," *BMJ Case Reports*, vol. 2014, 2014.

[4] I. Tonogai, D. Hamada, T. Goto et al., "Retrograde intramedullary nailing with a blocking pin technique for reduction of periprosthetic supracondylar femoral fracture after total knee arthroplasty: technical note with a compatibility chart of the nail to femoral component," *Case Reports in Orthopedics*, vol. 2014, Article ID 856853, 5 pages, 2014.

[5] D. J. Hak, H. Wu, C. Dou, C. Mauffrey, and P. F. Stahel, "Challenges in subtrochanteric femur fracture management," *Orthopedics*, vol. 38, no. 8, pp. 498–502, 2015.

[6] E. Shane, D. Burr, B. Abrahamsen et al., "Atypical subtrochanteric and diaphyseal femoral fractures: second report of a task force of the American society for bone and mineral research," *Journal of Bone and Mineral Research*, vol. 29, no. 1, pp. 1–23, 2014.

[7] J. Schilcher, O. Sandberg, H. Isaksson, and P. Aspenberg, "Histology of 8 atypical femoral fractures: remodeling but no healing," *Acta Orthopaedica*, vol. 85, no. 3, pp. 280–286, 2014.

[8] M. B. Banffy, M. S. Vrahas, J. E. Ready, and J. A. Abraham, "Non-operative versus prophylactic treatment of bisphosphonate-associated femoral stress fractures," *Clinical Orthopaedics and Related Research*, vol. 469, no. 7, pp. 2028–2034, 2011.

[9] C.-W. Oh, J.-K. Oh, K.-C. Park, J.-W. Kim, and Y.-C. Yoon, "Prophylactic nailing of incomplete atypical femoral fractures," *The Scientific World Journal*, vol. 2013, Article ID 450148, 4 pages, 2013.

[10] Y.-C. Ha, M.-R. Cho, K. H. Park, S.-Y. Kim, and K.-H. Koo, "Is surgery necessary for femoral insufficiency fractures after long-term bisphosphonate therapy?" *Clinical Orthopaedics and Related Research*, vol. 468, no. 12, pp. 3393–3398, 2010.

[11] Y.-K. Lee, Y.-C. Ha, B. J. Kang, J. S. Chang, and K.-H. Koo, "Predicting need for fixation of atypical femoral fracture," *Journal of Clinical Endocrinology and Metabolism*, vol. 98, no. 7, pp. 2742–2745, 2013.

[12] A. Saleh, V. V. Hegde, A. G. Potty, R. Schneider, C. N. Cornell, and J. M. Lane, "Management strategy for symptomatic bisphosphonate-associated incomplete atypical femoral fractures," *HSS Journal*, vol. 8, no. 2, pp. 103–110, 2012.

[13] S. De Das, T. Setiobudi, L. Shen, and S. De Das, "A rational approach to management of alendronate-related subtrochanteric fractures," *Journal of Bone and Joint Surgery—Series B*, vol. 92, no. 5, pp. 679–686, 2010.

[14] M. Angelini, M. D. McKee, J. P. Waddell, G. Haidukewych, and E. H. Schemitsch, "Salvage of failed hip fracture fixation," *Journal of Orthopaedic Trauma*, vol. 23, no. 6, pp. 471–478, 2009.

[15] A. Combes, H. Migaud, J. Girard, A. Duhamel, and M. H. Fessy, "Low rate of dislocation of dual-mobility cups in primary total hip arthroplasty," *Clinical Orthopaedics and Related Research*, vol. 471, no. 12, pp. 3891–3900, 2013.

[16] T. Baba, Y. Homma, I. Morohashi, Y. Maruyama, K. Shitoto, and K. Kaneko, "Is internal fixation using a reversed condylar locking plate useful for treating Vancouver type B1 periprosthetic femoral fractures?" *European Orthopaedics and Traumatology*, vol. 6, no. 3, pp. 137–143, 2015.

[17] T. Wakayama, Y. Saita, T. Baba, H. Nojiri, and K. Kaneko, "Pathological relationship of osteomalacia at the site of atypical periprosthetic femoral shaft fracture after typical femoral neck fracture occurred in the patient with rheumatoid arthritis: a case report," *Journal of Rheumatic Diseases and Treatment*, vol. 1, article 017, 2015.

[18] A. Unnanuntana, A. Saleh, K. A. Mensah, J. P. Kleimeyer, and J. M. Lane, "Atypical femoral fractures: what do we know about them? AAOS exhibit selection," *The Journal of Bone & Joint Surgery—American Volume*, vol. 95, no. 2, article e8, 2013.

[19] G. I. Im and S. H. Lee, "Effect of teriparatide on healing of atypical femoral fractures: a systemic review," *Journal of Bone Metabolism*, vol. 22, no. 4, pp. 183–189, 2015.

[20] S. J. Warden, D. E. Komatsu, J. Rydberg, J. L. Bond, and S. M. Hassett, "Recombinant human parathyroid hormone (PTH 1-34) and low-intensity pulsed ultrasound have contrasting additive effects during fracture healing," *Bone*, vol. 44, no. 3, pp. 485–494, 2009.

25

The Role of Dynamic Contrast-Enhanced MRI in a Child with Sport-Induced Avascular Necrosis of the Scaphoid

Baris Beytullah Koc,[1] **Martijn Schotanus,**[1] **Bob Jong,**[2] **and Pieter Tilman**[1]

[1]*Department of Orthopedic Surgery, Zuyderland Medical Centre, Dr. H. van der Hoffplein 1, 6162 BG Sittard-Geleen, Netherlands*
[2]*Department of Radiology, Zuyderland Medical Centre, Dr. H. van der Hoffplein 1, 6162 BG Sittard-Geleen, Netherlands*

Correspondence should be addressed to Baris Beytullah Koc; baris.koc1991@gmail.com

Academic Editor: Johannes Mayr

Avascular necrosis (AVN) of the scaphoid in children is very rare and there is currently no consensus when conservative or operative treatment is indicated. A 10-year-old boy, practicing karate, presented with acute pain in his left wrist after falling on the outstretched hand. Imaging showed a scaphoid waist fracture with signs of an ongoing AVN. The diagnosis of AVN was confirmed with signal loss of the scaphoid on MRI T1. A dynamic contrast-enhanced MRI was performed for further assessment of the proximal pole vascularity and treatment planning. As dynamic contrast-enhanced MRI showed fair perfusion of the proximal pole, an adequate healing potential with conservative treatment was estimated. We achieved union and good function with cast immobilization for fourteen weeks. This case study showed dynamic contrast-enhanced MRI to be a valuable tool in assessing whether conservative or operative treatment is indicated to achieve union and good functional outcome.

1. Introduction

Cases of avascular necrosis (AVN) of the scaphoid are very rare with only six cases regarding the management of AVN in children reported [1–3]. Because of the limited reports there is currently no consensus when conservative or operative treatment is indicated. We report a case of a child with sport-induced AVN of the scaphoid in whom a dynamic contrast-enhanced MRI was performed for further treatment planning. The patient and his parents were informed about this report and agreed to its publication.

2. Case Presentation

A 10-year-old boy, practicing karate since the age of six, presented with acute pain in his left wrist after falling on the outstretched hand. On physical examination, there was tenderness in the anatomical snuffbox and a painful range of motion of the wrist. Plain radiograph showed a fracture of the scaphoid waist with sclerosis, central cystic bone alteration, and deformity of the proximal pole suggesting an ongoing AVN (Figure 1(a)). Additional CT scan supported the radiographic findings with a more pronounced central cystic bone alteration and irregularity of the fracture border (Figure 1(b)). The diagnosis of AVN was confirmed with signal loss of the scaphoid on MRI T1 (Figure 1(c)). A dynamic contrast-enhanced MRI was performed for further assessment of the proximal pole vascularity and treatment planning. Therefore, a region of interest was placed on the proximal and distal scaphoid poles. Time-signal intensity curves were recorded and were considered to represent the degree of vascularity. The time-signal intensity curves are classified into good, fair, or poor vascularity based on their shape and maximal enhancement comparing proximal pole with the distal pole [4, 5]. In this study, the time-signal intensity curve on the proximal pole was lower than the distal pole with a maximum enhancement of 50%, defining fair perfusion of the proximal pole. The fair perfusion of the proximal pole on dynamic contrast-enhanced MRI was with the account of measuring associated fibroblasts in the cystic alteration in the distal pole (Figure 2). Because of fair

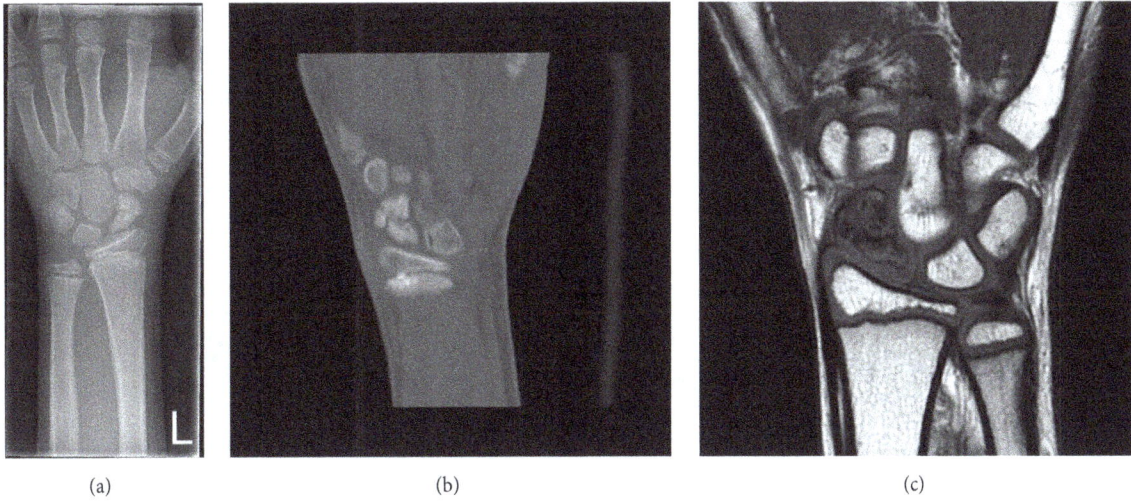

FIGURE 1: (a) Plain radiograph at acute presentation showing a fracture of the scaphoid waist with sclerosis, central cystic bone alteration, and deformity of the proximal pole. (b) CT scan 1 week after the initial injury showing a more pronounced central cystic bone alteration and irregularity of the fracture border. (c) MRI T1 showing signal loss of the whole scaphoid.

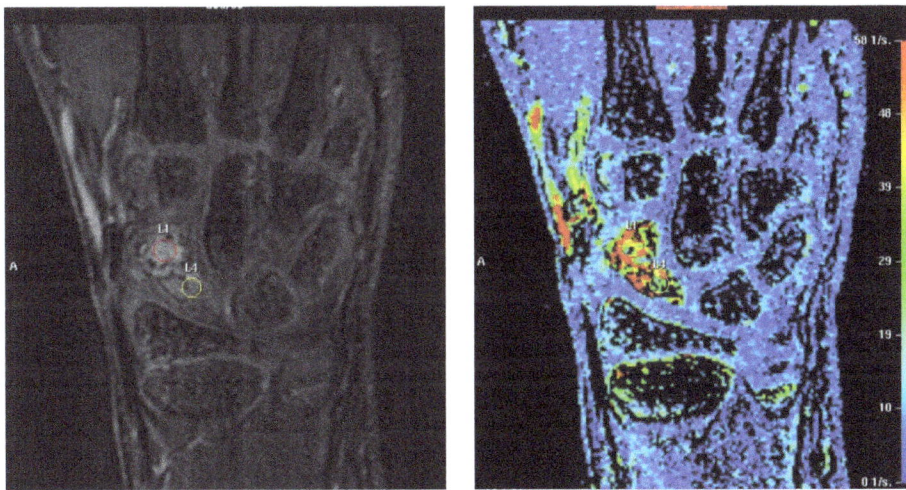

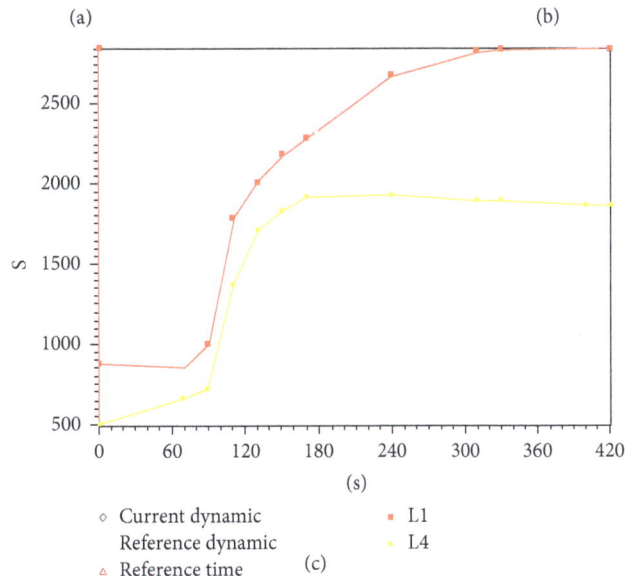

FIGURE 2: To assess the vascularity with dynamic contrast-enhanced MRI, a region of interest was placed on the proximal and distal scaphoid poles and time-signal intensity curves were recorded. The dynamic contrast-enhanced MRI showed fair perfusion of the proximal pole with account of measuring associated fibroblasts in the cystic alteration in the distal pole. The time-signal intensity curve on the proximal pole (yellow curve) was lower than the distal pole (red curve) with a maximum enhancement of 50%.

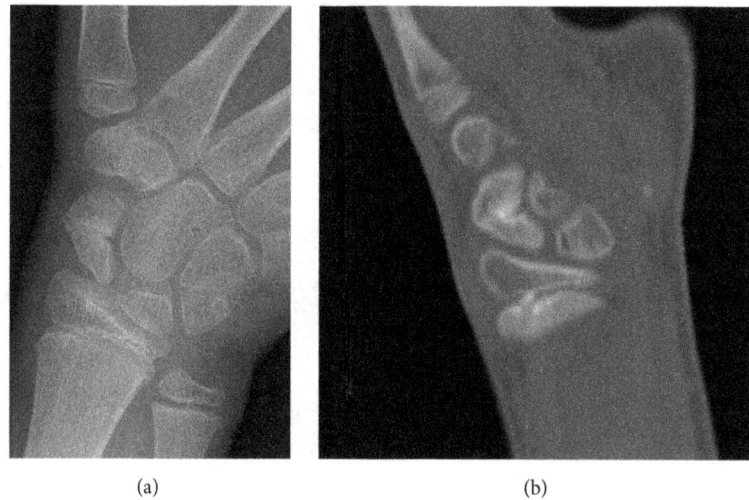

FIGURE 3: (a) Plain radiograph at the end of cast immobilization showing improved consolidation. (b) CT scan be performed one month after the end of cast immobilization showing union of the fracture.

perfusion of the proximal pole, an adequate healing potential with conservative treatment was estimated. The wrist was immobilized with a short arm cast for fourteen weeks and at the end of cast immobilization the patient was pain-free and had no tenderness and there was no restriction in range of motion. Plain radiograph showed improved consolidation and CT scan performed one month later confirmed union of the fracture (Figures 3(a) and 3(b)).

3. Discussion

Scaphoid fractures are rare, accounting for 0.4% of all fractures in the pediatric population [6]. Contrary to adults, scaphoid fractures in children involved mainly the distal pole [6]. However, it is believed that the grown intensive sport participation among children has caused a shift in the presentation of pediatric scaphoid fractures, resembling the adult pattern with mainly involvement of the scaphoid waist [7]. The retrograde perfusion of the scaphoid makes the scaphoid waist more susceptible for AVN than the distal pole [8]. Thereby, the diagnosis of AVN of the scaphoid is made by signal loss on MRI T1 [9]. In this case study, AVN was confirmed in the presence of a scaphoid waist fracture. Although a recent traumatic event occurred, the radiographic findings indicate the result of a longer existing disorder. A sport-induced stress fracture of the scaphoid waist is believed to have contributed to AVN of the scaphoid in a child practicing an intensive sport as karate. Stress fracture of the scaphoid is the result of repetitive dorsiflexion of the wrist, with the waist as the weakest point in the scaphoid [10]. Furthermore, the risk of sport-induced AVN is supposed to increase as a result of the grown sport participation among children [7]. However, there is currently no consensus when conservative or operative treatment is indicated. Gunal and Altay reported good results of two children with AVN treated by immobilization for several weeks [2]. Waters and Stewart achieved union and good function with vascularized bone

grafting and internal fixation after failure of immobilization [3]. Barthel et al. reported one case of AVN treated with vascularized bone grafting and internal fixation, obtaining union and pain relief [1]. The initial diagnosis and management in these studies were based on signal loss of the scaphoid on MRI T1 [2–4]. In our case study, a dynamic contrast-enhanced MRI was used for further treatment planning, as it is believed to be superior to contrast-enhanced MRI in assessing the vascularity of the scaphoid [4]. As dynamic contrast-enhanced MRI showed fair perfusion of the proximal pole, an adequate healing potential with conservative treatment was estimated. Subsequently, we achieved union and good functional outcome with cast immobilization for fourteen weeks.

In conclusion, this study showed dynamic contrast-enhanced MRI to be a valuable tool in assessing whether conservative or operative treatment is indicated to achieve union and good functional outcome in a child with sport-induced AVN of the scaphoid. If dynamic contrast-enhanced MRI had shown poor perfusion of the proximal pole, primary operative intervention would be indicated. Further studies are necessary to confirm the decision algorithm used in this study.

Competing Interests

The authors declare that there is no conflict of interests regarding the publication of this paper.

References

[1] P. Y. Barthel, A. Blum, and G. Dautel, "Avascular osteonecrosis of the scaphoid (Preiser's disease) in a 13-year-old boy treated with vascularized bone graft," Journal of Hand Surgery: European Volume, vol. 37, no. 2, pp. 180–182, 2012.

[2] I. Gunal and T. Altay, "Avascular necrosis of the scaphoid in children treated by splint immobilisation: a report of two cases,"

The Journal of Bone & Joint Surgery—British Volume, vol. 93, no. 6, pp. 847–848, 2011.

[3] P. M. Waters and S. L. Stewart, "Surgical treatment of nonunion and avascular necrosis of the proximal part of the scaphoid in adolescents," *The Journal of Bone & Joint Surgery—American Volume*, vol. 84, no. 6, pp. 915–920, 2002.

[4] A. W. H. Ng, J. F. Griffith, M. S. Taljanovic, A. Li, W. L. Tse, and P. C. Ho, "Is dynamic contrast-enhanced MRI useful for assessing proximal fragment vascularity in scaphoid fracture delayed and non-union?" *Skeletal Radiology*, vol. 42, no. 7, pp. 983–992, 2013.

[5] T. Konishiike, E. Makihata, H. Tago, T. Sato, and H. Inoue, "Acute fracture of the neck of the femur. An assessment of perfusion of the head by dynamic MRI," *The Journal of Bone & Joint Surgery—British Volume*, vol. 81, no. 4, pp. 596–599, 1999.

[6] A. G. Christodoulou and C. L. Colton, "Scaphoid fractures in children," *Journal of Pediatric Orthopaedics*, vol. 6, no. 1, pp. 37–39, 1986.

[7] J. J. Gholson, D. S. Bae, D. Zurakowski, and P. M. Waters, "Scaphoid fractures in children and adolescents: contemporary injury patterns and factors influencing time to union," *The Journal of Bone & Joint Surgery—American Volume* , vol. 93, no. 13, pp. 1210–1219, 2011.

[8] R. V. Grend, P. C. Dell, and F. Glowczewskie, "Intraosseous blood supply of the capitate and its correlation with aseptic necrosis," *Journal of Hand Surgery*, vol. 9, no. 5, pp. 677–680, 1984.

[9] R. Schmitt, G. Christopoulos, M. Wagner et al., "Avascular necrosis (AVN) of the proximal fragment in scaphoid nonunion: is intravenous contrast agent necessary in MRI?" *European Journal of Radiology*, vol. 77, no. 2, pp. 222–227, 2011.

[10] M. Majima, E. Horii, H. Matsuki, H. Hirata, and E. Genda, "Load transmission through the wrist in the extended position," *The Journal of Hand Surgery—American Volume*, vol. 33, no. 2, pp. 182–188, 2008.

26

Acute Failure of a Glenoid Component in Anatomic Shoulder Arthroplasty

William E. Daner, III and Norman D. Boardman, III

Department of Orthopaedic Surgery, Virginia Commonwealth University Health System, Richmond, VA 23298, USA

Correspondence should be addressed to William E. Daner, III; williamdaner@gmail.com

Academic Editor: Stephan Vogt

Glenoid loosening is the most common cause of failure in primary total shoulder arthroplasty (TSA) and often occurs years after the initial surgery. It is rare for a glenoid component to fail acutely. Several case reports of complete glenoid dissociation appear in the literature. It is important to report these failures to identify technical errors or component design flaws to improve outcomes in TSA. In this case report, we present an unrecognized acute failure of a cemented hybrid glenoid component at the time of surgery.

1. Introduction

Total shoulder arthroplasty (TSA) is an increasingly common procedure in the treatment of omarthrosis, with more than 50,000 total shoulder arthroplasties being performed annually in the United States [1]. This number has been on the rise since the early 1990s, particularly since FDA approval of reverse total shoulder arthroplasty (RTSA) for use beginning in 2004 [2]. Anatomic TSA comprises the majority of these cases, the most common indication being primary osteoarthritis [2]. TSA has proven to be an excellent pain relieving procedure that can improve range of motion and restore function. The overall complication rate has been reported to range from 12 to 39.8%, and the majority of these complications are related to glenoid component loosening [3–5]. Patients with a failed TSA may present with a painful, stiff shoulder with decreased range of motion, with or without associated symptoms of instability.

Several case reports of complete glenoid dissociation appear in the literature [6–9]. Among these failures were metal-backed components in which the polyethylene liner dissociated from the glenoid baseplate anywhere from 7 to 50 months postoperatively [7–9]. One report involved failure of a cemented all-polyethylene component 12 months after primary TSA [6]. Analogous failures have occurred through the pegs of all-polyethylene patella components in total knee

arthroplasty, none acutely [10–12]. To the best of the authors' knowledge, there are no reported cases of acute failure of a cemented glenoid component at the time of surgery.

2. Case Report

The patient is a 65-year-old man referred to the senior author's clinic with persistent right shoulder pain and severely restricted range of motion approximately 10 months after a primary anatomic TSA. The indication for the primary procedure was longstanding severe osteoarthritis with an intact cuff. The Exactech Equinoxe (Exactech Inc., Gainesville, FL) shoulder system was used for the index procedure, with a pegged, caged glenoid (model number 314-02-04). Utilizing a standard deltopectoral approach, a 15 mm press fit humeral stem with a 47 × 18 humeral head, offset with a 4.5 mm replicator plate and a large beta curvature, pegged glenoid with cage was implanted. No complications had been noted at the time of the primary procedure. The patient had an uneventful, atraumatic postoperative course, but he failed to progress. His range of motion was severely restricted to about 15 degrees in all planes 8 months after surgery. A CT arthrogram was ordered to evaluate if there was a rotator cuff tear but instead found that the glenoid component had dissociated and was sitting posterior to the humeral head (Figure 1). The polyethylene glenoid component had

(a)

(b)

(c)

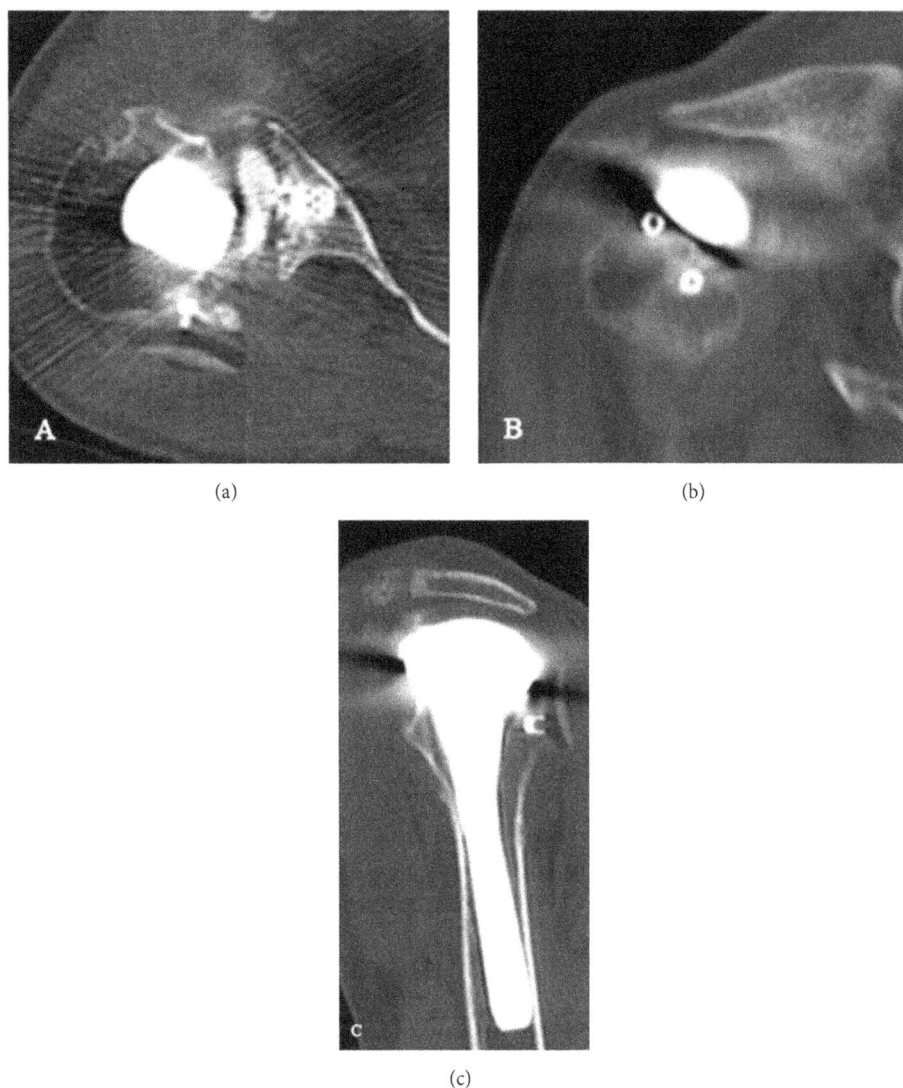

FIGURE 1: Selected axial (a), coronal (b), and sagittal (c) cuts of CT demonstrating dissociated glenoid component with cage remaining seated in the glenoid.

disengaged from its metallic cage and one of the three metallic peg caps, which remained seated in the glenoid. Close inspection of the postoperative films, as early as those immediately following surgery in the postanesthesia care unit, confirmed that the glenoid had in fact failed acutely (Figure 2).

The patient was subsequently referred to the senior author and underwent revision TSA. The glenoid component was retrieved from the posterior capsule. The component failure occurred at the interface between one of the pegs and its metallic cap as well as at the cage component, which had disengaged from the polyethylene (Figure 3). Inspection of the native glenoid revealed a region of proud bone, consistent with inadequate reaming of the glenoid. The retained glenoid cage and peg were extracted and the glenoid was prepared for the new implant. A new pegged glenoid was cemented into place and the humeral head was downsized.

Six months later, the patient was progressing well. He regained 90 degrees of pain-free forward flexion (110 passive)

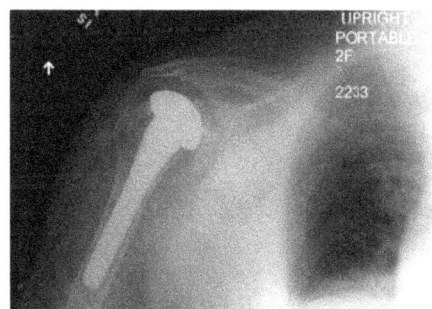

FIGURE 2: Postoperative X-ray, day of primary TSA.

with good rotation. He planned to continue to work on strength and range of motion with physical therapy. However, after the 6 month visit the patient was lost to follow-up. A good faith effort was made to contact the patient, but he could not be reached.

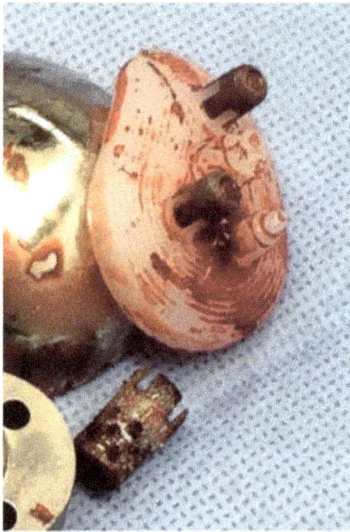

FIGURE 3: Explanted glenoid component. Note that one of the pegs and the cage have dissociated from the remainder of the glenoid component.

3. Discussion

Glenoid loosening is the most common cause of failure of contemporary TSA, comprising 32% of all complications and 7% of all indications for revision [3]. Failure most often occurs years after the initial surgery.

A variety of glenoid designs exist which have had varying degrees of success. A cemented, pegged all-polyethylene glenoid is presently the gold standard [13–17], though it is at risk for aseptic loosening. Because of concern for long-term survival of these implants, metal-backed components—including those utilizing trabecular metal to promote bone ingrowth—have been developed with the hope of improving glenoid fixation. Yet despite a greater percentage of peri-implant radiolucency in cemented all-polyethylene versus metal-backed components (42.5% versus 34.9%), the revision rate remains three times as great for metal-backed components [18]. Metal-backed glenoids have been unsuccessful for several reasons, including polyethylene dissociation from the metal baseplate, increased wear rates resulting in osteolysis of relatively thin polyethylene components, and potential metallosis due to extensive polyethylene wear and secondary metal on metal articulation. Metal-backed glenoids also rely on screw fixation for the metal base plate, which may fatigue and fail over time. Additionally, metal-backed components may cause more stress shielding and associated glenoid bone loss due to significant differences in stiffness between the metal and bone (Young's modulus of <10 GPa in bone versus >100 GPa in metal) [9, 19]. Material properties of all-polyethylene components more closely resemble those of the native glenoid bone, which improves stress transmission and thereby causes less shielding.

Nonetheless, the differences in stiffness between bone and polyethylene (Young's modulus <1 GPa) can create a stress riser across the cement mantle leading to aseptic loosening of all-polyethylene glenoid components. This is the most common point of late failure with this type of implant. To address this issue, glenoid components have been modified to hybrid designs with a central cage component in which bone graft is placed to promote bone ingrowth. The cemented pegs impart rotational stability and initial fixation while the central cage promotes bone ingrowth to improve late fixation. These implants have shown some promise with mid-term results [20–23]. The glenoid component that is the subject of this case report is a variation of this design. What is unique about this particular component is that the central cage is composed of plasma coated titanium to further promote ingrowth. The peripheral pegs are titanium and grit blasted to accommodate potential cementless technique. Based on early results of an Exactech consultant, this glenoid design is showing some promise. At two-year follow-up of 127 TSAs by one surgeon using this system, 3 patients showed radiographic evidence of loosening, 2 of which required revision [23].

It is rare for a component to suffer an acute mechanical failure. Most of the acute glenoid failures described in the literature have been due to late traumatic events. Polyethylene inserts have dissociated from their metal base plates [7–9]. One reported case involved a cemented polyethylene glenoid failure through its pegs with subsequent dissociation into the posterior subcutaneous tissue following a "minor trauma" [6]. In one of the revised failures of the Exactech Equinoxe system noted previously, the central cage locking mechanism failed [23]. There is an additional failure of this system registered with the MAUDE Database (Manufacturer and User Facility Device Experience Database) in which the glenoid component became "prematurely loose" one year after implantation [24].

The cause of acute glenoid failure in the subject of this case report was likely multifactorial and in all likelihood related to inadequate glenoid exposure. The glenoid component failed through the cement-implant interface as well as within the implant itself. The metal cage and one of the three metal peg caps dissociated from the polyethylene and remained seated in the patient's glenoid, while the remainder of the component dissociated posteriorly. The cement mantle failed acutely, which may have been due to premature cement hardening before the glenoid was impacted or improper component positioning secondary to poor exposure. Less likely, the cement may not have adequately set when compression was released and the shoulder reduced. However, with this implant, it has been reported that holding compression while the cement sets is an unnecessary step.

The dissociation of the metallic peg caps and cage from the polyethylene is not without precedence. In the two revised failures of the Exactech Equinoxe system noted previously, the central cage locking mechanism failed as well. Especially for this implant, glenoid exposure is paramount. The component requires "straight line" glenoid impaction. It must be directly perpendicular to the face of the glenoid to prevent damage to the locking mechanism of the central peg as it engages the drilled hole. Failure to do so may disengage the central peg from the polyethylene [23]. This technical point is likely the cause of the failure in this patient.

4. Conclusion

Glenoid component failure remains the most common cause of TSA failure and has been the focus of recent implant design modifications. The design rationale behind this hybrid glenoid component is intriguing, but it remains to be seen if it is a durable solution for glenoid failure. Further investigation with long-term outcome and comparative studies are necessary. Regardless of which TSA system is being used, it is imperative that the surgeon achieve adequate exposure for proper component placement. Poor glenoid exposure was likely the biggest factor in the component failure presented here. Delay in detection of failure in TSA can lead to poor outcomes. Postoperative monitoring of the patient's clinical progress and close radiographic evaluation of implant position, glenoid tilt, and peri-implant osteolysis will aid in catching failures early. Ultimately, good implant design, surgical technique with adequate exposure, and vigilant postoperative surveillance give patients the best chance for a successful long-term outcome with TSA.

Competing Interests

Each author has reviewed any potential conflict of interests. Dr. Daner has nothing to declare. Dr. Boardman is a paid consultant of DePuy Synthes, DePuy Orthopaedics Inc., Warsaw, Indiana. Dr. Boardman is also a paid consultant of Biomet Orthopaedics, LLC, Warsaw, Indiana.

References

[1] Agency for Healthcare Research and Quality, http://www.ahrq.gov/.

[2] S. H. Kim, B. L. Wise, Y. Zhang, and R. M. Szabo, "Increasing incidence of shoulder arthroplasty in the United States," *The Journal of Bone & Joint Surgery—American Volume*, vol. 93, no. 24, pp. 2249–2254, 2011.

[3] K. I. Bohsali, M. A. Wirth, and C. A. Rockwood Jr., "Complications of total shoulder arthroplasty," *The Journal of Bone & Joint Surgery—American Volume*, vol. 88, no. 10, pp. 2279–2292, 2006.

[4] P. Y. K. Chin, J. W. Sperling, R. H. Cofield, and C. Schleck, "Complications of total shoulder arthroplasty: are they fewer or different?" *Journal of Shoulder and Elbow Surgery*, vol. 15, no. 1, pp. 19–22, 2006.

[5] J.-F. Gonzalez, G. B. Alami, F. Baque, G. Walch, and P. Boileau, "Complications of unconstrained shoulder prostheses," *Journal of Shoulder and Elbow Surgery*, vol. 20, no. 4, pp. 666–682, 2011.

[6] W. F. Scully, D. A. Crawford, S. C. Brugman, and M. W. Manoso, "Glenoid component failure after total shoulder arthroplasty with migration of the component into posterior subcutaneous tissue: a case report," *Journal of Surgical Orthopaedic Advances*, vol. 22, no. 3, pp. 241–244, 2013.

[7] R. P. Driessnack, D. C. Ferlic, and J. D. Wiedel, "Dissociation of the glenoid component in the Macnab/English total shoulder arthroplasty," *Journal of Arthroplasty*, vol. 5, no. 1, pp. 15–18, 1990.

[8] A. Y. Feldman and T. D. Bunker, "Rotational dissociation of glenoid components in a total shoulder prosthesis: an indication that sagittal torque forces may be important in glenoid component design," *Journal of Shoulder and Elbow Surgery*, vol. 8, no. 3, pp. 279–280, 1999.

[9] A. L. Wallace, W. R. Walsh, and D. H. Sonnabend, "Dissociation of the glenoid component in cementless total shoulder arthroplasty," *Journal of Shoulder and Elbow Surgery*, vol. 8, no. 1, pp. 81–84, 1999.

[10] M. Shafi, Y. Y. Kim, Y. S. Lee, J. Y. Kim, and C. W. Han, "Patellar polyethylene peg fracture: a case report and review of the literature," *Knee Surgery, Sports Traumatology, Arthroscopy*, vol. 13, no. 6, pp. 472–475, 2005.

[11] C.-H. Huang, Y.-M. Lee, J.-H. Lai, J.-J. Liau, and C.-K. Cheng, "Failure of the all-polyethylene patellar component after total knee arthroplasty," *Journal of Arthroplasty*, vol. 14, no. 8, pp. 940–944, 1999.

[12] E. I. Francke and P. F. Lachiewicz, "Failure of a cemented all-polyethylene patellar component of a press-fit condylar total knee arthroplasty," *Journal of Arthroplasty*, vol. 15, no. 2, pp. 234–237, 2000.

[13] B. L. Norris and P. F. Lachiewicz, "Modern cement technique and the survivorship of total shoulder arthroplasty," *Clinical Orthopaedics and Related Research*, no. 328, pp. 76–85, 1996.

[14] P. Boileau, C. Avidor, S. G. Krishnan, G. Walch, J.-F. Kempf, and D. Molé, "Cemented polyethylene versus uncemented metal-backed glenoid components in total shoulder arthroplasty: a prospective, double-blind, randomized study," *Journal of Shoulder and Elbow Surgery*, vol. 11, no. 4, pp. 351–359, 2002.

[15] A. D. Boyd Jr., W. H. Thomas, R. D. Scott, C. B. Sledge, and T. S. Thornhill, "Total shoulder arthroplasty versus hemiarthroplasty: indications for glenoid resurfacing," *Journal of Arthroplasty*, vol. 5, no. 4, pp. 329–336, 1990.

[16] B. C. Brenner, D. C. Ferlic, M. L. Clayton, and D. A. Dennis, "Survivorship of unconstrained total shoulder arthroplasty," *The Journal of Bone & Joint Surgery—American Volume*, vol. 71, no. 9, pp. 1289–1296, 1989.

[17] T. J. Fox, A. Cil, J. W. Sperling, J. Sanchez-Sotelo, C. D. Schleck, and R. H. Cofield, "Survival of the glenoid component in shoulder arthroplasty," *Journal of Shoulder and Elbow Surgery*, vol. 18, no. 6, pp. 859–863, 2009.

[18] A. Papadonikolakis and F. A. Matsen III, "Metal-backed glenoid components have a higher rate of failure and fail by different modes in comparison with all-polyethylene components: a systematic review," *The Journal of Bone & Joint Surgery—American Volume*, vol. 96, no. 12, pp. 1041–1047, 2014.

[19] K. D. Stone, J. J. Grabowski, R. H. Cofield, B. F. Morrey, and K. N. An, "Stress analyses of glenoid components in total shoulder arthroplasty," *Journal of Shoulder and Elbow Surgery*, vol. 8, no. 2, pp. 151–158, 1999.

[20] G. I. Groh, "Survival and radiographic analysis of a glenoid component with a cementless fluted central peg," *Journal of Shoulder and Elbow Surgery*, vol. 19, no. 8, pp. 1265–1268, 2010.

[21] R. S. Churchill, C. Zellmer, H. J. Zimmers, and R. Ruggero, "Clinical and radiographic analysis of a partially cemented glenoid implant: five-year minimum follow-up," *Journal of Shoulder and Elbow Surgery*, vol. 19, no. 7, pp. 1091–1097, 2010.

[22] L. De Wilde, N. Dayerizadeh, F. De Neve, C. Basamania, and A. Van Tongel, "Fully uncemented glenoid component in total shoulder arthroplasty," *Journal of Shoulder and Elbow Surgery*, vol. 22, no. 10, pp. e1–e7, 2013.

[23] S. G. Grey, "Use of a caged, bone ingrowth, glenoid implant in anatomic total shoulder arthroplasty: technique and early results," *Bulletin of the Hospital for Joint Disease*, vol. 71, supplement 2, pp. S41–S45, 2013.

[24] Manufacturer and User Facility Device Experience Database, http://www.accessdata.fda.gov/scripts/cdrh/cfdocs/cfmaude/search.cfm.

27

Effect of Long-Term Use of Bisphosphonates on Forearm Bone: Atypical Ulna Fractures in Elderly Woman with Osteoporosis

Yusuf Erdem,[1] Zafer Atbasi,[2] Tuluhan Yunus Emre,[3] Gülis Kavadar,[4] and Bahtiyar Demiralp[5]

[1]*Orthopedics and Traumatology Department, Girne Military Hospital, Kyrenia, Cyprus*
[2]*Orthopedics and Traumatology Department, Ankara Military Hospital, Ankara, Turkey*
[3]*Orthopedics and Traumatology Department, Memorial Hizmet Hospital, Istanbul, Turkey*
[4]*Physical Medicine and Rehabilitation Department, Medicine Hospital, Istanbul, Turkey*
[5]*Orthopedics and Traumatology Department, Medipol University Hospital, Istanbul, Turkey*

Correspondence should be addressed to Yusuf Erdem; dryusufoguzerdem@gmail.com

Academic Editor: Werner Kolb

Osteoporosis is a common musculoskeletal disease of the elderly population characterized by decreased bone mineral density and subsequent fractures. Bisphosphonates are a widely accepted drug therapy which act through inhibition of bone resorption and prevent fractures. However, in long-term use, atypical bisphosphonate induced fractures may occur, particularly involving the lower weight bearing extremity. Atypical ulna fracture associated with long-term bisphosphonate use is rarely reported in current literature. We present a 62-year-old woman with atypical ulna due to long-term alendronate therapy without a history of trauma or fall. Clinicians should be aware of stress fracture in a patient who has complaints of upper extremity pain and history of long-term bisphosphonate therapy.

1. Introduction

Osteoporosis is a common musculoskeletal disease of the elderly population characterized by decreased bone mineral density and subsequent fractures. The prevalence of osteoporosis is frequent among the subjects older than 75 years, and almost one-third of this population is affected [1]. Due to the higher prevalence, osteoporosis-related fractures gained importance as both the population of the world is expanding and life expectancy is rising [2, 3].

Although there are several treatment modalities used in osteoporosis, bisphosphonates (alendronate, risedronate, ibandronate, and zoledronic acid) are a widely accepted drug therapy which inhibit bone resorption [4]. On the other hand, long-term use of bisphosphonates may cause atypical insufficiency fractures. Bisphosphonate associated fractures commonly involve lower extremities particularly seen in femur subtrochanteric location [5–7]. However, bisphosphonate induced ulnar fractures are rarely reported in relevant literature [8–14]. Herein, we present a case of bifocal ulnar fracture that occurred twice within a period of two years.

2. Case Report

A 62-year-old female was admitted to our outpatient clinic with pain on the ulnar side of the right (dominant) forearm which began suddenly after lifting a light object (grocery bag) seven days ago. There was no other history of trauma or fall. On examination, there was pain over the ulnar shaft on palpation, and elbow and wrist range of motion was painful. Neurovascular examination revealed no abnormality. Plane radiographic examination revealed a fracture at the proximal one-third of the ulna. Moreover, there was a hypertrophic callus formation on the distal ulna. The fracture was a transverse fracture and there was marked bony sclerosis at the fracture line (Figure 1).

Her past medical history revealed that she had type 2 diabetes mellitus, rheumatoid arthritis, and hypertension

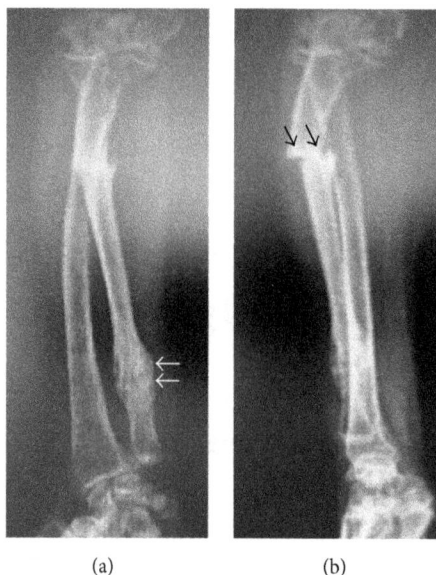

FIGURE 1: Anteroposterior (a) and lateral radiographs (b) of the patient's forearm at initial admission. Black arrows show the atypical fracture line. White arrows show the previous healed fracture.

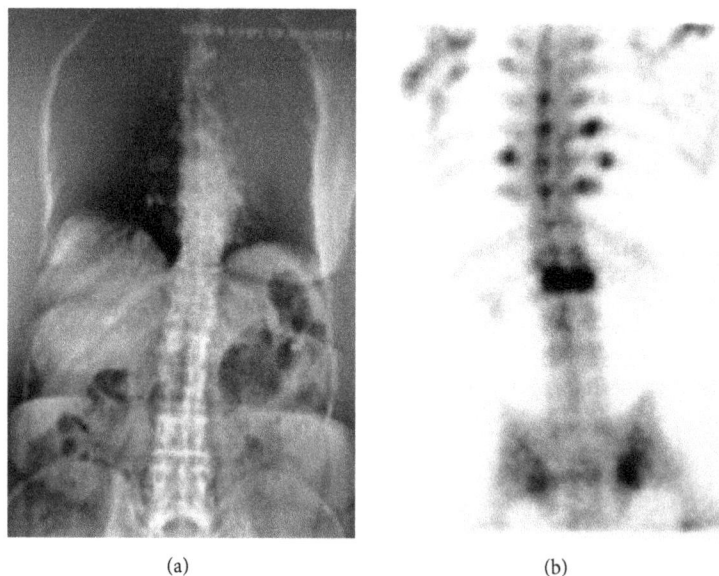

FIGURE 2: (a) Plane radiography and (b) scintigraphy showing L1 osteoporotic vertebra fracture.

diagnosed 12 years ago. Moreover, 7 years ago she had low back pain and radiodiagnostic studies detected L1 osteoporotic vertebrae fracture (Figure 2). Osteoporosis was diagnosed based on low T-score in DEXA, and bisphosphonate therapy was initiated (70 mg alendronate sodium/week). She was still using bisphosphonate, approximately for a 7-year duration. Three years ago, she underwent bilateral sequential total hip arthroplasty due to marked coxarthrosis secondary to rheumatoid arthritis and used a walking cane for the duration of one year. During the rehabilitation period, when the patient was still using the walking cane, a distal ulnar stress fracture occurred and was treated with conservative treatment.

With the prolonged use of bisphosphonates, substantial amount could be accumulated over the skeletal binding sites which could cause nonunion or delayed union by conservative treatment and by being the dominant hand fracture, so aiming to enhance the early mobilization, operative treatment (open reduction and plate/screw fixation) was offered to the patient for enhancement, but the patient denied the surgical intervention. Bisphosphonate treatment was ceased and a long-arm plaster cast was applied to the patient. Laboratory blood tests including serum calcium, phosphate, alkaline phosphatase, vitamin D, thyroid, and parathyroid hormone levels were all normal to evaluate whether to use bisphosphonates after bone healing.

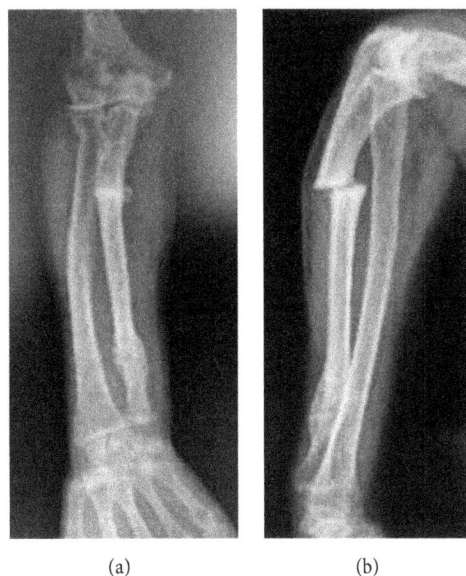

(a)   (b)

FIGURE 3: Forearm radiographs at the 6th week follow-up demonstrating the nonunion.

At the 4th week, long-arm cast was changed to short arm cast and continued for two more weeks. At the end of 6 weeks, the plaster cast was removed and the pain subsided, but there was no sign of bony union at the fracture site (Figure 3). The patient continued to deny the operative treatment. After the last visit at the 6th week, the patient was lost to follow-up.

3. Discussion

Either fatigue (related to overuse) or insufficiency (related to failure in bone structure) type of stress fractures is rarely seen in upper extremities [8]. In particular, ulna stress fractures are the least among them. These fractures are mostly reported in athletes. Sujino et al. and Steunebrink et al. reported bilateral ulnar fractures in a Kendo player and a weight-lifter, respectively [15, 16]. Other than overuse related to sports, ulnar stress fractures may be related to crutch use as Grace et al. have reported recently [17]. This fracture can also be accepted as overuse due to repetitive loading to upper extremity.

In current literature, there are few cases that report ulna fractures due to long-term bisphosphonate therapy [8–14]. In a recent systematic review, Tan et al. could document only seven patients with ulnar fractures secondary to long-term bisphosphonate use [8]. They emphasized that fractures due to long-term use of bisphosphonates have characteristic changes in plane radiography and common risk factors. According to their analysis, all patients were on bisphosphonate therapy for 7 to 15 years and predisposing factors included elderly females requiring walking aids. Similarly, our patient had a history of 7 years' bisphosphonate therapy and crutch use. Furthermore, dominant upper extremity was affected in most of the cases like our case. In contrast to femoral fractures, ulnar fractures occur without any type of trauma. Thus, clinicians may miss the diagnosis due to atraumatic nature of these fractures.

Neviaser et al. reported 25 bisphosphonate induced femoral fractures and analyzed the fracture pattern in these patients. 20 out of 25 patients demonstrated similar fracture patterns, namely, transverse fracture, cortical thickening, and sclerosis [7]. Similarly, Tan et al. reported that ulnar fractures are transverse, located in proximal ulna, and noncomminuted and had localized periosteal or endosteal thickening at the fracture site and generalized cortical thickening of the diaphysis [8]. Although the exact mechanisms that caused this typical fracture pattern are not clearly understood, it is believed that abnormal bone turnover results in brittle bone structure similar to osteopetrosis [13].

The treatment of these fractures can present several problems. First, there may be difficulties in fracture fixation such as proving enough primary stability. Second, fracture union cannot be achieved or delayed. If the patient is still on bisphosphonate therapy, it should be immediately stopped; thus bisphosphonates accumulation on fracture surface had been prevented to break the resistance to fracture site resorption [10–13]. Early diagnosis of undisplaced occult fractures is crucial and prophylactic surgical fixation is recommended due to difficulties in fracture site fixation. In case of ulnar fractures, open reduction and fixation should be chosen even if the fracture is nondisplaced or incomplete. Tang and Kumar reported a case of nonunion upon conservative treatment (plaster cast for 2 months) which had happened like in our case [12].

In conclusion, this case has some important messages for the readers. First, bisphosphonates should be ceased once the increase in BMD and decrease in biochemical bone turnover markers (urine cross-linked N-telopeptides of type 1 collagen, cross-linked C-telopeptides of type 1 collagen, bone-specific alkaline phosphatase, osteocalcin, and propeptide of type 1 collagen) compared to initial levels are achieved to prevent atypical fractures. We believe that patients should be individually reevaluated by using fracture risk assessment system (FRAX) before making a decision on whether a drug holiday is necessary [18, 19]. Second, clinicians should suspect a possible insufficiency fracture even in upper extremity in patients under long-term bisphosphonate therapy.

Consent

Informed consent was obtained from the patient to present and publish the medical documents.

Competing Interests

The authors declare that they have no competing interests.

References

[1] A. D. Manthripragada, C. D. O'Malley, U. Gruntmanis, J. W. Hall, R. B. Wagman, and P. D. Miller, "Fracture incidence in a large cohort of men age 30 years and older with osteoporosis," *Osteoporosis International*, vol. 26, no. 5, pp. 1619–1627, 2015.

[2] Z. A. Cole, E. M. Dennison, and C. Cooper, "Osteoporosis epidemiology update," *Current Rheumatology Reports*, vol. 10, no. 2, pp. 92–96, 2008.

[3] S. R. Cummings and L. J. Melton III, "Osteoporosis I: epidemiology and outcomes of osteoporotic fractures," *The Lancet*, vol. 359, no. 9319, pp. 1761–1767, 2002.

[4] R. P. Tonino, P. J. Meunier, R. Emkey et al., "Skeletal benefits of alendronate: 7-year treatment of postmenopausal osteoporotic women," *Journal of Clinical Endocrinology and Metabolism*, vol. 85, no. 9, pp. 3109–3115, 2000.

[5] K. Wang, A. Moaveni, A. Dowrick, and S. Liew, "Alendronate-associated femoral insufficiency fractures and femoral stress reactions," *Journal of Orthopaedic Surgery*, vol. 19, no. 1, pp. 89–92, 2011.

[6] S. Çakmak, M. Mahiroğulları, K. Keklikçi, E. Sarı, B. Erdik, and O. Rodop, "Bilateral low-energy sequential femoral shaft fractures in patients on long-term bisphosphonate therapy," *Acta Orthopaedica et Traumatologica Turcica*, vol. 47, no. 3, pp. 162–172, 2013.

[7] A. S. Neviaser, J. M. Lane, B. A. Lenart, F. Edobor-Osula, and D. G. Lorich, "Low-energy femoral shaft fractures associated with alendronate use," *Journal of Orthopaedic Trauma*, vol. 22, no. 5, pp. 346–350, 2008.

[8] S. H. Tan, S. Saseendar, B. H. Tan, A. Pawaskar, and V. P. Kumar, "Ulnar fractures with bisphosphonate therapy: a systematic review of published case reports," *Osteoporosis International*, vol. 26, no. 2, pp. 421–429, 2015.

[9] G. S. Chiang, K. W. Koh, T. W. Chong, and B. Y. Tan, "Stress fracture of the ulna associated with bisphosphonate therapy and use of walking aid," *Osteoporosis International*, vol. 25, no. 8, pp. 2151–2154, 2014.

[10] J. Moon, N. Bither, and T. Lee, "Atypical forearm fractures associated with long-term use of bisphosphonate," *Archives of Orthopaedic and Trauma Surgery*, vol. 133, no. 7, pp. 889–892, 2013.

[11] B. F. H. Ang, J. S. B. Koh, A. C. M. Ng, and T. S. Howe, "Bilateral ulna fractures associated with bisphosphonate therapy," *Osteoporosis International*, vol. 24, no. 4, pp. 1523–1525, 2013.

[12] Z. H. Tang and V. P. Kumar, "Alendronate-associated ulnar and tibial fractures: a case report," *Journal of Orthopaedic Surgery*, vol. 19, no. 3, pp. 370–372, 2011.

[13] K. Bjørgul and A. Reigstad, "Atypical fracture of the ulna associated with alendronate use," *Acta Orthopaedica*, vol. 82, no. 6, pp. 761–763, 2011.

[14] K. D. Stathopoulos, C. Kosmidis, and G. P. Lyritis, "Atypical fractures of the femur and ulna and complications of fracture healing in a 76-years-old woman with Sjögren's syndrome," *Journal of Musculoskeletal Neuronal Interactions*, vol. 11, no. 2, pp. 208–211, 2011.

[15] T. Sujino, T. Ohe, and M. Shinozuka, "Bilateral stress fractures of the ulnae in a Kendo (Japanese fencing) player," *British Journal of Sports Medicine*, vol. 32, no. 4, pp. 340–342, 1998.

[16] M. Steunebrink, D. de Winter, and J. L. Tol, "Bilateral stress fracture of the ulna in an adult weightlifter: a case report," *Acta Orthopaedica Belgica*, vol. 74, no. 6, pp. 851–855, 2008.

[17] C. S. H. Grace, K. W. B. Kelvin, C. T. Wei, and T. B. Yeow, "Stress fracture of the ulna associated with bisphosphonate therapy and use of walking aid," *Osteoporosis International*, vol. 25, no. 8, pp. 2151–2154, 2014.

[18] S. M. Ott, "What is the optimal duration of bisphosphonate therapy?" *Cleveland Clinic Journal of Medicine*, vol. 78, no. 9, pp. 619–630, 2011.

[19] D. L. Diab and N. B. Watts, "Bisphosphonate drug holiday: who, when and how long," *Therapeutic Advances in Musculoskeletal Disease*, vol. 5, no. 3, pp. 107–111, 2013.

28

Primary Ewing's Sarcoma of the Spine in a Two-Year-Old Boy

Ali J. Electricwala and Jaffer T. Electricwala

Electricwala Hospital and Clinics, Himalayan Heights, Pune, Maharashtra 411013, India

Correspondence should be addressed to Ali J. Electricwala; ali.electricwala@gmail.com

Academic Editor: Ali F. Ozer

Ewing's Sarcoma (ES) is a highly malignant bone tumour. It may involve any part of the skeleton but the most frequent parts are the ilium and diaphysis of femur and tibia (Alfeeli et al., 2005; Zhu et al., 2012). Primary ES of the spine is extremely rare (Yan et al., 2011). It accounts for only 3.5 to 14.9 percent of all primary bone sarcomas. The age of presentation ranges from 12 to 24 years (median 21 years) (Ferguson, 1999; Sharafuddin et al., 1992; Klimo Jr. et al., 2009). We report an unusual case of primary ES of the spine in a two-year-old boy, who presented to us with paraparesis and features of cauda equina syndrome. MRI scan showed a tumour mass arising from the pedicle of L4 vertebra invading the spinal canal. Tc-99 bone scan showed increased tracer uptake in L4 vertebra and normal tracer uptake elsewhere in the skeleton. After reaching the diagnosis of a space occupying lesion invading the lumber spinal canal, we performed a decompressive laminectomy and a biopsy was sent which confirmed the diagnosis of ES. Immunohistochemistry showed tumour cells staining positive for CD-99 (specific stain for ES). Gene testing showed an EWS-FLI 1 chimera. Surgery was followed by good improvement in motor signs. The child was then referred to a specialized oncotherapy centre for further treatment, radiation, and chemotherapy. To the best of our knowledge, we are the first to report primary ES of the spine at the age of two years.

1. Introduction

Ewing's Sarcoma (ES) is a highly malignant bone tumour. It may involve any part of the skeleton but the most frequent parts are the ilium and diaphysis of femur and tibia [1, 2]. Primary ES of the spine is extremely rare [3]. It accounts for only 3.5 to 14.9 percent of all primary bone sarcomas. The age of presentation ranges from 12 to 24 years (median 21 years) [4–6].

2. Case History

A two-year-old male child, first issue of a nonconsanguineous marriage, was brought with a 15-day history of progressive weakness of both the lower extremities, difficulty in standing and walking, and progressive loss of bowel and bladder function. He had no history of trauma, back pain, and failure to thrive. No constitutional symptoms were present. He had no significant past, personal, or family history. All developmental milestones were achieved for his age.

On clinical examination there was paraspinal fullness and complete loss of power below the level of the knee joint in both lower extremities. (Hip flexion and knee extension was grade 5; ankle dorsiflexion, great toe extension, and ankle planter flexion were grade zero.) Bulk was normal and tone was reduced. There were decreased sensations below the level of L3 dermatome in both the lower limbs. Perianal sensations were reduced. Ankle reflex and planter (Babinskis) response were absent bilaterally.

His laboratory parameters were normal except for a raised erythrocyte sedimentation rate (48 mm/hour). X-rays of the whole spine, chest, and abdomen were normal. Ultrasonography of the abdomen and pelvis showed abnormal distension of the bladder suggestive of the possibility of neurogenic bladder.

MRI of the lumbosacral spine (Figures 1(a) and 1(b)) revealed a soft tissue mass arising from the pedicle of L4 vertebral body invading the spinal canal, posterior elements, and Right Psoas muscle with destruction of the L4 vertebral body.

The patient was without the evidence of metastasis at presentation as found by chest and abdominal radiographs, chest computed tomography scan, and Tc-99 bone scan (Figures 2(a) and 2(b)).

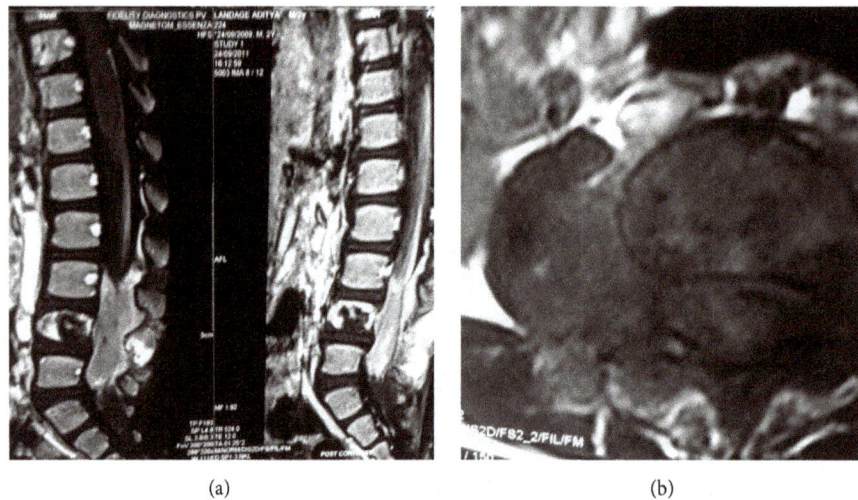

FIGURE 1: Sagittal projection of postcontrast T1 and T2 images demonstrating destruction of L4 vertebral body and tumour mass invading the spinal canal and posterior elements at L3, L4, and L5 vertebral levels. Axial projection of postcontrast T2 MRI image demonstrating tumour mass arising from the pedicle of L4 vertebra invading the spinal canal and the Right Psoas muscle.

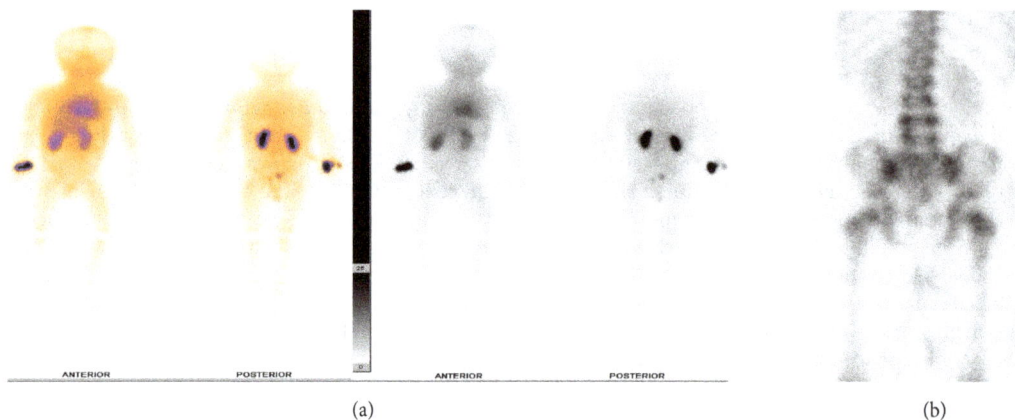

FIGURE 2: Tc-99 labelled bone scan.

The child underwent a decompressive laminectomy (Figure 3) as the first line of management.

The diagnosis of Ewing's Sarcoma was confirmed on histopathology, immunohistochemistry, and cytogenetic analysis. Histopathology showed small round cells packed in nests (Figures 4(a) and 4(b)). Immunohistochemistry showed tumour cells staining positive for CD-99: specific stain for ES (Figure 5). Gene testing showed an EWS-FLI 1 chimera.

Following decompressive surgery the patient had a good initial improvement in motor weakness. On postoperative day 15 the patient was referred to a specialized oncotherapy centre for radiation and combination chemotherapy.

3. Discussion

Ewing's Sarcoma (ES) is a small round cell tumour and accounts for one quarter of all primary bone tumours during childhood. Its peak incidence is during the second decade of life and it is very rare after 30 years of life [7]. ES usually presents with pain and swelling of the affected bone and vertebral involvement occurs in less than 5 percent of cases [8]. It has a poor prognosis but multimodality chemotherapy has increased life expectancy by 40 percent. Primary ES of the spine is a very rare condition [9]. Our case report is an extremely rare case of primary ES of the spine in a two-year-old boy. Our case was diagnosed 3 days after presentation. The initial interpretation of the MRI scan by the radiologist was that of a destructive lesion in the vertebral body of the fourth lumber vertebra most likely to be due to an infective process like tuberculosis.

In a retrospective study of Widhe et al., at the first visit, a bone tumour was suspected in only 19 percent of the cases of primary ES of the spine [10, 11]. A high index of suspicion and careful physical examination is required for the diagnosis of this condition. Signs of spinal cord compression may be the only initial indicators for primary ES of the spine [11–13].

Histopathology is the mainstay of diagnosis of small round cell tumours. The differential diagnoses of small round

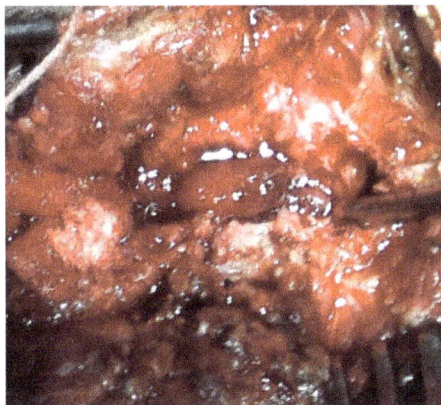

FIGURE 3: Decompressive laminectomy done revealing the tumour mass invading the spinal canal.

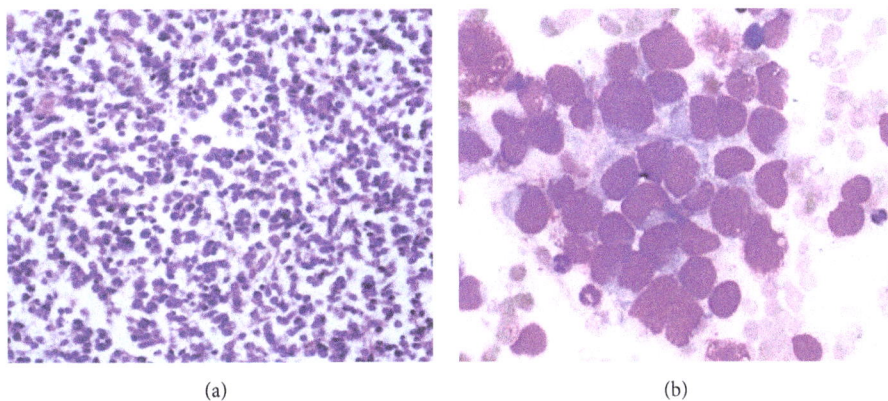

| (a) | (b) |

FIGURE 4: Low power view showing small round cells uniformly packed in nests. High power view showing tumour cells.

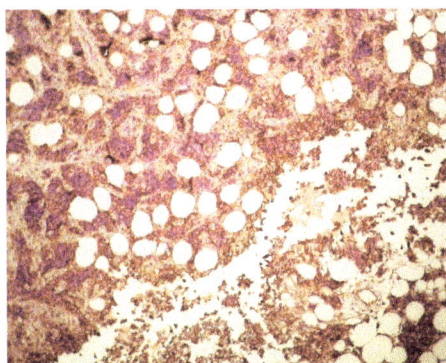

FIGURE 5: Immunohistochemistry stain showing tumour cells staining positive for CD-99.

cell tumours include neuroblastoma, primitive neuroectodermal tumours of bone (PNET), malignant lymphoma, rhabdomyosarcoma, and ES. The differentiation between these tumours on the basis of light microscopy alone is not accurate.

Current standards require evaluation by immunohistochemistry (CD-99) and cytogenetic analysis for the diagnosis of ES [14–17]. Chromosomal data from ES reveals a remarkably consistent chromosomal anomaly: the reciprocal translocation t(11;22)(q24;q12) involving chromosome 22 located on EWS-FLI 1 in more than or equal to 90% of the cases [18, 19]. The child in this case report satisfied both the histological and cytogenetic criteria required for the diagnosis.

Radiographs usually show a lytic lesion but sometimes sclerotic changes are also seen. However these findings on X-ray appear late usually after neurological signs have become obvious [15].

MRI scan is more sensitive than CT in the early detection on ES [20, 21]. Bone scan before staging is an important step to rule out other foci and in the follow-up treatment of primary ES of the spine [22].

These tumours have variable sensitivity to radiation and chemotherapy due to biological heterogenecity [23]. The classical chemotherapy regimen followed in ES consists of VAC-A (vincristine sulfate, dactinomycin, cyclophosphamide, and doxorubicin hydrochloride) [24, 25].

4. Conclusion

The purpose of this study was to report the incidence of such a rare tumour in a very young child. To the best of our knowledge, we are the first to report primary ES of the spine at the age of two years. Orthopaedic surgeons may encounter such a condition and should have a high index of suspicion to diagnose this rare tumour at its early stage for a better prognosis.

Competing Interests

The authors declare that there is no conflict of interests.

References

[1] M. A. Alfeeli, S. Y. Naddaf, and G. M. S. Syed, "Ewing sarcoma of the rib with normal blood flow and blood pool imagings on a 3-phase bone scan," *Clinical Nuclear Medicine*, vol. 30, no. 9, pp. 610–611, 2005.

[2] Q. Zhu, J. Zhang, and J. Xiao, "Primary dumbbell-shaped Ewing's sarcoma of the cervical vertebra in adults: four case reports and literature review," *Oncology Letters*, vol. 3, no. 3, pp. 721–725, 2012.

[3] Y. Yan, T. Xu, J. Chen, G. Hu, and Y. Lu, "Intraspinal Ewing's sarcoma/primitive neuroectodermal tumors," *Journal of Clinical Neuroscience*, vol. 18, no. 5, pp. 601–606, 2011.

[4] W. S. Ferguson, "Chronic leg pain in an adolescent male," *Medicine and health, Rhode Island*, vol. 82, no. 11, pp. 407–409, 1999.

[5] M. J. A. Sharafuddin, F. S. Haddad, P. W. Hitchon, S. F. Haddad, and G. Y. El-Khoury, "Treatment options in primary Ewing's sarcoma of the spine: report of seven cases and review of the literature," *Neurosurgery*, vol. 30, no. 4, pp. 610–619, 1992.

[6] P. Klimo Jr., P. J. Codd, H. Grier, and L. C. Goumnerova, "Primary paediatric intraspinal sarcomas. Report of 3 cases," *Journal of Neurosurgery: Pediatrics*, vol. 4, no. 3, pp. 222–229, 2009.

[7] L. I. Dini, R. Mendonça, and P. Gallo, "Primary Ewings sarcoma of the spine: case report," *Arquivos de Neuro-Psiquiatria*, vol. 64, no. 3, pp. 654–659, 2006.

[8] Y. Mori, H. Tsuchiya, T. Tsuchida, N. Asada, T. Nojima, and K. Tomita, "Disappearance of Ewing's sarcoma following bacterial infection: a case report," *Anticancer Research*, vol. 17, no. 2, pp. 1391–1397, 1997.

[9] M. R. Grubb, B. L. Currier, D. J. Pritchard, and M. J. Ebersold, "Primary Ewing's sarcoma of the spine," *Spine*, vol. 19, no. 3, pp. 309–313, 1994.

[10] B. Widhe and T. Widhe, "Initial symptoms and clinical features in osteosarcoma and Ewing sarcoma," *Journal of Bone and Joint Surgery—Series A*, vol. 82, no. 5, pp. 667–674, 2000.

[11] F. A. Paul, "Ewings sarcoma as an etiology for persistent back pain in a 17-year-old girl after trauma to the back," *Journal of the American Osteopathic Association*, vol. 95, no. 1, pp. 58–61, 1995.

[12] M. Kogawa, T. Asazuma, K. Iso et al., "Primary cervical spinal epidural Extra-osseous Ewing's sarcoma," *Acta Neurochirurgica*, vol. 146, no. 9, pp. 1051–1053, 2004.

[13] P. Mukhopadhyay, M. Gairola, M. C. Sharma, S. Thulkar, P. K. Julka, and G. K. Rath, "Primary spinal epidural extraosseous Ewing's sarcoma: report of five cases and literature review," *Australasian Radiology*, vol. 45, no. 3, pp. 372–379, 2001.

[14] A. S. Goktepe, R. Alaca, H. Mohur, and U. Coskun, "Paraplegia: an unusual presentation of Ewing's sarcoma," *Spinal Cord*, vol. 40, no. 7, pp. 367–369, 2002.

[15] L. I. Dini, R. Mendonça, and P. Gallo, "Primary Ewings sarcoma of the spine: case report," *Arquivos de Neuro-Psiquiatria*, vol. 64, no. 3, pp. 654–659, 2006.

[16] D. Schmidt, D. Harms, and V. A. Pilon, "Small-cell pediatric tumors: histology, immunohistochemistry, and electron microscopy," *Clinics in Laboratory Medicine*, vol. 7, no. 1, pp. 63–89, 1987.

[17] T. J. Triche, "Diagnosis of small round cell tumors of childhood," *Bulletin du Cancer*, vol. 75, no. 3, pp. 297–310, 1988.

[18] C. Turc-Carel, I. Philip, M.-P. Berger, T. Philip, and G. M. Lenoir, "Chromosome study of Ewing's Sarcoma (ES) cell lines. Consistency of a reciprocal translocation t(11;22)(q24;q12)," *Cancer Genetics and Cytogenetics*, vol. 12, no. 1, pp. 1–19, 1984.

[19] C. Turc-Carel, A. Aurias, F. Mugneret et al., "Chromosomes in Ewing's sarcoma: I. An evaluation of 85 cases of remarkable consistency of t(11;22)(q24;q12)," *Cancer Genetics and Cytogenetics*, vol. 32, pp. 229–238, 1988.

[20] B. K. Lawson, H. J. Goldstein, R. K. Hurley, R. L. Hutton, E. R. Anderson III, and J. F. Alderete, "Pelvic Ewing sarcoma: a radiologic and histopathologic correlation," *The Spine Journal*, vol. 16, no. 2, pp. e1–e3, 2016.

[21] D. Vanel, D. Couanet, J. Leclere, and C. Patte, "Early detection of bone metastases of Ewing's sarcoma by magnetic resonance imaging," *Diagnostic Imaging in Clinical Medicine*, vol. 55, no. 6, pp. 381–383, 1986.

[22] D. N. Estes, H. L. Magill, E. I. Thompson, and F. A. Hayes, "Primary Ewing sarcoma: follow-up with Ga-67 scintigraphy," *Radiology*, vol. 177, no. 2, pp. 449–453, 1990.

[23] J. D. Bruckner and E. U. Conrad III, "Spine," in *Surgery for Bone and Soft-Tissue Tumors*, M. A. Simon and D. Springfield, Eds., pp. 435–450, Lippincott-Raven, Philadelphia, Pa, USA, 1998.

[24] E. O. Burgert Jr., M. E. Nesbit Jr., L. A. Garnsey et al., "Multimodal therapy for the management of nonpelvic, localized Ewing's sarcoma of bone: Intergroup study IESS-II," *Journal of Clinical Oncology*, vol. 8, pp. 1514–1524, 1990.

[25] J. S. Miser, T. J. Kinsella, T. J. Triche et al., "Preliminary results of treatment of Ewing's sarcoma of bone in children and young adults: six months of intensive combined modality therapy without maintenance," *Journal of Clinical Oncology*, vol. 6, no. 3, pp. 484–490, 1988.

29

A Case of Implant Failure in Partial Wrist Fusion Applying Magnesium-Based Headless Bone Screws

Alice Wichelhaus, Judith Emmerich, and Thomas Mittlmeier

Department of Trauma, Hand and Reconstructive Surgery, University Faculty of Medicine Rostock, Schillingallee 35, 18057 Rostock, Germany

Correspondence should be addressed to Alice Wichelhaus; alice.wichelhaus@med.uni-rostock.de

Academic Editor: Zbigniew Gugala

This article presents a case of implant failure resulting in mechanical instability of a scaphotrapezotrapezoideal arthrodesis using magnesium-based headless bone screws. During revision surgery osteolysis surrounding the screws was observed as well as degraded screw threads already in existence at 6 weeks after implantation. The supposed osseous integration attributed to magnesium-based screws could not be reproduced in this particular case. Thus, it can be reasoned that the use of magnesium-based screws for partial wrist arthrodesis cannot be encouraged, at least not in dual use.

1. Introduction

Triscaphoid arthrodesis is an established treatment option for symptomatic osteoarthritis of the scaphotrapezotrapezoideal joint [1, 2]. Long-term effects of the hereby diverted force transmission can be arthritic changes of the adjacent carpal joints [2, 3], so that the younger the patient is, the more probable the need for revision surgery is. The use of biodegradable implants has the basic advantage to render implant removal unnecessary. In the last decade, biodegradable magnesium-based implants have been tested in clinical trials with promising results [4, 5]. A case of a severe adverse event using magnesium-based screws for partial wrist fusion is reported.

2. Case Presentation

The patient is a 42-year-old, right-hand dominant manual worker who presented himself after a fall on the extended right hand. Previous trauma could not be recalled. Preexisting medical conditions, smoking, long-term medication, allergic diathesis, or the like were negated.

At initial presentation a subtle swelling of the right wrist was stated as well as tenderness on palpation in the scaphoid region, especially the snuff box. Peripheral sensorimotor deficits were not detected. Radiographic imaging revealed a scaphoid fracture, classified as B2 according to the Herbert-classification [6]. Both the native radiographs and the computed tomography showed a preexistent scaphotrapezotrapezoidal (STT) arthritis and the configuration of static dorsally intercalated segmental instability (DISI) (Figures 1(a)–1(c)).

The patient insisted on having been completely free of pain and practicing undisturbed skilled manual work prior to the accident. Therefore he gave his informed consent to only address the scaphoid fracture operatively although it was well explained that persistent discomfort was probable due to the preexisting osteoarthritis. Fracture reduction was achieved via palmar approach and retained with a cannulated headless bone screw (KLS Martin, Tuttlingen, Germany). Postoperatively a wrist-cast manumitting the metacarpophalangeal joint was applied for 6 weeks. After fracture consolidation was ensured by CT-scan (Figure 2(a)), the patient still suffered from significant pain on load bearing of the affected wrist and, respectively, the base of the thumb. Plain radiographs visualized progression of the preexistent osteoarthritis of the STT-joint.

MRI-scans excluded circulatory disorders of the scaphoid (Figure 2(b)).

Despite functional training and physiotherapy, wrist function remained restricted and painful. To minimize the handicap and restore the ability to work, arthrodesis of

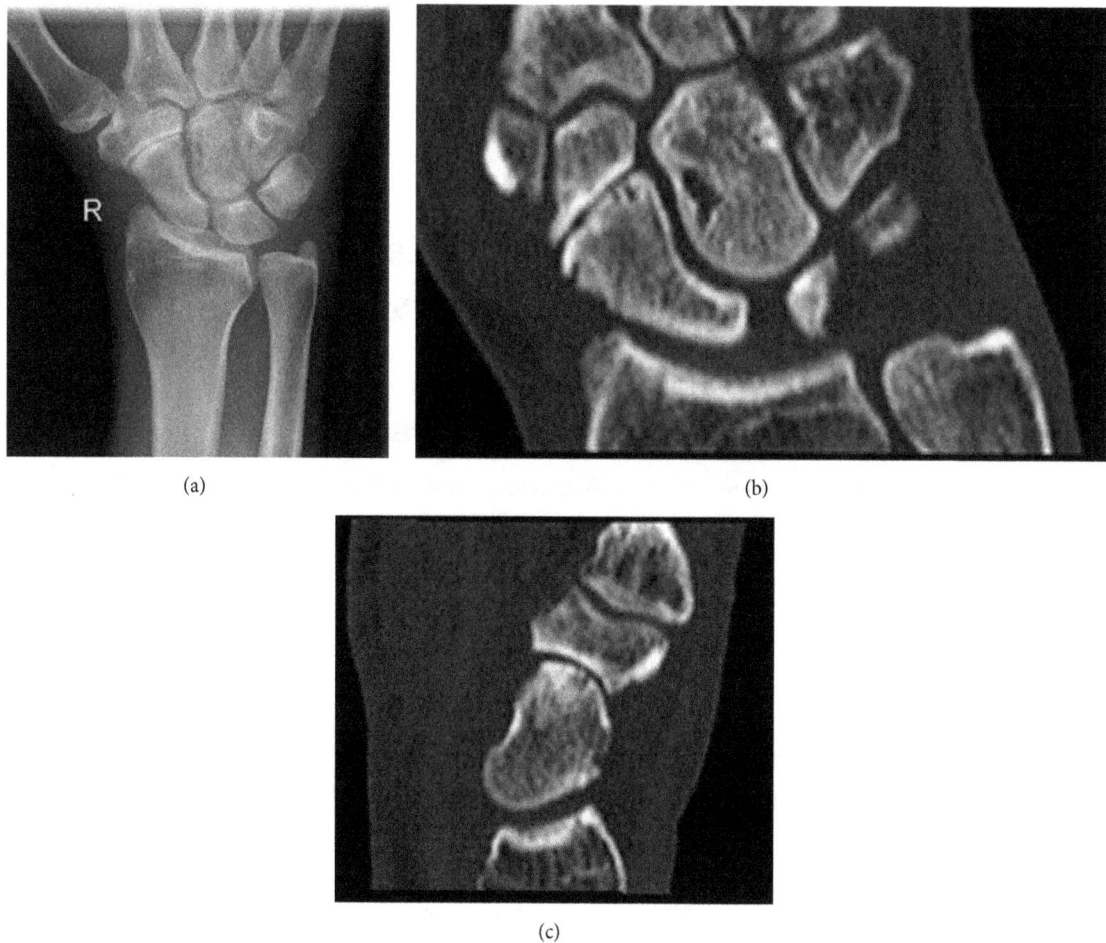

(a)

(b)

(c)

FIGURE 1: (a) X-ray of right wrist showing fracture of the scaphoid and preexistent osteoarthritis of the STT-joint. (b, c) Preoperative CT-scan demonstrating fracture of scaphoid classified as Herbert B2 but also clearly demonstrating degenerative changes of the carpal bones.

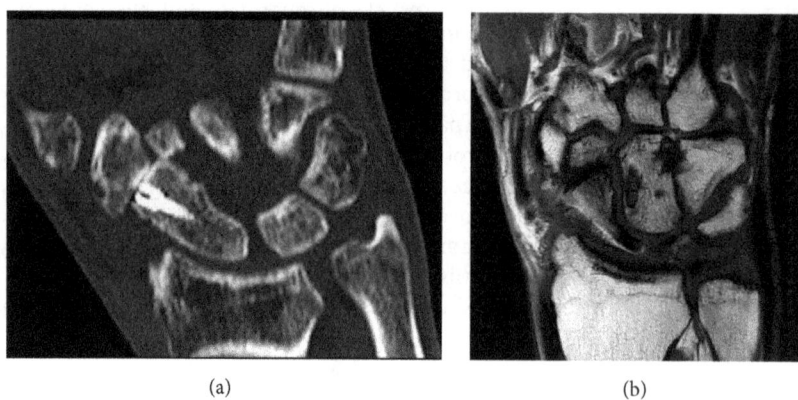

(a)

(b)

FIGURE 2: (a) CT-scan showing consolidated fracture of the scaphoid and progression of osteoarthritis in STT-joint. (b) MRI-scan showing healed fracture of the scaphoid with regular perfusion.

the STT-joint was performed in February 2014 (Figure 3). As further revision surgery is not unlikely after partial wrist fusion, two biodegradable magnesium-based headless bone screws (Magnezix®, Syntellix, Hannover, Germany) were used along with autologous bone grafting from the iliac crest.

Magnesium-based implants have been successfully applied by the authors for corrective surgery of the forefoot including revision surgery and in two cases for reconstruction of comminuted distal humerus fractures. After the operation cast immobilization was maintained for 6 weeks. Several

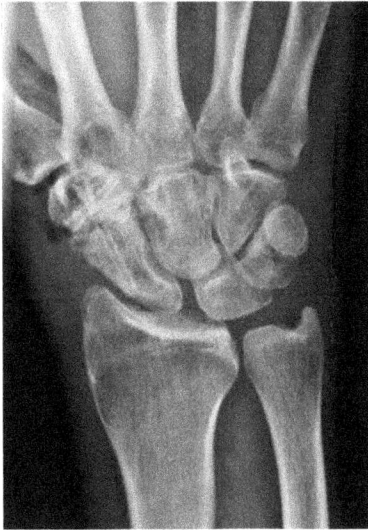

FIGURE 3: X-ray right wrist a.p. following STT-fusion with magnesium-based screws.

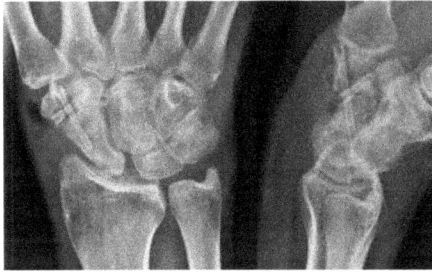

FIGURE 4: X-ray of the same wrist as in Figure 3, 6 weeks after arthrodesis showing loosening and backing out of both screws.

days after removal of the plaster cast, the patient complained about painful paraesthesia in the dorsal thumb region. He developed severe swelling of the radial and dorsal aspect of the wrist. X-rays of the wrist in two planes revealed loosening and backing out of the screws causing irritation to the dorsal ramus of the superficial radial nerve (Figure 4).

CT-scans showed osteolytic seams around both screws with cystic formations in the scaphoid, trapezium, and trapezoid (Figures 5(a)–5(d)).

Subcutaneous gas accumulations could not be palpated. During revision surgery large voids around the inserted screws were found. The two screws could be removed with tweezers without using a drill. The screw threads were barely recognizable; the tissue surrounding the screws was discolored blackish. The surrounding soft tissue showed severe synovitis with anthracite pigmentation. Unfortunately, no tissue was retained for histological assessment. As the arthrodesis was not consolidated by any means, rearthrodesis was necessary using Kirschner-wires.

In autumn 2014 progressive DISI-deformity and symptomatic periscaphoid osteoarthritis called for midcarpal arthrodesis with extirpation of the scaphoid as a salvage procedure. During the course of this operation, synovia was sampled for histological examination. Microscopy revealed signs of chronical hyperplastic synovitis with a wide range of proliferated synoviocytes throughout the whole sample. Hemosiderin pigment in macrophages was detected as well as multinucleated giant cells equaling foreign body reaction. Extraneous material could not be visualized under plane polarising light. Pigment due to metallic abrasive wear was not found any more than signs for pigmented villonodular synovitis.

The 4-corner fusion consolidated in time (Figure 6).

The patient has not been free of wrist pain ever since the first operation. Wrist range of motion remained restricted with ROM extension/flexion of 30–0–15° and ulnar/radial deviation of 15–0–10°. Grip strength measured with a Jamar-dynamometer achieved 1/3 of the uninjured contralateral side. So far, the patient did not settle for total wrist arthrodesis considering the hitherto conflicted devolution of disease. Till today resumption of manual work has not been possible.

3. Discussion

STT-fusions are performed for degenerative arthritic changes of the STT-joint, scaphoid instability, and advanced necrosis of the lunate [3, 7]. Triscaphoid arthrodesis has been proposed to redirect force transmission away from the lunate in way of stabilizing the radial column. The altered joint surfaces are uncoupled. Different stabilization techniques have been described using K-wires, headless bone screws, or anatomically shaped angular stable plates. Regardless of the technique, good results in terms of function and pain reduction are reported accompanied by a loss of grip strength of 20–40%. Nonunion is reported in up to 15% of the cases irrespective of the used material [3, 7]. For carpal arthrodesis a consolidation period of 8–12 weeks is assumed. In the reported case, the observable migration of the screws was caused by loss of retention force due to heavy corrosion of the screw threads present six weeks after implantation of the screws. Based on the published data on the magnesium-based screws, a slower degradation of the bolts had to be expected [8–10]. In animal studies, good biocompatibility has been described [8–11] for the magnesium-based screws. The degradation process of the magnesium material is said to have no adverse effect on bone healing but rather to promote bone formation at the screw-bone interface [8–11]. The mechanical strength of magnesium screws was tested to be equal to titanium-based screws [5]. A higher mechanical strength was determined for magnesium-based screws compared to other biodegradable polymer-based interference screws [12]. Reviewing the literature, reports of allergic reactions to magnesium-containing implants could not be found. Quite the contrary, magnesium-based implants attested little allergenic potential [13, 14]. Some authors even suggest to resign from using conventional metal alloys in patients with known allergic diathesis since their corrosion products showed cytotoxic and proinflammatory effects. In contrast the magnesium-based substitutes are said to deliver ions during their degradation that are needed for the physiological metabolism [14].

Despite the reported good osseointegration properties of magnesium screws, severe osteolysis surrounding the

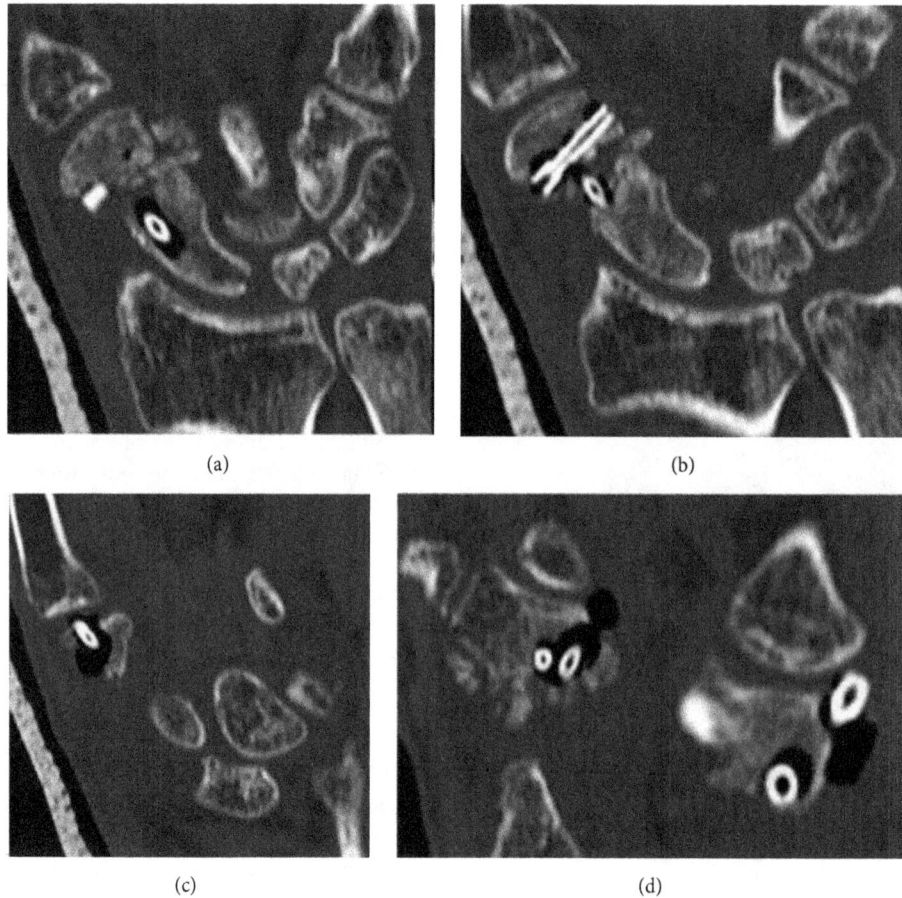

(a)

(b)

(c)

(d)

FIGURE 5: CT-scan taken 6 weeks after triscaphoid arthrodesis.

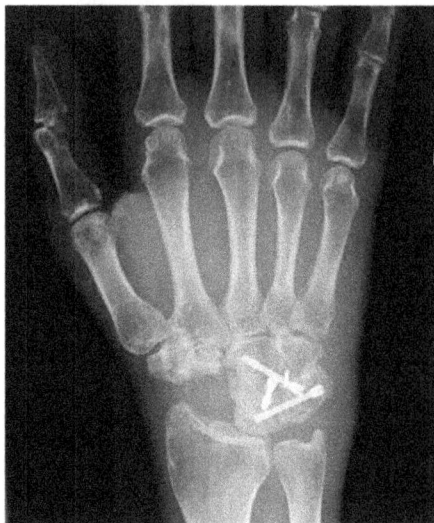

FIGURE 6: X-ray right wrist a.p. showing consolidated 4-corner fusion.

implants occurred in the present case. In a clinical application study good results were reported using magnesium-based headless bone screws for Chevron osteotomy [5]. However these good results could not be reproduced in the partial wrist fusion in this case. After revision surgery using titanium-based implants, solid osseous consolidation of the fusion could be achieved. Since headless bone screws were used in both operations, it can be assumed that the initial treatment failure is not due to the nature of the screws but to their metallic composition. Our observations are supported by an animal study which also stated poor osseointegration when using magnesium-based screws resulting in mechanical instability [15].

4. Conclusion

Early degradation of the screws leads to mechanical instability resulting in nonunion and osteolysis of the three carpal bones. Due to this disappointing result of the operation with premature mechanical instability, we cannot support the use of magnesium-based screws for partial wrist arthrodesis, at least not in dual use.

Consent

By means of the presented information the concerned patient is not identifiable. Nevertheless, the patient has given written consent for publication of the material in the presented form. The signed form is available on request.

Disclosure

External funding was not provided. Expenses were covered by institutional budget.

Competing Interests

The authors declare no competing interests.

Authors' Contributions

Alice Wichelhaus carried out all necessary operations, is responsible for the conception and design of the case report, and wrote the manuscript. Judith Emmerich and Thomas Mittlmeier were involved in drafting the manuscript. All authors read and approved the final manuscript.

References

[1] J.-N. Goubier, B. Bauer, J.-Y. Alnot, and F. Teboul, "Scapho-trapezio-trapezoidal arthrodesis for scapho-trapezio-trapezoidal osteoarthritis," *Chirurgie de la Main*, vol. 25, no. 5, pp. 179–184, 2006.

[2] K. Kalb, V. Fuchs, U. Bartelmann, R. Schmitt, and B. Landsleitner, "Experiences with scapho-trapezio-trapezoid arthrodesis. A retrospective analysis," *Handchirurgie Mikrochirurgie Plastische Chirurgie*, vol. 33, no. 3, pp. 181–188, 2001.

[3] R. Meier, M. Busche, C. Krettek et al., "Force distribution in the wrist following scaphotrapeziotrapezoid arthrodesis," *Der Unfallchirurg*, vol. 108, pp. 456–460, 2005.

[4] K. F. Farraro, K. E. Kim, S. L.-Y. Woo, J. R. Flowers, and M. B. McCullough, "Revolutionizing orthopaedic biomaterials: the potential of biodegradable and bioresorbable magnesium-based materials for functional tissue engineering," *Journal of Biomechanics*, vol. 47, no. 9, pp. 1979–1986, 2014.

[5] H. Windhagen, K. Radtke, A. Weizbauer et al., "Biodegradable magnesium-based screw clinically equivalent to titanium screw in hallux valgus surgery: short term results of the first prospective, randomized, controlled clinical pilot study," *BioMedical Engineering OnLine*, vol. 12, article 62, 2013.

[6] P. C. Amadio and S. L. Moran, "Fractures of the carpal bones," in *Operative Hand Surgery*, D. P. Green, Ed., pp. 711–768, Elsevier/Churchill Livingstone, Philadelphia, Pa, USA, 2005.

[7] R. Meier, K. J. Prommersberger, and H. Krimmer, "Scapho-trapezio-trapezoid arthrodesis (triscaphe arthrodesis)," *Handchirurgie, Mikrochirurgie, Plastische Chirurgie*, vol. 35, pp. 323–327, 2003.

[8] A. Chaya, S. Yoshizawa, K. Verdelis et al., "In vivo study of magnesium plate and screw degradation and bone fracture healing," *Acta Biomaterialia*, vol. 18, pp. 262–269, 2015.

[9] J. Diekmann, S. Bauer, A. Weizbauer et al., "Examination of a biodegradable magnesium screw for the reconstruction of the anterior cruciate ligament: a pilot in vivo study in rabbits," *Materials Science and Engineering C*, vol. 59, pp. 1100–1109, 2016.

[10] H. Waizy, J. Diekmann, A. Weizbauer et al., "In vivo study of a biodegradable orthopedic screw (MgYREZr-alloy) in a rabbit model for up to 12 months," *Journal of Biomaterials Applications*, vol. 28, no. 5, pp. 667–675, 2014.

[11] P. Han, P. Cheng, S. Zhang et al., "In vitro and in vivo studies on the degradation of high-purity Mg (99.99wt%) screw with femoral intracondylar fractured rabbit model," *Biomaterials*, vol. 64, pp. 57–69, 2015.

[12] M. Ezechieli, M. Ettinger, C. König et al., "Biomechanical characteristics of bioabsorbable magnesium-based (MgYREZr-alloy) interference screws with different threads," *Knee Surgery, Sports Traumatology, Arthroscopy*, 2014.

[13] F. Witte, I. Abeln, E. Switzer, V. Kaese, A. Meyer-Lindenberg, and H. Windhagen, "Evaluation of the skin sensitizing potential of biodegradable magnesium alloys," *Journal of Biomedical Materials Research Part A*, vol. 86, no. 4, pp. 1041–1047, 2008.

[14] F. Witte, T. Calliess, and H. Windhagen, "Biodegradable synthetic implant materials: clinical applications and immunological aspects," *Der Orthopäde*, vol. 37, no. 2, pp. 125–130, 2008.

[15] U. Thormann, V. Alt, L. Heimann et al., "The biocompatibility of degradable magnesium interference screws: an experimental study with sheep," *BioMed Research International*, vol. 2015, Article ID 943603, 15 pages, 2015.

30

Preservation and Tissue Handling Technique on Iatrogenic Dural Tear with Herniated Nerve Root at Cauda Equina Level

Ahmad Jabir Rahyussalim,[1] **Yoshi Pratama Djaja,**[1] **Ifran Saleh,**[1] **Ahmad Yanuar Safri,**[2] **and Tri Kurniawati**[3]

[1]*Department of Orthopaedic and Traumatology, Faculty of Medicine, Universitas Indonesia,*
Dr. Cipto Mangunkusumo General Hospital, Jakarta 10320, Indonesia
[2]*Neurophysiology Division, Neurology Department, Faculty of Medicine, Universitas Indonesia,*
Dr. Cipto Mangunkusumo General Hospital, Jakarta 10320, Indonesia
[3]*Stem Cell and Tissue Engineering Cluster, MERC Faculty of Medicine, University of Indonesia,*
Dr. Cipto Mangunkusumo Hospital, Jakarta, Indonesia

Correspondence should be addressed to Ahmad Jabir Rahyussalim; rahyussalim71@ui.ac.id

Academic Editor: Eyal Itshayek

Iatrogenic or incidental dural tear is a relatively common complication in lumbar decompression surgery. Although mostly there are no changes that occurred in long-term result following an incidental durotomy, the sequelae are not always benign especially when the herniated nerve root is involved. Preservation and tissue handling is paramount in order to prevent further injury. Two cases of dural tear with herniated nerve root complicating the lumbar decompression surgery are presented. Direct watertight repair was performed using the preservation and tissue handling concept. Assessing the relative size between the dural tear and the root mass is the key in determining whether enlargement of tear is needed. Whenever feasible, the tear will not be enlarged. Opening the vent by using a suture anchor and manually repositioning the nerve root with a fine instrument is the key for an atraumatic handling of the herniated nerve root. Clinical and neurophysiology examination was performed postoperatively and no further neurologic deficit occurred despite the iatrogenic injury. Although some debate on a few intraoperative and postoperative details still persists, tissue handling and preservation concept should be applied in all cases.

1. Introduction

Iatrogenic or incidental dural tear is a relatively common complication in lumbar decompression surgery. The incidence varies and ranges from 1% to 17% [1–4]. The increased incidence of incidental durotomy (ID) is related to epidural fibrosis, which is induced by previous operation and advanced spinal degenerative changes, such as ossified yellow ligament [1, 3, 4]. Beside direct dural laceration, other intraoperative mechanisms causing dural tear are excessive nerve root traction during removal of the disc extrusion and excessive force during removal of the adherent yellow ligament [2].

Some authors reported that there are no changes that occurred in long-term results following a spine surgery complicated by an incidental durotomy [1, 4, 5]. However,

the sequelae after a dural tear are not always benign. In several cases, the direct complications of dural tear include postural headache, meningeal pseudocyst, arachnoiditis, or meningeal infection. Indirect complications associated with prolonged bed rest frequently required in these cases are pneumonia, pressure ulcer, deep venous thrombosis, and pulmonary embolism.

Therefore, in order to reduce the risk of these complications, direct dural repair is recommended. The objectives of dural repair are containment of the nerve roots and creation of watertight closure to allow early mobilization of the patients, even though a period of bed rest is usually recommended after the repair of durotomy [6].

Various dural repair techniques have been described, such as direct primary suture using either simple interrupted suture or running locked suture, sealants such as fibrin glue, hydrogel or cyanoacrylate, bioabsorbable staples, and various types of grafts and patches [6]. Among these techniques, direct primary suture using simple interrupted suture is considered as the gold standard for achieving microsurgical anastomosis.

Despite the achievement of a watertight dural closure, several cases with herniated nerve roots are commonly associated with poor outcomes [7]. Accordingly, atraumatic tissue handling is paramount in order to avoid further injury to the nerve [8].

2. Case Illustration

2.1. Case 1. Female, 63-year-old, came with chronic back and leg pain, especially on her right side, due to spondylolisthesis at L4-5 and lumbar degenerative disc disease. On initial presentation, minor sensory deficit was found at the dermatomes of L4 and L5. Decreased motor power also occurred in ankle dorsiflexion (L4) and long toe extensor (L5). The diagnosis was confirmed by radiological examination and MRI images that showed degenerative changes at lumbar region, including scoliosis de novo along with degenerative spondylolisthesis at L4-5 compressing the spinal cord, that is, the L4 and L5 nerve roots, especially on the right side. After a series of failed conservative treatments consisting of oral medication and physiotherapy, the patient finally underwent a lumbar decompression surgery.

Posterior stabilization using pedicle screw and rod system were performed to restore the lumbar coronal and sagittal balance prior to performing L4-5 laminectomy. During the laminectomy and flavectomy, iatrogenic durotomy occurred as an adherence of yellow ligament to the spinal cord. The lesion occurred at the left dorsolateral region of L4 with herniated nerve root.

To repose the herniated nerve root, one anchor suture of 6-0 polypropylene monofilament (Premilene; B Braun, Melsungen, Germany) was placed on the lateral edge of the vent. The anchor suture was pulled carefully to the lateral side in order to open the vent without increasing the size. The herniated nerve root was then manually reposed gently into the vent by using the tip of nontoothed fine forceps. Unfortunately, the extent of the herniated nerve root was greater than the size of the vent. Therefore, additional incision on the dura was required to allow gentle attempt to repose the herniated nerve root.

Simple interrupted suture of 6-0 polypropylene was performed to create a watertight dural closure. Subfascial drainage was placed and controlled in order to prevent excessive drainage.

The patient was recommended to remain in postoperative bed rest for 48 hours. There were no complaints associated with the sequelae of the dural tear, such as dizziness or headache. Additional neurologic deficit did not occur. On the contrary, sensory improvement occurred at the dermatomes of L4 and L5.

Three months after the surgery, nerve conduction velocity study yielded an improvement in the right peroneal nerve motor but there was some decrease in the right sural sensory nerve compared to the preoperative evaluation (Figure 3). EMG evaluation cannot be performed due to preoperative massive radiculopathy.

2.2. Case 2. Female, 60-year-old, presented with back pain that radiated to both of her lower extremities for about one year. From physical examination, no motoric deficit was found and only a minor sensory deficit over the dermatomes of L4-5 and L5-S1 was found. The diagnosis was confirmed by MRI images showing canal stenosis of L4-5 and L5-S1 due to degenerative disc disease.

Similar to the first case, conservative therapy was first applied for a minimum of 2 months. After 3 months, there was no significant improvement that it was decided to perform posterior stabilization along with minimal decompression surgery by partial laminectomy.

Intraoperatively, during performing partial laminectomy, an iatrogenic durotomy occurred when removing the lamina and yellow ligament using a kerrison rongeur. To clearly expose the site and tear area, partial laminectomy was converted to total laminectomy. It was discovered later that the tear was at the dorsal region accompanied with herniated nerve root (Figure 1(a)).

Similar technique with the first case was performed by using an anchor suture to open the vent and insert the herniated nerve root by using a root dissector in order to minimize further injury to the nerve root. Watertight closure procedure was performed by using a simple interrupted suture of 6-0 polypropylene.

The protocol was continued with bed rest for the first 48 hours after the surgery. On the followup, there was no headache or postural dizziness, the wound healed without any complications, and the sensory deficit found before the operation was improved.

3. Preservation and Tissue Handling Technique

In order to achieve optimal care in dural repair, preservation and tissue handling are paramount. There are five general steps that should be taken into consideration (Figure 2). The first one is assessing the size of the tear and the ratio to the size of the herniated nerve root in order to determine whether or not the tear size should be enlarged. Second, preparation of microsurgery tools before the operation is essential in all lumbar decompression surgeries. Sealants are also needed in cases where tears are not repairable or watertight closures are not achieved.

Third, ensuring a sterile environment by gently cleansing the tear site before the repair should be done. Blood clot around the tear site may interfere with the dural repair process. Fourth, a watertight dural repair is performed whenever possible and the use of sealant is recommended as an adjunct. Fifth, the final step is ensuring the quality of the repair either by using valsalva maneuver or by neurophysiology assessment.

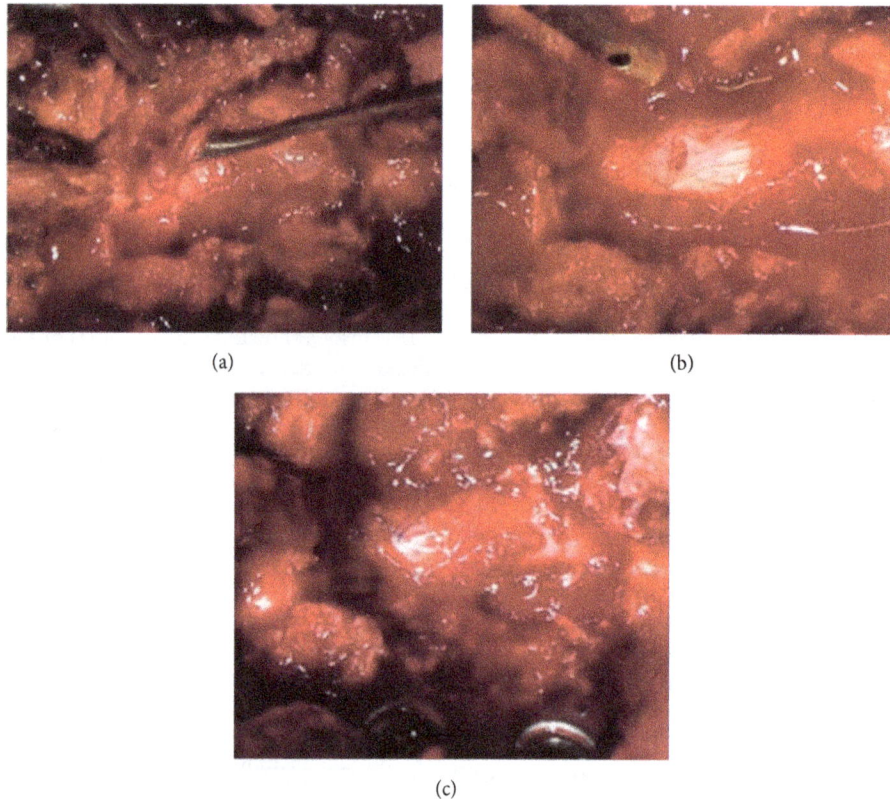

FIGURE 1: (a) Dorsal incidental durotomy with herniated nerve root (marked by root dissector). (b) Anchor suture to open the vent and reposing the herniated nerve root. (c) Watertight closure using simple interrupted 6-0 polypropylene.

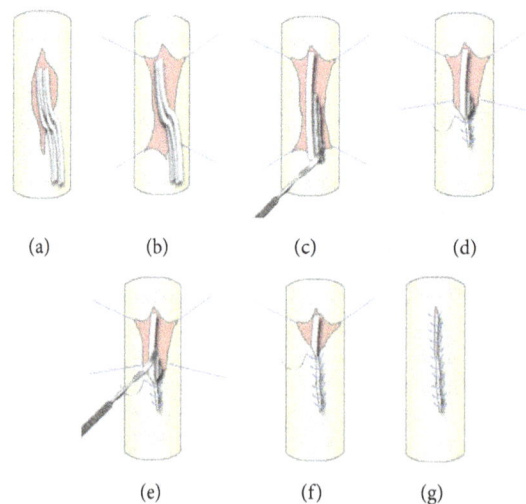

FIGURE 2: Tissue handling and preservation technique. (a) Assessment of the herniated nerve root; (b) putting the suture anchor at the edge of the vent; (c) reposing the nerve root at the top of the vent using blunt instrument; (d) gentle traction at the anchor to swallow the herniated nerve root and continuous suture were performed; (e) using the blunt edge of the root dissector to give a gentle push for the remaining herniated nerve root; (f) continuous suture was performed to the cephalad part of the vent; (g) final result shows that all nerves were into dural sac and the tear was recovered.

4. Discussion

As mentioned above, the incidence of incidental durotomy (ID) varies from 1% to 17%. However, herniation and incarceration of nerve roots due to the tear are quite rare,

especially on nontrauma cases [9]. Herniated nerve roots in iatrogenic durotomy cases are commonly associated with poor prognosis [7]. Chang et al. summarize 7 reported cases of herniated nerve roots following a discectomy. Five out of the seven cases had their neurological deficit completely

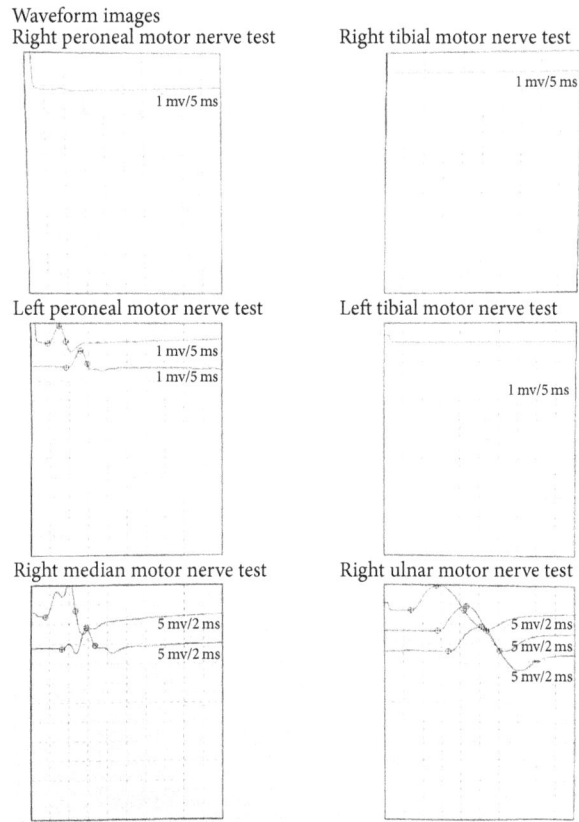

(a)

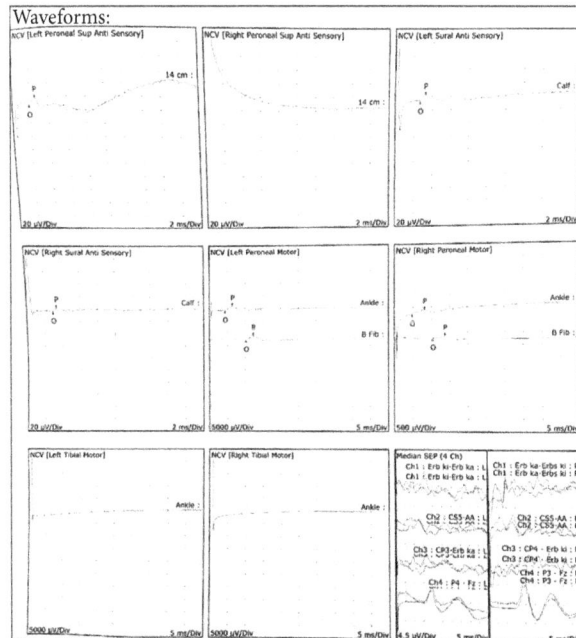

(b)

FIGURE 3: (a) Preoperative waveform images of nerve conduction velocity test in the first patient; (b) postoperative (3 months) waveform images showing improvements in the right peroneal nerve motor test and decrease in amplitude in the right sural nerve sensory test.

recovered and the remaining two were left with permanent neurologic deficit. Both cases had dural defects at the ventral side, in which surgical repair was quite challenging [9]. Fortunately, both cases of the present study had the tears at the dorsal and dorsolateral region of the cord, which were easier to repair and had more favorable outcomes compared to the above-mentioned series.

Gentle manipulation to the herniated nerve roots is mandatory to prevent further neurologic injury. The use of nontoothed fine forceps is commonly acknowledged to repose nerve roots. However, the use of a more concave side of the nerve root dissector is believed to be less traumatic in guiding the nerve roots back inside the vent. Further study is required to justify this concept.

Limited size of vent is also a problem when reposing the nerve roots. The dorsal dural vent was primarily repaired, surgically, by increasing the vent, and manually, by reposing the nerve roots. However, enlarging the vent is controversial and should be used as a last resort. Tewari and Gupta proposed another method to repose these nerve roots by using the "no touch hip flexion technique." Without touching the nerve root or enlarging the vent, the herniated nerve roots are reposed indirectly by flexing the hip joint. By flexing the hip, intrathecal stretching of the nerves caused the herniated nerve roots to go inside spontaneously [10]. This technique will minimize further damage to the roots; however, it requires changing the position of the patient to semiprone on Jackson table or Wilson frame during the surgery, which could be quite troublesome for the surgical team members who are not familiar with this technique. Another alternative is by using a suture anchor on the edge of the vent as mentioned in the present series. The concept of this technique is maximizing the opening of the vent without increasing the size, so the herniated nerve root can be reposed manually and gently. However, in certain cases with the size of the herniated nerve roots being too large, in order to allow gentle and minimal manipulation to the nerve roots, an additional incision of the dura is unavoidable.

Watertight closure of the dural tear is mandatory whenever possible, by using either simple interrupted suture or continuous locked suture technique. Similar outcomes between these two suture techniques were found [11]. Cain Jr et al. [12] showed that there was no significant difference in the leak pressure in a dural repair model. A 6-0 prolene suture is a recommended product in dural repair. Using a suture with the closest diameter in relation to the needle's diameter is important to minimize leakage from the needle hole [6].

If a tight suture cannot be performed or the location is not accessible (ventral dural tear), the use of sealant, such as collagen patch, fibrin glue, or hydrogel, is recommended [6, 13]. Sealants are effective in reducing leak, especially when applied in the presence of suture.

Drainage is controversial in dural tear cases. Some recommend the absence of drainage to prevent excessive draining of CSF. Others recommend controlled drainage to prevent meningoceles and extradural hematomas [14]. In a protocol proposed by Wolff et al., the use of controlled drainage is recommended only if the suture is watertight. In nonclosed breaches, it is not clear whether drainage will result in fewer

revisions. Furthermore, the low complication rate makes the value of drainage questionable when compared to the risk of cerebral complication due to excessive drainage of CSF [13].

Postoperative 48-hour bed rest is recommended following an iatrogenic durotomy repair. Bed rest is thought to reduce hydrostatic pressure on the repaired dura. According to postoperative protocol proposed by Khan et al., a trial of a brief bed rest (48 hours) followed by early mobilization was an effective strategy and was successful in 98.2% of their series [15]. Previous study by Wang et al. also stated similar outcome. In their study, an average bed rest period of 2.9 days resulted in only 2.3% reoperation rate (2 out of 88 patients) [4].

Postoperative neurophysiology evaluation was performed to evaluate the extent of the nerve injury/recovery related to the surgery (and iatrogenic durotomy). Improvement that was found in right peroneal nerve (motor) resulted from the decompression surgery. Meanwhile, there was some decrease in sural nerve (S1, 2) conductivity, which is possibly related to the injury. The limitation of this examination is that evaluation on the nerve conduction that innervates the autonomic element in accordance with the patient's complaint cannot be performed. Another limitation of this study is the minimal number of cases. Further evaluation, such as MRI and serial clinical evaluation, should be performed in the future.

5. Conclusion

When encountering an incidental durotomy with herniated nerve root during lumbar decompression surgery, preservation of the existing structure should be the first priority. This may be done by using a preservation and tissue handling technique by first assessing the size of the vent and, whenever feasible, opening the vent by anchoring using suture and reposing the nerve root by using a fine instrument. This way, further neurological damage can be prevented. Intraoperative and postoperative protocols are equally important to optimize the outcome and prevent future complications.

Competing Interests

The authors declare that there is no conflict of interests regarding the publication of this paper.

References

[1] F. P. Cammisa Jr., F. P. Girardi, P. K. Sangani, H. K. Parvataneni, S. Cadag, and H. S. Sandhu, "Incidental durotomy in spine surgery," Spine, vol. 25, no. 20, pp. 2663–2667, 2000.

[2] S. K. Kalevski, N. A. Peev, and D. G. Haritonov, "Incidental Dural Tears in lumbar decompressive surgery: incidence, causes, treatment, results," Asian Journal of Neurosurgery, vol. 5, no. 1, pp. 54–59, 2010.

[3] N. E. Epstein, "The frequency and etiology of intraoperative dural tears in 110 predominantly geriatric patients undergoing multilevel laminectomy with noninstrumented fusions," Journal of Spinal Disorders and Techniques, vol. 20, no. 5, pp. 380–386, 2007.

[4] J. C. Wang, H. H. Bohlman, and K. D. Riew, "Dural tears secondary to operations on the lumbar spine. Management and results after a two-year-minimum follow-up of eighty-eight patients," *Journal of Bone and Joint Surgery A*, vol. 80, no. 12, pp. 1728–1732, 1998.

[5] A. A. M. Jones, J. L. Stambough, R. A. Balderston, R. H. Rothman, and R. E. Booth, "Long-term results of lumbar spine surgery complicated by unintended incidental durotomy," *Spine*, vol. 14, no. 4, pp. 443–446, 1989.

[6] E. E. Dafford and P. A. Anderson, "Comparison of dural repair techniques," *Spine Journal*, vol. 15, no. 5, pp. 1099–1105, 2015.

[7] Y. Ahn, H. Y. Lee, S.-H. Lee, and J. H. Lee, "Dural tears in percutaneous endoscopic lumbar discectomy," *European Spine Journal*, vol. 20, no. 1, pp. 58–64, 2011.

[8] V. K. Tewari and H. K. D. Gupta, "Reposing the herniated spinal nerves following accidental iatrogenic dural tear in spine surgery-the 'no touch hip flexion technique'," *Journal of Neurosciences in Rural Practice*, vol. 5, no. 5, pp. 106–107, 2014.

[9] M.-Y. Chang, J.-Y. Chan, C.-T. Huang, Y.-K. Liu, and J.-S. Huang, "Cauda equina incarceration secondary to dural tears after lumbar microsurgical discectomy," *Formosan Journal of Surgery*, vol. 45, no. 1, pp. 37–40, 2012.

[10] V. K. Tewari and H. K. D. Gupta, "Reposing the herniated spinal nerves following accidental iatrogenic dural tear in spine surgery-The 'no touch hip flexion technique'," *Journal of Neurosciences in Rural Practice*, vol. 5, no. 5, supplement 1, pp. S106–S107, 2014.

[11] B. Schlechter and B. Guyuron, "A comparison of different suture techniques for microvascular anastomosis," *Annals of Plastic Surgery*, vol. 33, no. 1, pp. 28–31, 1994.

[12] J. E. Cain Jr., R. F. Dryer, and B. R. Barton, "Evaluation of dural closure techniques. Suture methods, fibrin adhesive sealant, and cyanoacrylate polymer," *Spine*, vol. 13, no. 7, pp. 720–725, 1988.

[13] S. Wolff, W. Kheirredine, and G. Riouallon, "Surgical dural tears: prevalence and updated management protocol based on 1359 lumbar vertebra interventions," *Orthopaedics and Traumatology: Surgery and Research*, vol. 98, no. 8, pp. 879–886, 2012.

[14] S. I. Tafazal and P. J. Sell, "Incidental durotomy in lumbar spine surgery: incidence and management," *European Spine Journal*, vol. 14, no. 3, pp. 287–290, 2005.

[15] M. H. Khan, J. Rihn, G. Steele et al., "Postoperative management protocol for incidental dural tears during degenerative lumbar spine surgery: a review of 3,183 consecutive degenerative lumbar cases," *Spine*, vol. 31, no. 22, pp. 2609–2613, 2006.

31

A Rare Case of Tuberculosis with Sacrococcygeal Involvement Miming a Neoplasm

Walid Osman,[1] **Meriem Braiki,**[2] **Zeineb Alaya,**[3] **Thabet Mouelhi,**[1] **Nader Nawar,**[1] **and Mohamed Ben Ayeche**[4]

[1]*Department of Orthopedic Surgery, MES Medical College, Sahloul University Hospital, 4051 Sousse, Tunisia*
[2]*MES Medical College, Sahloul University Hospital, 4051 Sousse, Tunisia*
[3]*Department of Rheumatology, MES Medical College, University Farhat Hached Hospital, 4051 Sousse, Tunisia*
[4]*Department of Orthopedics, MES Medical College, Sahloul University Hospital, 4051 Sousse, Tunisia*

Correspondence should be addressed to Meriem Braiki; m-braiki@live.fr

Academic Editor: Ali F. Ozer

Infection of the lumbosacral junction by tuberculosis is quite rare and occurs in only 1 to 2% of all cases of spinal tuberculosis; moreover, isolated sacrococcygeal or coccygeal tuberculosis is much rarer. Failure to identify and treat these areas of involvement at an early stage may lead to serious complications such as vertebral collapse, spinal compression, and spinal deformity. In the present paper, we report an uncommon case of spinal tuberculosis with sacrococcygeal location revealed by a chronic low back pain that was successfully managed. Computed tomography scan and magnetic resonance imaging of the pelvis revealed a lytic lesion affecting both of sacrum and coccyx causing osseous destruction and suggesting a malignant process. A surgical biopsy was performed to establish the tissue diagnosis. Histopathological report confirmed the diagnosis of skeletal tuberculosis. The patient was treated with antibacillary chemotherapy for a period of 9 months. The follow-up period was of 36 months. There was a full recovery and the patient was asymptomatic.

1. Introduction

Tuberculosis (TB) has been described as an ancient infectious disease, with evidence being discovered in centuries-old skeletal remains [1, 2].

The proportion of spinal tuberculosis (TB) to all TB cases varied from 1% to 5% [3, 4]. Involvement of the lumbosacral region in spinal tuberculosis is rare, with only few reported cases in the literature [5]. There is only one reported isolated sacrococcygeal lesion [6].

In the present paper, we report an uncommon case of spinal tuberculosis with sacrococcygeal location revealed by a chronic low back pain that was successfully managed.

2. Case Presentation

A 55-year-old woman without medical or surgical history of interest was referred to our team with 1-year history of isolated lower back pain. She reported neither fever nor recent weight loss; there was no tuberculosis contagion. On physical examination, the patient was afebrile. Palpation of the sacrococcygeal region was too painful. Respiratory, cardiovascular, and abdominal system examination was normal. Higher mental functions and cranial nerve examination were normal. There were no meningeal signs. Motor and sensory examination in the lower limbs was normal. There was no bowel or bladder incontinence. Biologic parameters were within normal limits. Chest X-ray was normal. These were followed up by AP and oblique X-ray of pelvis (Figure 1) which were not suggestive of any lesion and showed blurry margins of the sacrococcygeal region. Initial CT scan of the pelvis (Figure 2) revealed a large hypodense heterogeneous solid lesion with enhanced peripheral portions after contrast administration, affecting both of sacrum and coccyx causing osseous destruction and suggesting a malignant process. The magnetic resonance imaging (MRI) (Figure 3) was performed showing a process of hypointense signals in T1W images and hyperintense signals in T2W images. The lesion

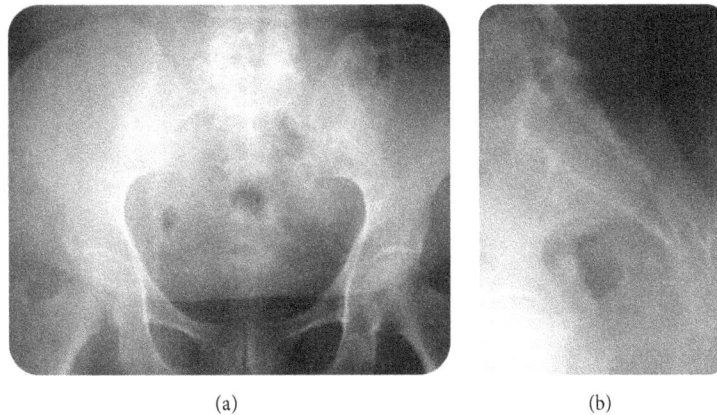

FIGURE 1: AP and oblique X-rays of pelvis showing fuzziness of the sacrococcygeal region with irregular margins.

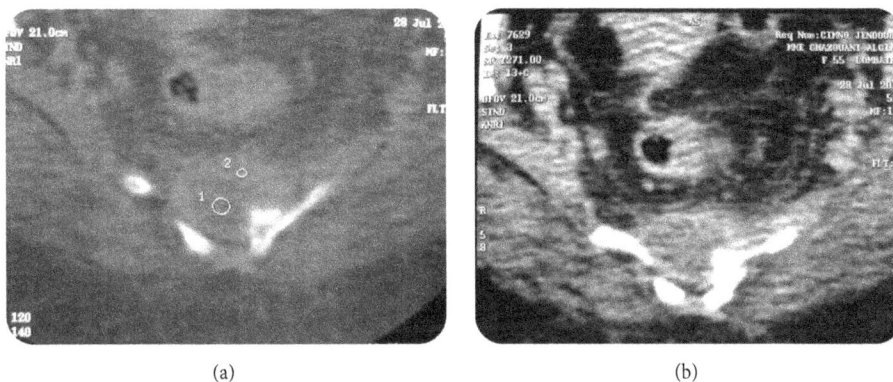

FIGURE 2: Contrast-enhanced computed tomography (CT) scans of the patient revealing presacrococcygeal lytic process.

was moderately enhanced in its periphery after gadolinium administration. The spread of lesion to right piriformis muscle and large gluteal muscles was noted.

Based on these radiological findings, a malignant process such as chordoma was suspected.

The patient underwent a surgical intervention and an open biopsy was performed to establish the tissue diagnosis. Histopathological report (Figure 4) confirmed the diagnosis of skeletal tuberculosis by showing tuberculous granuloma with central caseous necrosis surrounded by epithelioid cells and Langhans type giant cells. The patient was treated with antibacillary chemotherapy for a period of 9 months. Treatment was initiated with a four-drug antibiotic regimen (isoniazid, rifampicin, pyrazinamide, and ethambutol) for initial intensive phase of two months followed by continuation phase with two-drug regimen (isoniazid and rifampicin) for next 7 months with a favorable evolution. The follow-up period was of 36 months. There was a full recovery and the patient was asymptomatic at the last follow-up after 3 years with standard radiographs showing no evidence of recurrence (Figure 5).

3. Discussion

Tuberculosis still remains one of the most pressing health problems in the developing world, and tuberculosis of the spine occurs by hematogenous spread of infection from a pulmonary or extrapulmonary site; pulmonary infection is detected in around 50% of cases of spinal tuberculosis. More rarely, the condition may be encountered in the absence of a pulmonary infection [7].

The infection begins in subchondral bone and spreads slowly to the intervertebral disk space and the adjacent vertebral bodies, commonly in the lower dorsal and upper lumbar spine [8].

Failure to identify and treat these areas of involvement at an early stage may lead to serious complications such as vertebral collapse, spinal compression, and spinal deformity [8, 9].

Infection of the lumbosacral junction by tuberculosis is quite rare and occurs in only 1 to 2% of all cases of spinal tuberculosis; moreover, isolated sacrococcygeal or coccygeal tuberculosis is much rarer [7].

The sacrum is an uncommon site for tuberculosis involving the spine. In a review of 107 patients of tuberculous spondylitis by Lifeso et al. [10], no patient had lumbosacral and sacrococcygeal involvement. Dayras et al. [11] reported first case of isolated sacral tuberculosis with lower back pain. In 2004, Wellons et al. [12] presented a case of sacral tuberculosis with lower back pain and difficulty in walking with bilateral involvement of lower limbs.

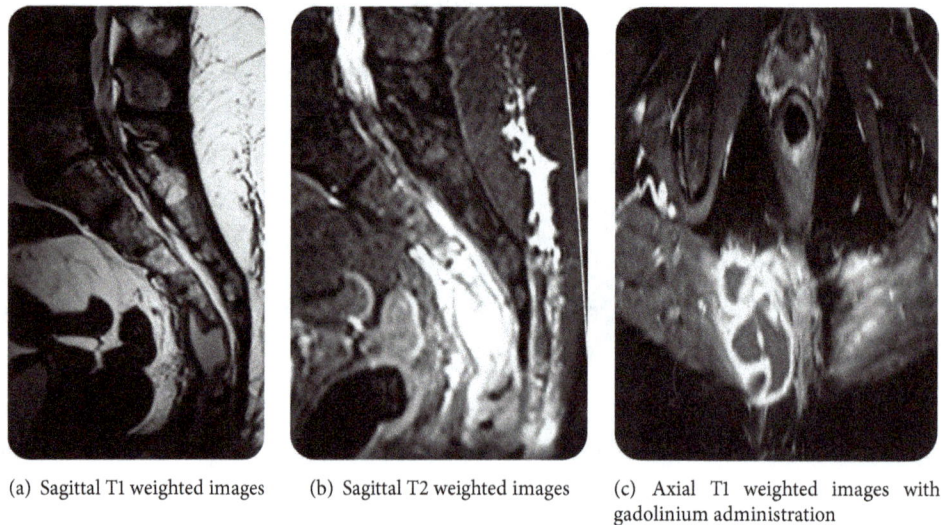

(a) Sagittal T1 weighted images   (b) Sagittal T2 weighted images   (c) Axial T1 weighted images with gadolinium administration

FIGURE 3: Magnetic resonance images of the patient. Revealing a process of hypointense signals in T1W images (a) and hyperintense signals in T2W images (b), the lesion was moderately enhanced in its periphery after gadolinium administration (c).

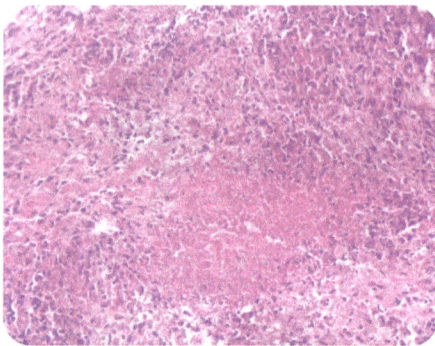

FIGURE 4: Histological examination revealing caseating granulomatous inflammation.

However, the reasons for the low incidence of lumbosacral or sacrococcygeal tuberculosis have not been exactly elucidated [7].

The single reported case of sacrococcygeal tuberculosis presented as an anal fistula [6]. Our patient with isolated sacrococcygeal involvement is probably the second described in the literature.

A confident diagnosis of skeletal involvement in tuberculosis is often difficult as the clinical presentation is nonspecific. Constitutional symptoms and nonspecific back pain are the predominant complaints. Thus, a delayed diagnosis is common [13]. Isolated sacral tuberculosis usually presents as chronic back pain in adults and discharging sinuses or abscess formation in children, with or without neurological deficit [7].

Briefly, in the literature, it was reported that isolated sacral or coccygeal tuberculosis is generally revealed by back pain without neurological deficit. That was compatible with the present case in which the patient was complaining of isolated chronic low back pain.

Neurological deficit is relatively uncommon in isolated sacral tuberculosis [14]. Because the sacral nerve roots are protected by bone, the incidence of neurological symptoms is relatively low [7].

Imaging findings in musculoskeletal TB are often nonspecific: in fact, plain radiographs are extremely insensitive and do not detect vertebral involvement until at least 50% of a vertebra is destroyed [7]. The first sign may be demineralization of the endplates with resorption and loss of dense margins [13]. Pre- and parasacral collection with destruction of the sacrum is seen on CT scan. MRI is the most sensitive modality for early diagnosis and complete delineation of the disease [8]. It usually reveals diffuse marrow edema which is hypointense on T1 and hyperintense on T2 weighted images; gadolinium contrast-enhanced MRI shows the enhancement of granulation tissue [14]. However, the MRI appearance of infection caused by *M. tuberculosis* is similar to the appearance of spinal neoplasms [15]. Consequently, bone imaging can notably be prone to miss this disease: pyogenic osteomyelitis and neoplasm such as chordoma or osteogenic sarcoma were included in the differential diagnosis [7].

As tuberculosis lesions may be mistaken for other infectious diseases or neoplasms, fresh tissue should be obtained for culture and biopsy [7].

The diagnosis of tuberculosis is confirmed by the histopathological study [16]. We presented a case of a neurologically intact patient with spinal tuberculosis because of the uncommon anatomical location of her lesion as well as radiological features suggesting a neoplasm such as chordoma. Surgical biopsy was indicated. Pathologic examination of biopsy specimens confirmed the diagnosis.

Regarding treatment of spinal tuberculosis, various chemotherapy protocols have been proposed. Medical treatment involves a combination of four drugs: rifampicin, isoniazid, pyrazinamide, and ethambutol for 2 months followed by bitherapy [3]. Thus, many workers prescribe chemotherapy

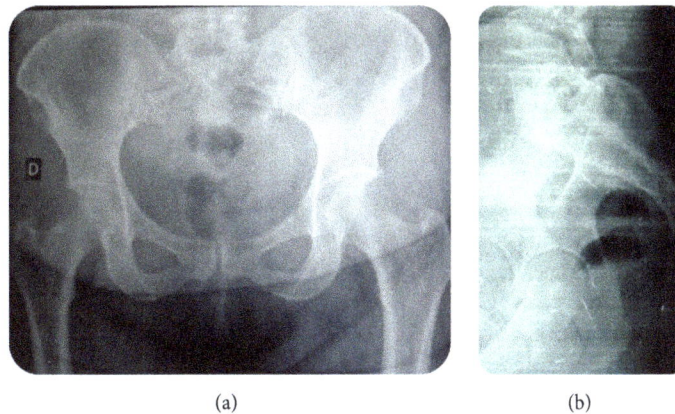

(a)　　　　　　　　　　　　　　　　(b)

FIGURE 5: Follow-up AP and oblique X-rays of pelvis at 3 years showing no evidence of recurrence.

for 6 months, while some continue it for 9 to 12 months [16, 17]. Excellent response of vertebral tuberculosis to multidrug therapy prevents the need for surgical management [16]. Our patient had a complete recovery with antitubercular treatment and bed rest.

Surgery may be necessary because of signs of neurological compression during extensive destruction of several vertebral bodies with spinal deformity or to evacuate an abscess that is resistant to medical treatment.

The prognosis of sacral tuberculosis is good, if a rapid and correct diagnosis is made and adequate treatment is provided [17].

This pathology should always be suspected in any process of the lytic sacrum or coccyx, especially in endemic areas of tuberculosis, to prevent or at least reduce the morbidity of this disease, which is generally curable [16].

4. Conclusion

Isolated sacrococcygeal tuberculosis is exceptional, and it should be kept in mind in isolated low back pain associated with any process of the lytic sacrum and coccyx. It is necessary to make a rapid and correct diagnosis in order to provide adequate management for this disease which has an excellent response to antitubercular treatment.

Competing Interests

The authors declare that they have no competing interests.

References

[1] N. Al-Khudairi and A. Meir, "Isolated tuberculosis of the posterior spinal elements: case report and discussion of management," *Journal of the Royal Society of Medicine*, vol. 5, no. 9, pp. 1–6, 2014.

[2] T. Hajdu, H. D. Donoghue, Z. Bernert, E. Fóthi, I. Kovári, and A. Marcsik, "A case of spinal tuberculosis from the middle ages in Transylvania (Romania)," *Spine*, vol. 37, no. 25, pp. E1598–E1601, 2012.

[3] O. Oniankitan, E. Fianyo, K. Kakpovi, L. K. Agoda-Koussema, and M. Mijiyawa, "Sacrum Pott's disease: a rare location of spine tuberculosis," *The Egyptian Rheumatologist*, vol. 36, no. 4, pp. 209–211, 2014.

[4] M. F. Ferrer, L. G. Torres, O. A. Ramírez, M. R. Zarzuelo, and N. Del Prado González, "Tuberculosis of the spine. A systematic review of case series," *International Orthopaedics*, vol. 36, no. 2, pp. 221–231, 2012.

[5] A. Agrawal, V. Shanthi, K. M. Mohan, and G. V. Reddy, "Lumbosacral spinal tuberculosis: a case report and review of literature," *The Egyptian Orthopaedic Journal*, vol. 50, no. 1, pp. 73–75, 2015.

[6] A. Kumar, M. K. Varshney, V. Trikha, and S. A. Khan, "Isolated tuberculosis of the coccyx," *The Journal of Bone & Joint Surgery—British Volume*, vol. 88, no. 10, pp. 1388–1389, 2006.

[7] D. U. Kim, S. W. Kim, and C. I. Ju, "Isolated coccygeal tuberculosis," *Journal of Korean Neurosurgical Society*, vol. 52, no. 5, pp. 495–497, 2012.

[8] E. Skoura, A. Zumla, and J. Bomanji, "Imaging in tuberculosis," *International Journal of Infectious Diseases*, vol. 32, pp. 87–93, 2015.

[9] M. Vorster, M. M. Sathekge, and J. Bomanji, "Advances in imaging of tuberculosis: the role of 18F-FDG PET and PET/CT," *Current Opinion in Pulmonary Medicine*, vol. 20, no. 3, pp. 287–293, 2014.

[10] R. M. Lifeso, P. Weaver, and E. H. Harder, "Tuberculous spondylitis in adults," *The Journal of Bone & Joint Surgery—American Volume*, vol. 67, no. 9, pp. 1405–1413, 1985.

[11] J. C. Dayras, J. Lorilloux, M. Hugonet, and P. Benichou, "Tuberculosis of the sacrum," *Annales de Pediatrie*, vol. 32, no. 3, pp. 289–293, 1985.

[12] J. C. Wellons, A. R. Zomorodi, A. T. Villaviciencio, C. W. Woods, W. T. Lawson, and J. D. Eastwood, "Sacral tuberculosis: a case report and review of the literature," *Surgical Neurology*, vol. 61, no. 2, pp. 136–139, 2004.

[13] P. Gupta, M. Prakash, N. Sharma, R. Kanojia, and N. Khandelwal, "Computed tomography detection of clinically unsuspected skeletal tuberculosis," *Clinical Imaging*, vol. 39, no. 6, pp. 1056–1060, 2015.

[14] A. Kumar, M. K. Varshney, and V. Trikha, "Unusual presentation of isolated sacral tuberculosis," *Joint Bone Spine*, vol. 73, no. 6, pp. 751–752, 2006.

[15] J. C. Wellons III, A. R. Zomorodi, A. T. Villaviciencio, C. W. Woods, W. T. Lawson, and J. D. Eastwood, "Sacral tuberculosis: a case report and review of the literature," *Surgical Neurology*, vol. 61, no. 2, pp. 136–139, 2004.

[16] F. Lazrak, F. E. Abourazzak, F. E. Elouzzani, M. Benzagmout, and T. Harzy, "A rare location of sacral tuberculosis: a report of three cases," *European Journal of Rheumatology*, vol. 1, pp. 78–80, 2014.

[17] V. P. S. Punia and S. Kumar, "Atypical manifestation of sacral tuberculosis as cauda-conus syndrome," *Journal, Indian Academy of Clinical Medicine*, vol. 9, no. 1, pp. 57–60, 2008.

32

Metallosis after Exchange of the Femoral Head and Liner following Ceramic Acetabular Liner Dissociation in Total Hip Arthroplasty with a Modular Layered Acetabular Component

Tomoya Takasago, Tomohiro Goto, Keizo Wada, Daisuke Hamada, Toshiyuki Iwame, Tetsuya Matsuura, Akihiro Nagamachi, and Koichi Sairyo

Department of Orthopedics, Institute of Biomedical Sciences, Tokushima University Graduate School, Tokushima, Japan

Correspondence should be addressed to Tomohiro Goto; gt510@tokushima-u.ac.jp

Academic Editor: Andreas Panagopoulos

The type of bearing material that should be used in revision surgery after the failure of ceramic-on-ceramic total hip arthroplasty (THA) remains controversial. In the case of ceramic fracture, the residual ceramic particles can cause consequent metallosis when metal implants are used for revision THA. On the other hand, in the case of THA failure without ceramic fracture, revision THA with a metal femoral head provides satisfactory results. We report an unusual case of progressive osteolysis due to metallosis that developed after revision THA for ceramic liner dissociation without a liner fracture performed using a metal femoral head and polyethylene liner. The residual metal debris and abnormal pumping motion of the polyethylene liner due to the breakage of the locking system or the aspherical metal shell being abraded by the ceramic head seemed to be the cause of the progressive osteolysis.

1. Introduction

Alumina ceramic components have been used in total hip arthroplasty (THA) for over 30 years. These implants were introduced to reduce wear and to increase long-term survivorship. A modular layered acetabular component, consisting of an alumina ceramic liner housed in an ultra-high-molecular-weight polyethylene shell (ABS liner) that is held in a titanium alloy metal shell (AMS HA shell), was developed in Japan (Kyocera, Kyoto, Japan) for use in alumina ceramic-on-ceramic THA. The main limitations of this component are the risk of ceramic liner fracture and failure of the ceramic liner fixation system [1–3]. Moreover, revision THA after ceramic liner fracture can be problematic. For example, in revision THA using a metal femoral head, metallosis may occur as a consequence of abrasive wear caused by ceramic particles deposited in periarticular tissues [4–6]. On the other hand, in the case of ceramic liner dissociation due to the breakage of the locking system between the socket and liner without ceramic fracture, revision THA with a metal femoral head may provide satisfactory results [7]. We

report here an unusual case of progressive osteolysis due to metallosis that developed after revision THA for ceramic liner dissociation without liner fracture in THA with a modular layered acetabular component.

2. Case Presentation

A 64-year-old man underwent primary THA with alumina-on-alumina bearings on the right side for the treatment of secondary osteoarthritis due to developmental dysplasia of the hip by posterolateral approach (Figure 1(a)). The implants used were a modular layered acetabular component, a titanium alloy stem, and a ceramic head (AMS HA shell with ABS liner 52 mm, PerFix HA stem size 11, and alumina ceramic head 28 mm with +4 mm offset; Kyocera, Kyoto, Japan). The postoperative course was uneventful. At the age of 74, 8 years after the last follow-up, he presented with right hip pain and crepitus during walking. Plain radiographs and computed tomography (CT) images of the hip revealed failure of the acetabular component, including liner dissociation from the metal shell, and osteolysis behind the cup was

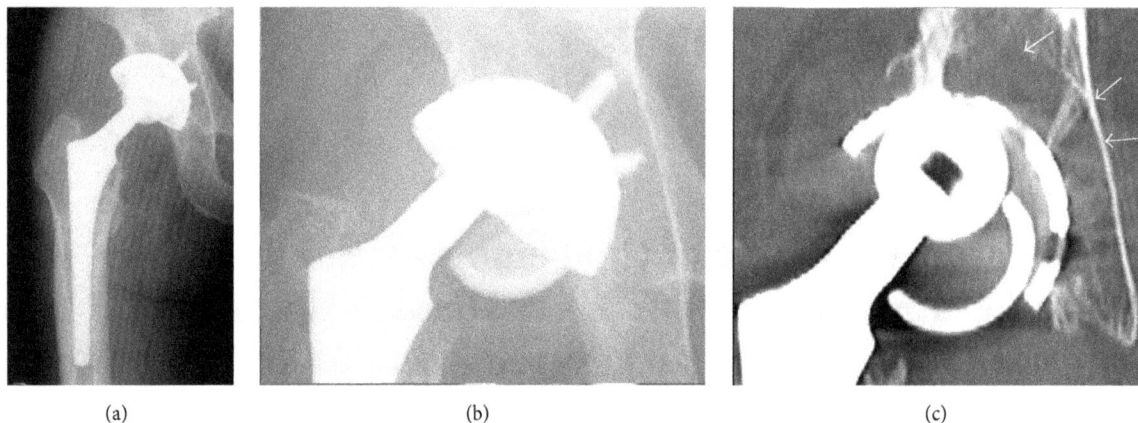

(a)   (b)   (c)

FIGURE 1: A postoperative anteroposterior radiographic image showing primary THA with alumina-on-alumina bearings on the right side for the treatment of secondary osteoarthritis due to developmental dysplasia of the hip (a). A plain radiograph and a computed tomography (CT) image, obtained 10 years after primary THA, showing the liner's dissociation from the metal shell along with retroacetabular osteolysis (white arrows) (b and c).

observed in DeLee and Charnley zones I and II (Figures 1(b) and 1(c)). At the time of the first revision surgery, no fracture or damage was observed at the alumina ceramic liner, ceramic head, or neck of the stem, but the polyethylene rotation prevention mechanism was observed to have failed. Pelvic osteolysis and black metallic debris behind the metal socket were observed through the screw holes. The cup and stem were well fixed and hence left in situ. We removed the granulomatous tissue and metallic debris around the cup as much as possible, and the backside debris was also debrided using screw holes. The liner and head were replaced with a highly cross-linked polyethylene and cobalt-chrome alloy head (910 MX liner CP, PHS metal ball 28 mm with +4 mm offset; Kyocera, Kyoto, Japan). At two years and five months following the first revision surgery, pain and swelling were noted over the right groin. Plain radiographs and CT images confirmed expanding retroacetabular osteolysis in all 3 zones and an intrapelvic pseudotumor, which is classified as fluid filled type, connecting to the right hip joint (Figures 2(a), 2(b), and 2(c)). Black synovial fluid was observed by puncture of the mass. A diagnosis of pseudotumor due to metallosis was made and the patient was referred to our hospital. Subsequently, rerevision THA was performed for managing the retroacetabular osteolysis and metallosis with direct lateral approach. Intraoperative findings included black pigmentation of metallic debris within the osteolytic lesions and around the joint capsule and acetabulum (Figure 2(d)). Bone ingrowth was noted only at the periphery of the cup, and it was easily removed by utilizing an explant device. The osteolytic lesions, synovial tissue, and joint capsule were debrided to remove the metal debris to the maximum possible extent. Acetabular reconstruction was performed with a Kerboull-type acetabular reinforcement device and bulk structural allograft (Figure 3). The well-fixed femoral stem was left in situ using a titanium sleeve on the trunnion with a new ceramic head (KT plate 480010, standard socket liner 44 mm, and alumina ball 28 mm with standard offset; Kyocera, Kyoto, Japan). There were no metal or ceramic particles on the

polyethylene liner articulation, and little damage on the cobalt-chrome alloy head was observed by scanning electron microscopy of the retrieved cup, polyethylene liner, and head. The inside of the metallic shell connecting to polyethylene liner had abraded, possibly resulting in direct contact with the alumina ceramic head before the first revision surgery performed for dissociation of the ceramic liner (Figure 2(e)). Furthermore, abnormal pumping movement between the polyethylene liner and the metallic shell and slight deformity and abrasion in the liner locking system were observed on inspection of the retrieved cup. A loose locking mechanism and the liner malseating to the metallic shell caused this abnormal pumping movement. After rerevision surgery, the postoperative course was uneventful. At the latest follow-up, that is, 4 years after the surgery, the patient was able to walk without an aid and was independent in all activities of daily living, with no evidence of osteolysis or loosening of the implant.

3. Discussion

The type of bearing that should be used after a fracture in ceramic-on-ceramic THA remains controversial, and there are no prospective studies since few patients suffer this complication. Revision THA with metal-on-polyethylene pairing is not feasible. Despite performing radical synovectomy and thorough washout of the hip joint, it may not be possible to remove all of the minute ceramic fragments following such ceramic fracture. While ceramic is a material with higher rigidity than metal, severe damage to the metal head and the polyethylene liner may occur due to wear from residual ceramic particles, resulting in early failure as metallosis [8, 9]. On the other hand, placing a new ceramic head on an undamaged trunnion has been shown to be effective. Hannouche et al. reported implantation of standard ceramic heads onto well-fixed stems in 61 cases of revision surgery with no ceramic head fractures after 7 years of follow-up [10]. However, it is difficult to exclude microscopic trunnion

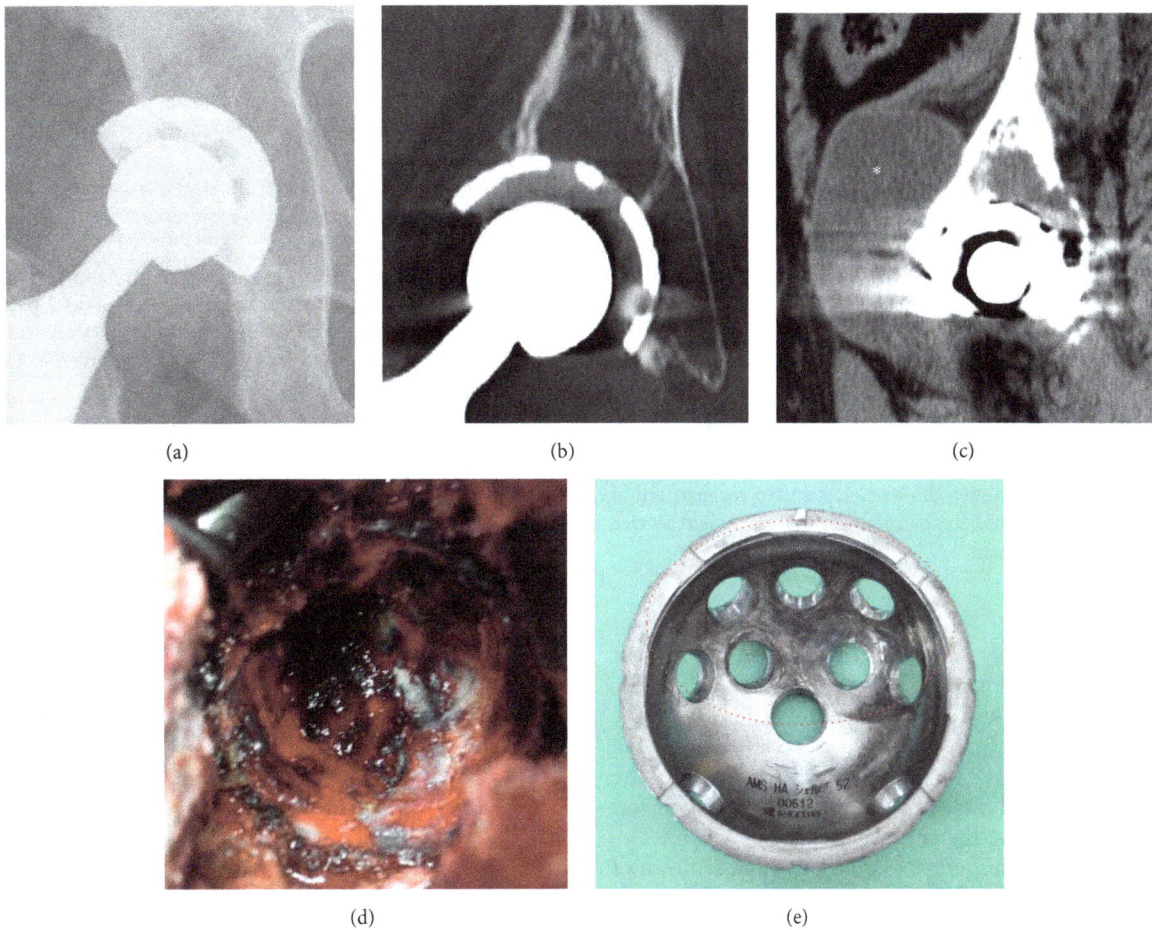

FIGURE 2: An anteroposterior view of plain radiograph (a) and a CT coronal image (b) showing the expanding retroacetabular osteolysis. A pseudotumor at the anterior aspect of the right hip (asterisk) connected to the hip joint was observed in a CT sagittal image (c). Pigmentation of metallic debris inside the osteolytic lesion and around the joint capsule and acetabulum was seen intraoperatively (d). A photograph of the retrieved cup (e) showing abrasion inside the metallic shell connecting to polyethylene liner (dotted circle).

damage during such revision surgery, and implanting a ceramic head on a damaged trunnion carries a certain risk of ceramic head fracture or earlier failure. In recent years, the use of a trunnion adaptor or sleeve, which ensures a pristine interface between ceramic and metal, has become common as a new option for minor trunnion damage. Jack et al. reported excellent survival rate and function after utilizing a sleeve on a used/damaged trunnion together with a ceramic head [11].

In the case of acetabular component failure without ceramic fracture, revision THA with a metal femoral head can be a reasonable treatment option because of the absence of residual ceramic particles in the joint [7]. In the present case, metallosis occurred unexpectedly after the first revision THA using a metal femoral head and a polyethylene liner although there was no ceramic fracture. At first, we speculated that ceramic particles existed within the articular surface leading to metallosis. However, the retrieved cup and head showed no metal or ceramic particles on the polyethylene liner articulation, and little damage was noted on the cobalt-chrome alloy head by scanning electron microscopy. In addition, no obvious damage at the trunnion of the well-fixed stem was observed intraoperatively. Maloney et al. reviewed 35 revision

THA cases for pelvic osteolysis after the primary cementless THA with a porous-coated acetabular component and reported that none of the osteolytic lesions had progressed after revision surgery involving the exchange of the liner [12]. In contrast, in the present case, retroacetabular osteolysis continued to expand after replacement of the liner and head. In the first revision THA, where the well-fixed shell was left in place, metal debris generated by direct impaction between the metallic shell and alumina ceramic head after liner dissociation might have remained. Moreover, an abnormal pumping movement between the polyethylene liner and the metallic shell was observed on inspection of the retrieved cup, which may have contributed to the abnormal expansion of the osteolysis. Several authors have suggested that the pumping movement between the polyethylene liner and the metallic shell may pump fluid and particles from the space between the liner and the shell through the screw holes to the retroacetabular bone [13–15]. Walter et al. documented two versions of the polyethylene pumping mechanism, namely, diaphragm pumping characterized by deformation of a noncongruent liner suspended at the rim of the shell and piston pumping characterized by pistoning of the liner in and out of the shell,

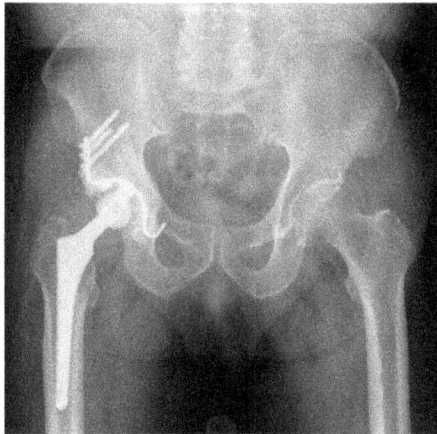

FIGURE 3: An anteroposterior plain radiograph, obtained 4 years after the rerevision surgery, showing acetabular reconstruction performed with a Kerboull-type acetabular reinforcement device and bulk structural allograft.

both of which probably coexist in vivo [16]. In the present case, these two pumping mechanisms might have occurred, leading to the flow of fluid in and out of the joint through the screw hole. As a result, some metal debris remained inside the retroacetabular osteolytic lesion, leading to expansion of the osteolysis along with diffusion around the periacetabular soft tissue, for example, into the intrapelvic space.

At the rerevision surgery, we considered that removal of the cup and radical debridement of the osteolytic lesion and pseudotumor were necessary. We performed rerevision THA using a reinforcement plate with bulk structural allograft. This technique is also useful for recovering bone stock and restoring the leg length and an adequate hip center [17].

We have presented a unique case of progressive osteolysis after revision surgery comprising exchange of the femoral head and liner due to ceramic acetabular liner dissociation in THA with a modular layered acetabular component. It is important to consider the possibilities of damage to the metal shell as well as the polyethylene liner locking mechanism in the case of ceramic articulation failure treated by such exchange of the liner and femoral head. In such cases, the removal of the entire implant and complete debridement of the metal debris may be required for reconstruction surgery.

Competing Interests

The authors declare that there are no competing interests regarding the preparation of this manuscript. The authors, their immediate families, and any research foundation with which they are affiliated did not receive any financial payments or other benefits from any commercial entity related to the subject of this article.

References

[1] M. Hasegawa, A. Sudo, H. Hirata, and A. Uchida, "Ceramic acetabular liner fracture in total hip arthroplasty with a ceramic sandwich cup," *Journal of Arthroplasty*, vol. 18, no. 5, pp. 658–661, 2003.

[2] M. Akagi, T. Nonaka, F. Nishisaka, S. Mori, K. Fukuda, and C. Hamanishi, "Late dissociation of an alumina-on-alumina bearing modular acetabular component," *Journal of Arthroplasty*, vol. 19, no. 5, pp. 647–651, 2004.

[3] K. Yamamoto, T. Shishido, T. Tateiwa et al., "Failure of ceramic THR with liner dislocation: a case report," *Acta Orthopaedica Scandinavica*, vol. 75, no. 4, pp. 500–502, 2004.

[4] J. Allain, F. Roudot-Thoraval, J. Delecrin, P. Anract, H. Migaud, and D. Goutallier, "Revision total hip arthroplasty performed after fracture of a ceramic femoral head: a multicenter survivorship study," *The Journal of Bone & Joint Surgery—American Volume*, vol. 85, no. 5, pp. 825–830, 2003.

[5] J. Allain, D. Goutallier, M. C. Voisin, and S. Lemouel, "Failure of a stainless-steel femoral head of a revision total hip arthroplasty performed after a fracture of a ceramic femoral head: a case report," *The Journal of Bone & Joint Surgery—American Volume*, vol. 80, no. 9, pp. 1355–1360, 1998.

[6] M. Hasegawa, A. Sudo, and A. Uchida, "Cobalt-chromium head wear following revision hip arthroplasty performed after ceramic fracture—a case report," *Acta Orthopaedica*, vol. 77, no. 5, pp. 833–835, 2006.

[7] M. Hasegawa, A. Sudo, and A. Uchida, "Alumina ceramic-on-ceramic total hip replacement with a layered acetabular component," *The Journal of Bone & Joint Surgery—British Volume*, vol. 88, no. 7, pp. 877–882, 2006.

[8] M. Pospischill and K. Knahr, "Strategies for head and inlay exchange in revision hip arthroplasty," *International Orthopaedics*, vol. 35, no. 2, pp. 261–265, 2011.

[9] I. Kempf and M. Semlitsch, "Massive wear of a steel ball head by ceramic fragments in the polyethylene acetabular cup after revision of a total hip prosthesis with fractured ceramic ball," *Archives of Orthopaedic and Trauma Surgery*, vol. 109, no. 5, pp. 284–287, 1990.

[10] D. Hannouche, J. Delambre, F. Zadegan, L. Sedel, and R. Nizard, "Is there a risk in placing a ceramic head on a previously implanted trunion?" *Clinical Orthopaedics and Related Research*, vol. 468, no. 12, pp. 3322–3327, 2010.

[11] C. M. Jack, D. O. Molloy, W. L. Walter, B. A. Zicat, and W. K. Walter, "The use of ceramic-on-ceramic bearings in isolated revision of the acetabular component," *The Journal of Bone & Joint Surgery—British Volume*, vol. 95, no. 3, pp. 333–338, 2013.

[12] W. J. Maloney, P. Herzwurm, W. Paprosky, H. E. Rubash, and C. A. Engh, "Treatment of pelvic osteolysis associated with a stable acetabular component inserted without cement as part of a total hip replacement," *The Journal of Bone & Joint Surgery—American Volume*, vol. 79, no. 11, pp. 1628–1634, 1997.

[13] O. L. Huk, M. Bansal, F. Betts et al., "Polyethylene and metal debris generated by non-articulating surfaces of modular acetabular components," *The Journal of Bone & Joint Surgery—British Volume*, vol. 76, no. 4, pp. 568–574, 1994.

[14] D. L. Scott, P. A. Campbell, C. D. McClung, and T. P. Schmalzried, "Factors contributing to rapid wear and osteolysis in hips with modular acetabular bearings made of hylamer," *Journal of Arthroplasty*, vol. 15, no. 1, pp. 35–46, 2000.

[15] A. M. Young, C. J. Sychterz, R. H. Hopper Jr., and C. A. Engh, "Effect of acetabular modularity on polyethylene wear and osteolysis in total hip arthroplasty," *The Journal of Bone & Joint Surgery—American Volume*, vol. 84, no. 1, pp. 58–63, 2002.

[16] W. L. Walter, J. Clabeaux, T. M. Wright, W. Walsh, W. K. Walter, and T. P. Sculco, "Mechanisms for pumping fluid through

cementless acetabular components with holes," *The Journal of Arthroplasty*, vol. 20, no. 8, pp. 1042–1048, 2005.

[17] Y. Kim, C. Tanaka, and H. Kanoe, "Long-term outcome of acetabular reconstruction using a kerboull-type acetabular reinforcement device with hydroxyapetite granule and structural autograft for AAOS type II and III acetabular defects," *Journal of Arthroplasty*, vol. 30, no. 10, pp. 1810–1814, 2015.

33

Thumb Reconstruction with Arthrodesis to the Second Metacarpal following Sarcoma Excision

Christopher Hein, Barry Watkins, and Lee M. Zuckerman

Department of Orthopaedic Surgery, Loma Linda University Medical Center, 11406 Loma Linda Drive, Suite 218, Loma Linda, CA 92354, USA

Correspondence should be addressed to Lee M. Zuckerman; lzuckerman@llu.edu

Academic Editor: Elke R. Ahlmann

Primary sarcomas of the thumb metacarpal are rare malignant lesions. Surgical treatment involves amputation versus tumor resection with thumb reconstruction. If complete tumor resection is possible, thumb preservation may be considered, as the thumb is vital to hand function. Following tumor resection, previous reports have described graft reconstruction with fusion to the trapezium or scaphoid. We present two cases of sarcoma necessitating resection of the thumb metacarpal that were reconstructed with an arthrodesis of the proximal phalanx to the second metacarpal shaft. Arthrodesis to the second metacarpal allows robust bony contact for fusion as well as improved resting position of the thumb. At 2- and 4-year follow-up, both patients have a stable, pain-free thumb without evidence of local recurrence.

1. Introduction

Primary bony tumors of the thumb metacarpal are a rare and challenging problem [1]. Chondrosarcoma is the most common malignant tumor of the hand but typically arises in the metacarpal or proximal phalanx of the index or small finger [2]. Synovial sarcoma is even less common in the fingers and usually presents in the wrist or hand. Historically, ray resection represented the foundation of treatment for malignant metacarpal lesions. However, ray resection of the thumb results in a greater functional deficit as compared with the resection of the other digits [3]. Thumb reconstruction with allograft or autograft has been shown to be a reasonable treatment option if acceptable margins are feasible and vital neurologic structures are spared [1, 3–8]. Previous descriptions of reconstructive efforts include iliac crest, fibula, and ulna autograft arthrodesis to the carpus. We report two cases of sarcoma that required resection of the entire thumb metacarpal, including one chondrosarcoma and one synovial cell sarcoma. Both were treated by resection and autograft arthrodesis of the proximal phalanx of the thumb to the shaft of the second metacarpal. To our knowledge, this technique has not been previously described after tumor resection.

2. Case Reports

2.1. Case 1. A 60-year-old male was referred to the orthopaedic clinic for an enlarging left hand mass (Figure 1). The hard, originally painless mass was located on the dorsum of the left thumb metacarpal and had been present for 6 years. The mass began enlarging and became painful. Its size began to affect the patient's thumb function. Physical examination showed a large, firm, minimally tender mass on the dorsoradial aspect of the hand over the thumb metacarpal which measured approximately 9 cm. Interphalangeal (IP) joint motion was decreased from 0 to 30 degrees, and thumb abduction and opposition were minimal. He had no lymphadenopathy, no systemic symptoms, and normal laboratory values.

Plain radiographs (Figure 2(a)) revealed a large, partially calcified mass arising from the thumb metacarpal. T1-weighted magnetic resonance imaging (MRI) (Figure 2(b)) showed a heterogeneous, expansile mass measuring 6 × 9 cm arising from the thumb metacarpal with complete involvement of the trapezium. T2-weighted imaging (Figure 2(c)) revealed a mass with increased signal and cystic, loculated regions without tendon sheath enhancement. A whole body bone scan and computed tomography (CT) scan of chest,

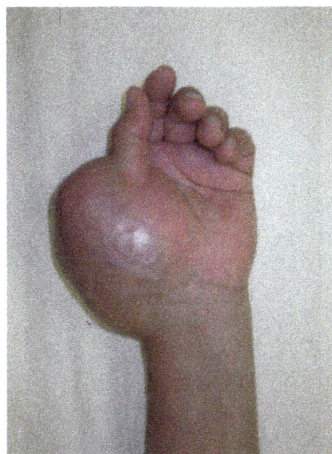

FIGURE 1: Preoperative photograph of the left hand demonstrating a large thumb mass.

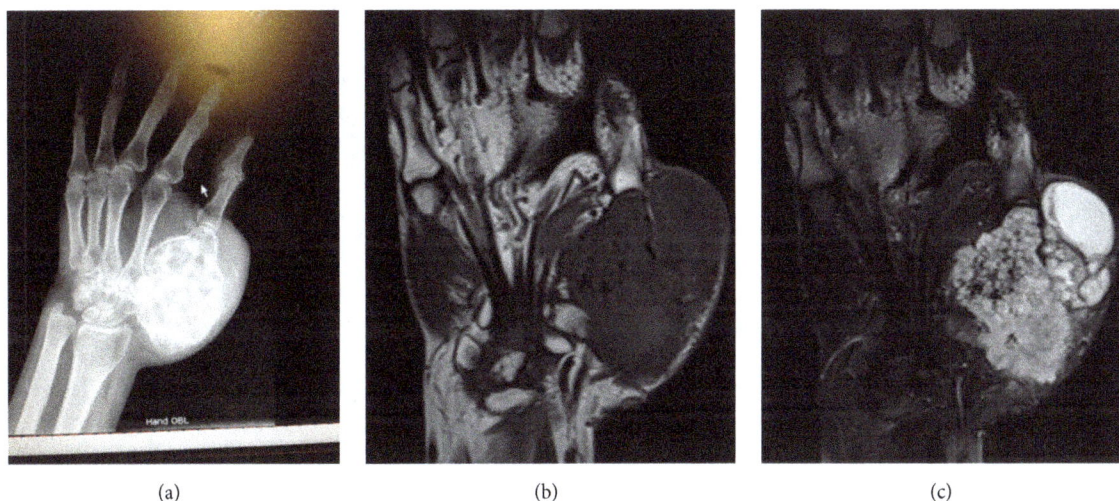

(a)　　　　　　　　　　　(b)　　　　　　　　　　　(c)

FIGURE 2: Preoperative imaging. (a) X-rays demonstrating a large, calcified tumor arising from the first metacarpal. (b) Coronal T1-weighted MRI of the left hand. (c) Coronal T2-weighted MRI of the left hand.

abdomen, and pelvis revealed no other lesions. A core biopsy was consistent with a Grade 2 chondrosarcoma.

Surgical treatment involved en bloc resection of the affected metacarpal with a portion of the proximal phalanx of the thumb and the entire trapezium in order to obtain negative margins. The extensor carpi radialis longus (ECRL), extensor pollicis longus (EPL), and flexor carpi radialis (FCR) were resected with the tumor. The flexor pollicis longus was uninvolved and therefore preserved. Tricortical iliac crest autograft was utilized for reconstruction of the proximal thumb and secured distally to the first proximal phalanx and proximally to the second metacarpal with two 2.7 mm locking plates and a lag screw in a position of opposition to the index finger. The EPL was reconstructed with free FCR autograft which was harvested proximally, away from the zone of tumor involvement. To prevent bowstringing of the extensor tendon, the ECRL was then harvested proximal to

the area of tumor involvement and was utilized to reconstruct the extensor retinaculum.

Postoperative pathology confirmed clear surgical margins. The postoperative course was complicated by necrosis of the skin and a wound dehiscence which resulted in exposed hardware. An irrigation and debridement were performed resulting in a wound measuring 9 × 6 cm. Coverage of the wound was obtained with a free fasciocutaneous flap from the dorsal forearm based on the posterior interosseous artery and anastomosed to the radial artery. Most recent follow-up at 4 years postoperatively revealed a stable, pain-free thumb. His IP joint had evidence of degenerative changes and his motion was limited from 0 to 5 degrees compared to 0 to 30 degrees preoperatively. There were no radiographic or clinical signs of recurrent disease. There was radiologic (Figure 3) and clinical evidence of a successful arthrodesis (Figures 4(a) and 4(b)). A Disabilities of the Arm, Shoulder and Hand (DASH) score

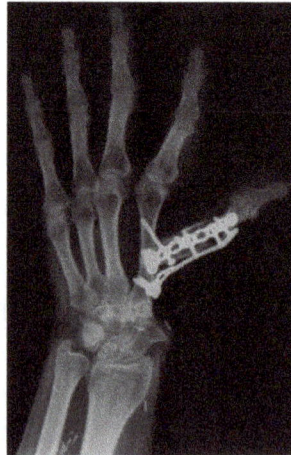

FIGURE 3: Postoperative X-ray of the left hand demonstrating fusion of the proximal phalanx of the thumb to the second metacarpal.

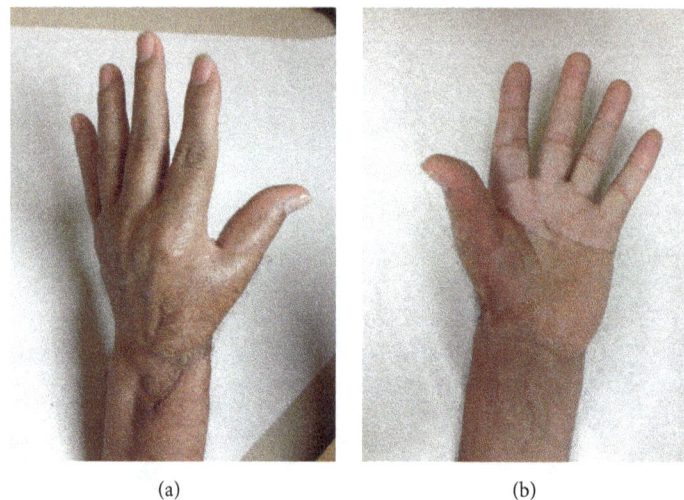

(a)   (b)

FIGURE 4: Postoperative clinical photographs. (a) Dorsal view. (b) Palmar view.

was 13.3 and the Musculoskeletal Tumor Society (MSTS) score was 25.

2.2. Case 2. A 39-year-old female was referred to the orthopaedic clinic for a left hand mass that had been enlarging over the past 9 months (Figure 5). Physical examination revealed a large, soft mass overlying the palmar and radial aspect of the thumb metacarpal with mild tenderness and intact thumb motion. Sensation and vascular status were normal. She had no fever or systemic symptoms and normal laboratory values.

Plain radiographs revealed a large, noncalcified soft tissue mass adjacent to the thumb metacarpal with some metacarpal erosion (Figure 6(a)). T1-weighted MRI sequences showed a large heterogeneous mass encompassing the thumb metacarpal with focal signal change in the metacarpal (Figure 6(b)). On T2-weighted imaging, the mass had increased signal and was multilobulated (Figure 6(c)). There was enhancement of the flexor pollicis longus and extensor tendon sheaths.

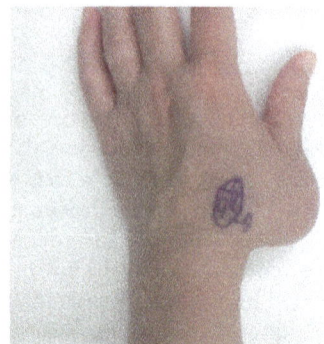

FIGURE 5: Preoperative photograph of the left hand demonstrating a large thumb mass.

A CT of the chest was normal and there was no lymphadenopathy. An open biopsy of the tumor revealed a highly cellular proliferation of spindle cells in sheets consistent with a high grade synovial cell sarcoma.

(a)

(b)

(c)

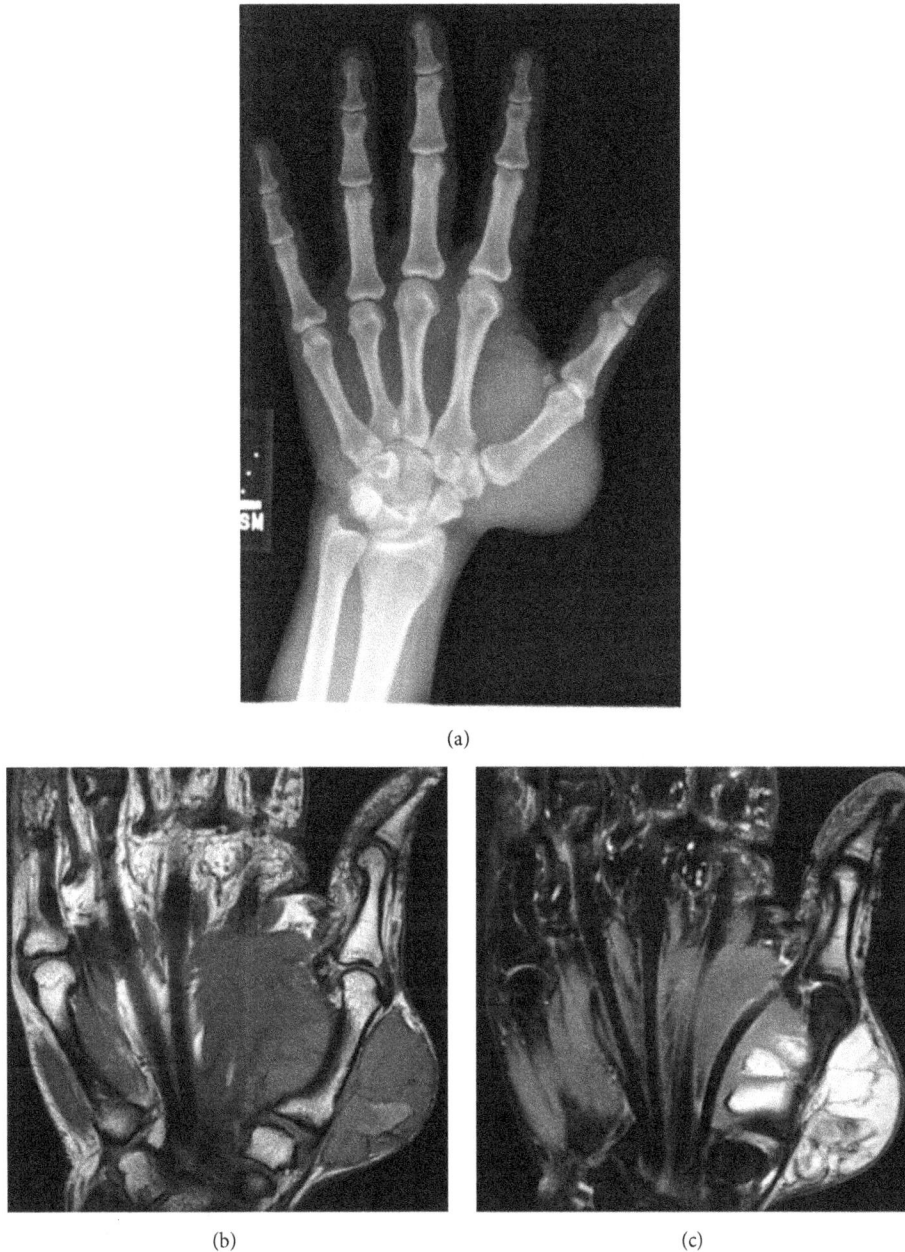

FIGURE 6: Preoperative imaging. (a) X-rays demonstrating a soft tissue mass with some underlying bony erosion of the first metacarpal. (b) Coronal T1-weighted MRI of the left hand demonstrating envelopment of the first metacarpal. (c) Coronal T2-weighted MRI of the left hand demonstrating involvement of the first metacarpal.

Surgical resection with a staged reconstruction was then performed. A staged reconstruction was chosen in this case to confirm negative margins prior to undergoing reconstruction. A vascularized autograft was chosen to optimize the chance of arthrodesis in the setting of planned adjuvant radiation therapy. The entire thumb metacarpal, trapezium, flexor pollicis longus, EPL, and first dorsal compartment tendons were resected and the wound was closed with provisional K-wire fixation of the thumb. Pathologic examination revealed negative margins. One week later, the patient returned to the operating room for reconstruction. The metacarpal

reconstruction was performed with a 5.5 cm distal radial osteofasciocutaneous flap vascularized by the radial artery. The graft was fixed proximally to the index metacarpal with a 2.4 mm locking plate and lag screw and distally to the proximal phalanx with a separate 2.4 mm locking plate. The graft was positioned to provide for index finger to thumb opposition with the thumb IP joint in flexion. Full flexion of the index finger to the palm was obtained when the thumb IP joint was extended. Approximately one-half of the distal radial shaft and metaphysis were utilized, and the defect was prophylactically stabilized with a contoured volar

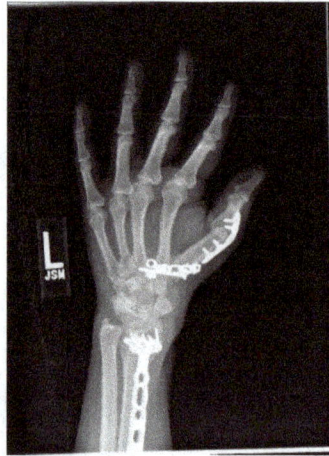

FIGURE 7: Postoperative X-ray of the left hand.

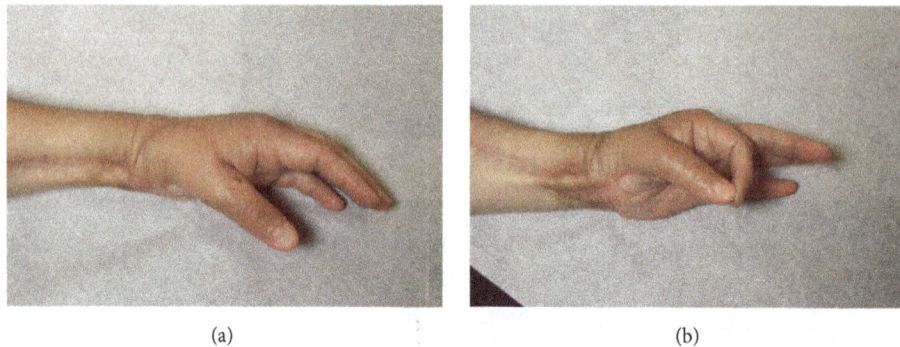

(a)

(b)

FIGURE 8: Postoperative clinical photographs. (a) Dorsal view of the thumb in a resting position. (b) Demonstration of the patient performing a functional pinch to the index finger.

locking plate (Figure 7). An extensor indicis proprius to EPL tendon transfer was then performed to restore extension of the thumb.

The patient received adjuvant radiation to the area with a total of 50 grays of radiation. At 2 years, thumb IP range of motion was 0–70 degrees compared to 0–80 degrees preoperatively. She had functional pinch strength and no evidence of local recurrence (Figures 8(a) and 8(b)). DASH and MSTS scores were 17.5 and 24, respectively. Clinical and radiographic arthrodesis has been achieved.

3. Discussion

Chondrosarcoma involvement of the hands and feet comprise 1–3.2% of all chondrosarcomas, and most of these are pha-langeal tumors [3, 9, 10]. Of 23 chondrosarcomas of the hand reported in the Scottish Bone Tumour Registry from 1954 to 1999, only one case involved the thumb metacarpal [10].

Synovial cell sarcoma is an uncommon soft tissue tumor that usually presents in the lower extremities. Deshmukh et al. reported only 5 synovial cell sarcomas occurring in the hand out of a total of 135 patients [11]. Successful treatment of these types of tumors with restoration of function is more complex then treating lesions of the other digits, as

the thumb is integral to hand function [3]. Amputation of the thumb, while highly successful in preventing local recurrence, results in a significant functional deficit that is greater than amputation of the other digits [12]. Therefore, a concerted effort to maintain function while still performing a resection with negative surgical margins is the goal when treating malignant tumors of the thumb metacarpal.

Iliac crest, fibular allograft, free fibular autograft, and distal ulna have all been described for reconstruction after tumor removal at the first metacarpal [1, 5, 7, 8]. In these reports, the graft was secured to the trapezium or scaphoid proximally. In our case series, the tumors were large and necessitated resection of the trapezium in order to obtain negative margins. The options for proximal arthrodesis were therefore limited to the scaphoid or index metacarpal. Auto-graft was used in both cases. As the treatment plan for the patient with the chondrosarcoma did not involve adjuvant radiation, iliac crest was chosen. A vascularized autograft was chosen when adjuvant radiation was used in order to increase the rate of fusion. Both options resulted in a successful arthrodesis.

Although described previously with good results, osteosynthesis to the scaphoid presents multiple potential problems [6]. First, the bony surface area for arthrodesis between graft and scaphoid is small, decreasing the chance of a successful fusion. Second, the distance from the proximal base of the graft to the tip of the thumb is increased with fixation to the scaphoid necessitating a larger graft. This creates a longer lever arm with increased torque at the fusion sites, which may result in a nonunion or failure of the hardware. In addition to this, resection of the thenar musculature and fusion of the thumb results in loss of the carpometacarpal motion. A fusion to the scaphoid fixes the base of the thumb in extension, which makes palmar adduction or abduction for grip more difficult.

The natural resting position of the thumb is in opposition to the distal phalanx of the index finger with the metacarpophalangeal (MCP) and IP joints flexed 10–15 degrees [13]. With grasp and key pinch activities, axial rotation at the trapeziometacarpal joint places the thumb out of the plane of the hand and in a position of function. This motion is lost following reconstruction with arthrodesis of the MCP and trapeziometacarpal joints. Therefore, the optimal position of fusion is one where the thumb can be placed in a position of maximum function, which is in slight palmar abduction and external rotation. In this position, the thumb is able to participate in power grip and pinch with IP flexion. Our reconstructive technique utilized a fusion site to the index metacarpal shaft. Due to the size and shape of the metacarpal, this position was able to be achieved without difficulty. Other benefits include the increased surface area for the arthrodesis to occur. There is also an increased area for placement of hardware to the metacarpal than to the carpus, providing for a higher likelihood of a successful fusion and a more stable base to allow earlier participation in rehabilitation. The position of the thumb at rest is also able to be placed further outside the plane of the hand, which more closely resembles the natural resting position of the thumb. This enhances the cosmesis of the reconstruction. Lastly, for functional activities, including key pinch and grasp, IP flexion in a plane perpendicular to the hand most closely resembles the anatomic position of function during key pinch and grasping activities.

In conclusion, we described two cases of sarcoma, necessitating resection of the thumb metacarpal that were reconstructed with an arthrodesis of the proximal phalanx of the thumb to the index metacarpal. Fusion was achieved in both cases and both patients had a pain-free, functional, and cosmetically acceptable thumb with no local recurrence. Arthrodesis of the thumb to the second metacarpal is a viable treatment option after tumor resection.

Ethical Approval

Each author certifies that his or her institution approved or waived approval for the reporting of this case and that all investigations were conducted in conformity with ethical principles of research.

Competing Interests

Each author certifies that he or she, or a member of his or her immediate family, has no funding or commercial associations (e.g., consultancies, stock ownership, equity interest, and patent/licensing arrangements) that might pose a conflict of interests in connection with the submitted paper.

References

[1] G. Pathak, W. B. Conolly, and S. W. McCarthy, "Chondrosarcoma of thumb metacarpal—a case report with literature review," *Hand Surgery*, vol. 6, no. 1, pp. 81–87, 2001.

[2] A.-M. Plate, G. Steiner, and M. A. Posner, "Malignant tumors of the hand and wrist," *Journal of the American Academy of Orthopaedic Surgeons*, vol. 14, no. 12, pp. 680–692, 2006.

[3] A. Miyake, H. Morioka, H. Yabe et al., "A case of metacarpal chondrosarcoma of the thumb," *Archives of Orthopaedic and Trauma Surgery*, vol. 126, no. 6, pp. 406–410, 2006.

[4] L. R. Ramos-Pascua, Ó. Fernández-Hernández, S. S. Herráez, J. Á. S. Sánchez, and T. F. Corral, "Ewing sarcoma of the first metacarpal with a 9-year follow-up: case report," *Journal of Hand Surgery—American Volume*, vol. 38, no. 8, pp. 1575–1578, 2013.

[5] B. S. Dhinsa, B. S. Mann, S. Z. Nawaz, A. Jalgaonkar, T. W. R. Briggs, and J. A. Skinner, "Free fibular graft reconstruction following resection of chondrosarcoma in the first metacarpal," *Hand Surgery*, vol. 16, no. 3, pp. 357–360, 2011.

[6] G. Biswas, A. Parashar, S. Ghosh, and N. Kakkar, "Extraosseous ewing's sarcoma of the thumb," *Journal of Hand Surgery: European Volume*, vol. 33, no. 5, pp. 667–669, 2008.

[7] P. T. Calvert, G. E. MacLellan, and M. F. Sullivan, "Chondrosarcoma of the thumb a case report of treatment with preservation of function," *Journal of Hand Surgery—British Volume*, vol. 10, no. 3, pp. 415–417, 1985.

[8] K. B. Jones, J. A. Buckwalter, and E. F. McCarthy, "Parosteal osteosarcoma of the thumb metacarpal: a case report," *The Iowa Orthopaedic Journal*, vol. 26, pp. 134–136, 2006.

[9] S. Patil, M. V. C. De Silva, J. Crossan, and R. Reid, "Chondrosarcoma of small bones of the hand," *Journal of Hand Surgery*, vol. 28, no. 6, pp. 602–608, 2003.

[10] K. K. Unni, *Dahlin's Bone Tumors: General Aspects and Data on 11087 Cases*, Lippincott-Raven, New York, NY, USA, 5th edition, 1996.

[11] R. Deshmukh, H. J. Mankin, and S. Singer, "Synovial sarcoma: the importance of size and location for survival," *Clinical Orthopaedics and Related Research*, vol. 419, pp. 155–161, 2004.

[12] M. E. Puhaindran, C. P. Rothrock, and E. A. Athanasian, "Surgical management for malignant tumors of the thumb," *Hand*, vol. 6, no. 4, pp. 373–377, 2011.

[13] W. P. Cooney III, M. J. Lucca, E. Y. S. Chao, and R. L. Linscheid, "The kinesiology of the thumb trapeziometacarpal joint," *The Journal of Bone & Joint Surgery—American Volume*, vol. 63, no. 9, pp. 1371–1381, 1981.

34

Traumatic Rupture of an Intermediate Tendon in a Patient with Patellar Duplication

Stéphane Pelet,[1,2] **Mathieu Hébert,**[2] **Amerigo Balatri,**[2] **and Pierre-Alexandre LeBlanc**[2]

[1]*Centre de Recherche FRSQ du CHU de Québec, Hôpital de l'Enfant-Jésus, 1401 18ème rue, Ville de Québec, QC, Canada G1J 1Z4*

[2]*Department of Orthopedic Surgery, CHU de Québec, Hôpital de l'Enfant-Jésus, 1401 18ème rue, Ville de Québec, QC, Canada G1J 1Z4*

Correspondence should be addressed to Amerigo Balatri; balatria@gmail.com

Academic Editor: Georg Singer

Patellar duplication is a rare asymptomatic condition. The diagnosis is often made following a traumatic event associated with an injury to the knee extensor mechanism. The treatment is often surgical and consists in removal of the smaller part of the patella with tendon reinsertion. The presence and rupture of an intermediate tendon between the two parts of the patella have not been reported in the modern literature. We present a traumatic rupture of an intermediate tendon in a patient with horizontal patellar duplication. The surgical management consisted of tenorrhaphy protected with a figure-of-eight tension band wire approximating the two parts of the patella. The patient recovered full knee range of motion and quadriceps strength at the last 8-month follow-up.

1. Introduction

Patellar duplication is a rare asymptomatic condition. The diagnosis is often accidentally stated after a traumatic event leading to a weak knee extensor mechanism. Most cases are reported during adolescence and are consecutive to either a powerful quadriceps tensing or a fall [1]. The size of both parts can differ from one case to another and influences the surgical management in case of disruption.

The presence of an intermediate tendon connecting the two patellar parts was only described by Petty [2]. The ruptured intermediate tendon was excised and healing achieved through bone fusion of the two patellar parts. The knee biomechanics is directly related to the restoration of its initial anatomy, including the extensor mechanism length. An anatomical repair should provide a better functional outcome.

We present a traumatic rupture of an intermediate tendon in a 47-year-old patient with horizontal patellar duplication. An anatomical repair of the ruptured tendon was performed with an excellent functional outcome.

2. Case Report

A 47-year-old woman presented at our emergency room with anterior right knee pain, one day after a fall at home on level surface. She was unable to stand on her right leg. No previous trauma or knee pain was reported. Past medical history was positive for pituitary dwarfism and epilepsy. Physical examination revealed knee effusion and anterior hematoma. The knee was stable in all directions. Passive range of motion was complete, but the patient was unable to actively extend her knee. A complete extension lag was observed.

Knee radiographs were obtained and demonstrated a significant diastasis between two patellar parts (Figures 1(a) and 1(b)). As both parts presented regular contours without evidence of acute fracture rims, further investigation was required. Magnetic resonance imaging (MRI) confirmed the presence of an intermediate ruptured tendon between the two patellar parts (Figure 1(c)).

The diagnosis of an intermediate tendon rupture in a duplicate patella was stated. In order to restore the integrity and length of the extensor mechanism, we proposed an

(a)　　　　　　　　(b)　　　　　　　　(c)

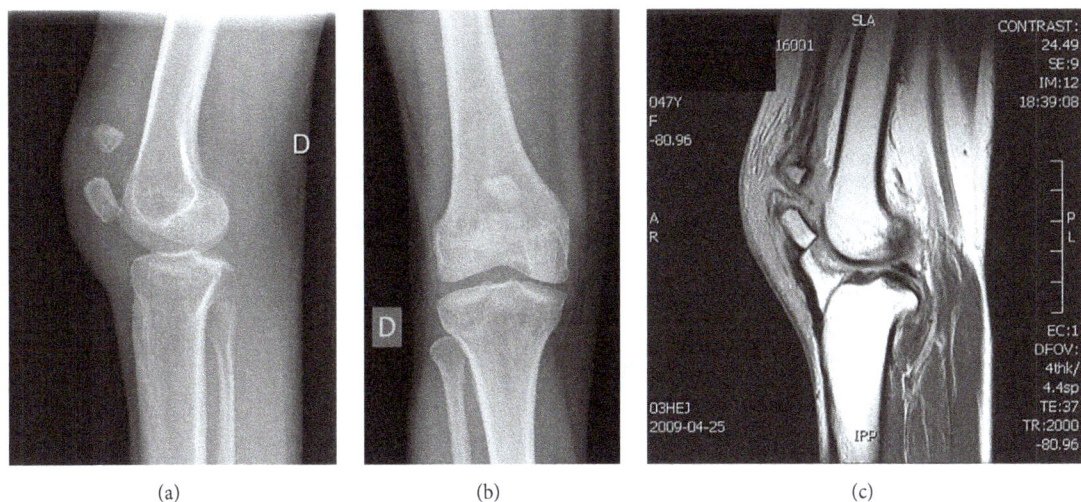

FIGURE 1: Lateral (a) and anteroposterior (b) knee views demonstrating a gap between the two parts of a duplicate patella. (c) Soft tissue is identified between the two parts of the patella (MRI T1 sagittal view).

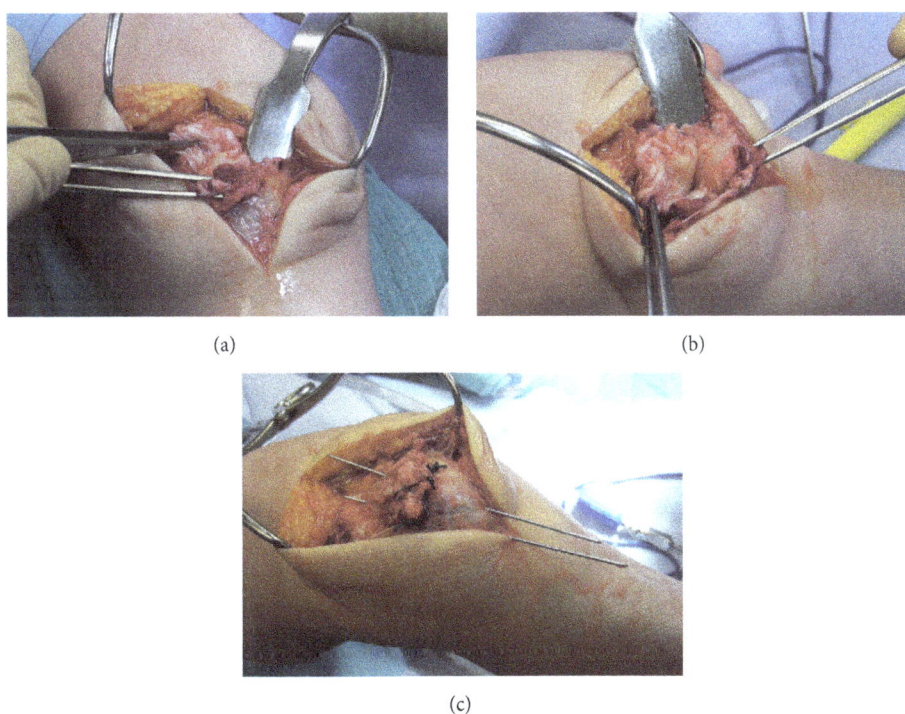

(a)　　　　　　　　(b)

(c)

FIGURE 2: Surgical pictures presenting (a) the proximal and distal stumps of the ruptured intermediate tendon, (b) the use of two 1.6 mm K-wires to reduce both patella parts, and (c) the tenorrhaphy protected with two K-wires.

anatomical repair of the intermediate tendon. The surgery was performed the same day.

2.1. Surgical Procedure. Surgery was performed under general anesthesia, standard intravenous antibiotic prophylaxis, and tourniquet. A longitudinal 10 cm incision was centered on the patellar parts. Immediately after skin opening a voluminous hematoma was discharged at the level between the two patellar parts. A ruptured tendon was observed at this level. The two patellar parts were identified, without evidence of an acute or old fracture. A strip of tendon with the characteristics of a fully developed insertion was observed at both the distal part of the proximal patellar piece and the proximal aspect of the distal patellar part (Figure 2(a)). The medial and lateral retinacula were ruptured. The knee was positioned at 60° of flexion, and the two patellar parts were brought closer with two 1.6 mm K-wires without removing any tissue at the interface (Figure 2(b)). Tenorrhaphy was performed (without any excessive tension or shortening

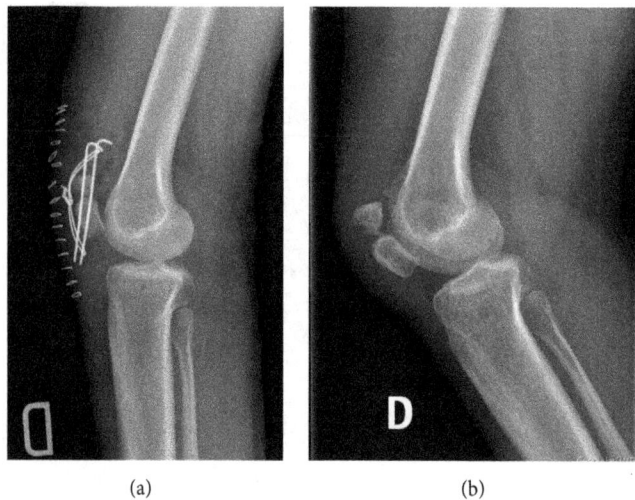

(a)   (b)

FIGURE 3: Immediate postoperative (a) and 8-month (b) lateral knee views.

of the tendon) through multiple sutures with Ethibond 1 (Figure 2(c)). A figure-of-eight tension band wire was added to protect the tenorrhaphy (Figure 3(a)).

Postoperative care consisted of full weight-bearing with a hinged brace (blocked in full extension) for six weeks. Passive knee flexion was limited to 60 degrees during the first ten days and progressively increased to achieve 90 degrees after six weeks. Isometric quadriceps contraction was initiated immediately after surgery. Active knee motion (flexion and extension) and isokinetic quadriceps contraction were authorized after six weeks.

The tension band was removed after 6 months for slight discomfort, although the patient had already recovered a full active knee range of motion. The patient presented for a final visit 8 months after the surgery. She had a painless knee with full range of motion and symmetric quadriceps extension strength (no extension lag). The last radiographs illustrate a typically healed duplicate patella with a free space between the two parts, as bone healing was not the goal (Figure 3(b)).

3. Discussion

Two etiological theories explain the development of a duplicate patella. The first hypothesis refers to a congenital malformation. This assertion is supported by the report of bilateral horizontal cases [1] and the observation of coronal [3] and frontal patellar duplication (also called double layer patella, reported in patients with multiple epiphyseal dysplasia) [4]. A fully developed tendon between the two patellar parts was described in these reports.

The second hypothesis considers the duplicate patella as the result of the natural healing of an undiagnosed sleeve fracture. This fracture occurs in skeletally immature patients and represents a traumatic avulsion of the extensor mechanism with a small sleeve of cartilage and periosteum. These fractures can occur at either the proximal or the distal pole of the patella. The treatment is mainly surgical;

however, some cases were successfully treated with braces [1]. The osteogenic potential of the cartilage sleeve explains the evolution towards a duplicate patella [5, 6].

The present case occurred in a patient with pituitary dwarfism. The two patellar parts have a significant size and the patient did not report any previous knee trauma. A previous sleeve fracture is unlikely. A duplicate patella is not commonly related to patients with dwarfism from any cause, and we were unable to find other reported cases in the literature with this kind of association. The duplicate patella's etiology remains unclear.

Most patellar duplications are asymptomatic [7] and surgery is reserved for cases when the continuity of the knee extensor mechanism is broken. The goal of the surgical management is to achieve good healing of the extensor mechanism with restoration of its initial length. Excessive shortening will result in a loss of knee flexion and lengthening in an extension lag.

The main surgical options are excision of the small fragment and tendon reinsertion into the remaining patellar part, rigid fixation of both parts in order to achieve bone healing, or anatomical repair of the intermediate tendon.

This case report is the first description of an intermediate tendon rupture in a patient with horizontal patellar duplication, treated with an anatomical repair. The treatment's choice was mainly influenced by the size of both fragments. An excision of the proximal patellar part and the resection of the intermediate tendon in order to achieve bone fusion would both result in a significant loss of flexion (we estimated in this case 2 to 3 cm extensor mechanism shortening with these options). An anatomical repair was temporarily protected by a tension band. The tendon suture was performed in 60-degree flexion in order to prevent overtightening. The original length of the extensor mechanism was restored, and the final outcome was excellent with a full knee range of motion and symmetrical complete quadriceps strength. The remaining gap between the two patellar parts on the final lateral knee view, with an anatomical patellar height, illustrates the characteristics of an intact horizontal duplicate patella with an intermediate tendon.

Petty reported a similar case in 1925, with rupture of an intermediate tendon in a horizontal duplicate patella [2]. The treatment consisted in bone fusion. However, the report did not describe the nature of the intermediate tendon. The final clinical outcome is unknown except that bone fusion was achieved.

Cipolla et al. reported six patients with rupture of the knee extensor mechanism and duplicate patella [8]. The treatment consisted in excision of the smaller patellar part and tendon reinsertion. The final clinical outcome was considered good with a 5-degree loss of knee flexion and some extension lag. All cases consisted of very small patellar parts (or even calcifications). The diagnostic etiology of a previous sleeve fracture was proposed. This small series differed from this case report as no cases were significant horizontal double patella. The presence and nature of the intermediate tendon were also not reported.

Patellar duplications should not be confused with bipartite patella. The development of bipartite patella is related to an anomaly in the ossification process. An original classification was proposed by Saupe [9]; type I is apical, type II lateral, and type III superolateral (the most frequent). Type I was excluded from bipartite patella by many authors since the presence of an apical ossification nucleus has never been demonstrated [10]. This type probably corresponds to a double patella. So-called bipartite patella fractures correspond to an injury to the intermediate tissue between the two patellar parts and have usually no influence on the knee extensor mechanism. Nonsurgical management is proposed for most cases [11] and surgery reserved for the rare cases with an injury of the extensor mechanism [12–16].

The need for complementary imaging is mandatory to diagnose the extensor mechanism rupture and identify an intermediate tendon in a patient with a painful double patella. We propose to request knee MRI in every patient presenting with a complete extension lag and a lateral knee radiograph describing a gap between two patellar parts with suspicious fracture rims.

This case illustrates the importance of a precise initial diagnosis. We should think of a double patella with intermediate tendon rupture in all cases when the two separated patellar fragments are atypical. Differential diagnosis with a bipartite patella is necessary. Complementary imaging helps to best understand the lesion. An anatomical tendon repair can provide an excellent clinical outcome.

Competing Interests

The authors have no conflict of interests to disclose.

References

[1] D. P. Grogan, T. P. Carey, D. Leffers, and J. A. Ogden, "Avulsion fractures of the patella," *Journal of Pediatric Orthopaedics*, vol. 10, no. 6, pp. 721–730, 1990.

[2] M. J. Petty, "Two cases of abnormal patellae," *British Journal of Surgery*, vol. 12, no. 48, pp. 799–800, 1925.

[3] J. Gasco, J. M. Del Pino, and F. Gomar-Sancho, "Double patella. A case of duplication in the coronal plane," *Journal of Bone and Joint Surgery B*, vol. 69, no. 4, pp. 602–603, 1987.

[4] H. Hodkinson, "Double patellae in MEDHM hodkinson," *The Journal of Bone and Joint Surgery. American*, vol. 3, p. 569, 1962.

[5] G. R. Houghton and C. E. Ackroyd, "Sleeve fractures of the patella in children. A report of three cases," *Journal of Bone and Joint Surgery—Series B*, vol. 61, no. 2, pp. 165–168, 1979.

[6] E. Yeung and J. Ireland, "An unusual double patella: a case report," *Knee*, vol. 11, no. 2, pp. 129–131, 2004.

[7] S. Weinberg, "Case report 177," *Skeletal Radiology*, vol. 7, no. 3, pp. 223–224, 1981.

[8] M. Cipolla, G. Cerullo, V. Franco, E. Gianní, and G. Puddu, "The double patella syndrome," *Knee Surgery, Sports Traumatology, Arthroscopy*, vol. 3, no. 1, pp. 21–25, 1995.

[9] H. Saupe, "Primare knochenmark seilerung der kniescheibe," *Deutsche z Chir*, pp. 228–386, 1943.

[10] Y. Oohashi, T. Koshino, and Y. Oohashi, "Clinical features and classification of bipartite or tripartite patella," *Knee Surgery, Sports Traumatology, Arthroscopy*, vol. 18, no. 11, pp. 1465–1469, 2010.

[11] S. R. Carter, "Traumatic separation of a bipartite patella," *Injury*, vol. 20, no. 4, p. 244, 1989.

[12] G. H. Canizares and F. H. Selesnick, "Bipartite patella fracture," *Arthroscopy - Journal of Arthroscopic and Related Surgery*, vol. 19, no. 2, pp. 215–217, 2003.

[13] G. W. Woods, D. P. O'Connor, and H. A. Elkousy, "Quadriceps tendon rupture through a superolateral bipartite patella," *The Journal of Knee Surgery*, vol. 20, no. 4, pp. 293–295, 2007.

[14] H. Tonotsuka and Y. Yamamoto, "Separation of a bipartite patella combined with quadriceps tendon rupture: a case report," *Knee*, vol. 15, no. 1, pp. 64–67, 2008.

[15] H. Okuno, T. Sugita, T. Kawamata, M. Ohnuma, N. Yamada, and Y. Yoshizumi, "Traumatic separation of a type I bipartite patella: a report of four knees," *Clinical Orthopaedics and Related Research*, no. 420, pp. 257–260, 2004.

[16] M. Tauber, N. Matis, and H. Resch, "Traumatic separation of an uncommon bipartite patella type: a case report," *Knee Surgery, Sports Traumatology, Arthroscopy*, vol. 15, no. 1, pp. 83–87, 2007.

35

Surgical Treatment for Occipital Condyle Fracture, C1 Dislocation, and Cerebellar Contusion with Hemorrhage after Blunt Head Trauma

Shigeo Ueda, Nobuhiro Sasaki, Miyuki Fukuda, and Minoru Hoshimaru

Shin-Aikai Spine Center, Katano Hospital, Katano City, Osaka, Japan

Correspondence should be addressed to Shigeo Ueda; uedashigeo@yahoo.co.jp

Academic Editor: Eyal Itshayek

Occipital condyle fractures (OCFs) have been treated as rare traumatic injuries, but the number of reported OCFs has gradually increased because of the popularization of computed tomography (CT) and magnetic resonance imaging (MRI). The patient in this report presented with OCFs and C1 dislocation, along with traumatic cerebellar hemorrhage, which led to craniovertebral junction instability. This case was also an extremely rare clinical condition in which the patient presented with traumatic lower cranial nerve palsy secondary to OCFs. When the patient was transferred to our hospital, the occipital bone remained defective extensively due to surgical treatment of cerebellar hemorrhage. For this reason, concurrent cranioplasty was performed with resin in order to fix the occipital bone plate strongly. The resin-made occipital bone was used to secure a titanium plate and screws enabled us to perform posterior fusion of the craniovertebral junction. Although the patient wore a halo vest for 3 months after surgery, lower cranial nerve symptoms, including not only neck pain but also paralysis of the throat and larynx, improved postoperatively. No complications were detected during outpatient follow-up, which continued for 5 years postoperatively.

1. Introduction

Head trauma can be accompanied by parenchymal brain damage; one study [1] reported that 4% of patients who experienced severe traumatic brain injuries, particularly with severely impaired consciousness (Glasgow Coma Scale scores of 3–6 on admission), developed occipital condylar fractures (OCFs). OCFs were considered rare traumatic injuries in the past, but, in recent years, they have been reported more frequently because of the popularization of computed tomography (CT) and magnetic resonance imaging (MRI) [1, 2]. OCFs rarely occurs sporadically, and, in many cases, they are associated with multiple traumas, especially cervical spine injury [3]. Patients exhibit various clinical symptoms of OCFs, but few are characteristic findings. However, it is known that OCFs lead to localized pain, limited range of motion, and severe nerve damage, especially lower cranial nerve (CN-IX to -XII) symptoms [4–6]. Clinical characteristics of lower cranial nerve palsy are hoarseness, difficulty swallowing (CN-IX and -X), and weakness in the shoulder and neck muscles (CN-XI). Hypoglossal nerve palsy

(CN-XII) causes swallowing disturbance and masticatory dysfunction, as well as dysarthria and anarthria. Proper diagnosis and treatment are critical because coexisting symptoms can result from undiagnosed or untreated OCFs, which sometimes can be fatal [7].

We experienced a case in which a patient return to normal activities of daily living after surgical treatment who experienced dislocation of the atlas (C1), fractures of the left occipital condyle, and a traumatic hemorrhagic cerebellar contusion in the left hemisphere caused by blunt head trauma. An extensive literature review revealed that there have been few reports of surgical treatment in patients with OCFs. Therefore, this is the first report of the simultaneous performance of cranioplasty and posterior fusion of the craniovertebral junction.

2. Case Presentation

A 57-year-old man, who fell off of a bicycle and bruised the back of his head, became comatose immediately after the accident and was transported to a medical emergency center. He had a score of 7 on the GCS at the time of ambulance transport. CT of the head revealed hemorrhagic cerebellar contusion in the left hemisphere, fractures of the left occipital condyle, and C1 dislocation. Brain herniation occurred due to cerebral edema associated with the hemorrhagic contusion of the left cerebellar hemisphere, which was a medical emergency (Figure 1). Physicians at the medical emergency center performed lifesaving left suboccipital craniotomy and removed the hematoma and a part of the cerebellar hemisphere damaged by the contusion. Two weeks after surgery, the physicians intended to perform extubation due to the patient's improved of consciousness, since airway narrowing caused by left-sided vocal cord paralysis was observed, tracheostomy was additionally performed. At that time, neurological findings revealed lower cranial nerve (CN-IX to -XII) palsy. The patient was referred to our hospital for OCF and C1 dislocation treatment. On admission, he had clear consciousness but required bed rest in the supine position because of prominent neck pain that occurred when he was in the seated position. Although he complained of muscle weakness, which resulted from the prolonged bed rest, no obvious motor paralysis of the four extremities or sensory impairment was observed; however, he experienced left trapezius weakness, as well as paralysis of the larynx and the left side of the throat, which were associated with lower cranial nerve (CN-IX to -XII) palsy.

2.1. Imaging in the Preoperative Evaluation. CT revealed OCFs associated with C1 dislocation. A fracture extended to the left jugular foramen and hypoglossal canal. The left and medial sides of the occipital bone were defective because of the left suboccipital craniotomy (Figure 2). The left vertebral artery, which normally runs through the vertebrae proceeding away from the C1 vertebra, was not revealed by CT angiography, indicating traumatic vertebral artery occlusion.

2.2. Preoperative Care. We found that the neck pain was largely due to craniovertebral junction instability because halo vest immobilization (HVI) relieved the pain. We adjusted the craniovertebral angles in a halo vest and optimized them to prevent airway narrowing and swallowing disturbance. We made sure that HVI did not interfere with everyday activities for the patient after the halo vest had been in place and positioned at this angle for several days.

2.3. Surgery. The patient was positioned prone in a halo ring after induction of general anesthesia. At the time of prone positioning, under lateral fluoroscopic guidance, we set the craniovertebral angles that had been optimized prior to surgery. We incised the skin along the marked median nuchal line from the external occipital protuberance to immediately above the seventh cervical (C7) spinous process and detached the posterior muscle group. A resin-made occipital bone was formed in accordance with the defective part of the occipital bone. Just before curing, the occipital bone plate and screws to be used for posterior fusion of the craniovertebral junction were also embedded together in resin. The resin-made occipital bone was placed in the defect's position and anchored with a titanium plate. We performed left-sided

occipital cervical fusion by connecting vertebral arch pedicle screws with the occipital bone plate that had been secured to the resin-made occipital bone. On the right side, this occipital bone plate was immobilized with screws of C2 and C3 lateral mass at the remaining area of occipital bone. We harvested the iliac crest bone and grafted it onto the tip of the decorticalized spinous process of the C2 vertebra and the dorsal part of the occipital bone. The spongy bone was used in order to avoid creating dead space. The grafted bone was fixed by an ultrahigh molecular weight polyethylene cable (Figure 3).

2.4. Postoperative Care. The patient underwent rehabilitation in the halo vest for 3 months after surgery. Initially, he required tube feeding but later could ingest food orally because of physical therapy and dysarthria therapy offered by a speech therapist, as well as of swallowing and breathing training. He had mild paralysis of the left side of his throat and larynx, but sealing the tracheostomy site was possible. He walked independently and left the hospital following 5 months of rehabilitation after surgery. One year later, he returned to work as a school principal. Outpatient follow-up continued for 5 years postoperatively, but there were no newly developed complications. We observed trapezius weakness associated with left spinal accessory nerve palsy but did not detect symptoms of other lower cranial nerve palsies. X-ray and CT examination showed good bone graft incorporation, and no displacement of the resin-made occipital bone was observed (Figure 4).

3. Discussion

After head trauma, cervical spine injuries require careful evaluation, particularly craniovertebral junction injuries, such as OCFs, which can potentially lead to fatal outcomes or significant partial disability [8]. Furthermore, patients with severely impaired consciousness associated with intracranial injuries require careful attention, because stability of the craniovertebral junction is not always assessed and both management and treatment are not always adequately provided, which can lead to unfortunate outcomes [3, 9]. In our case, however, because the original imaging findings clearly showed C1 dislocation and strongly indicated craniovertebral junction instability, we strictly managed the patient, with local rest, in order to prevent cervical cord injury and following spinal shock when changing position. As a result, we successfully avoided secondary conditions.

In 1988, Anderson and Montesano published a classification system of OCFs [10], which was revised by Tuli et al. in 1997 [11]. In the revised classification system, Tuli et al. divided OCFs into three types based on the following approaches: with or without ligament injuries according to CT and MRI findings and with or without rotation and displacement of the occipital bone-C1-C2 alignment. The three types of this classification system are type 1, which includes fractures without displacement; type 2A, which includes fractures without ligament injuries; and type 2B, which includes a clearly identified ligament injury in the craniovertebral junction or identified rotation and displacement in occipital bone-C1-C2 alignment. Tuli et al. further

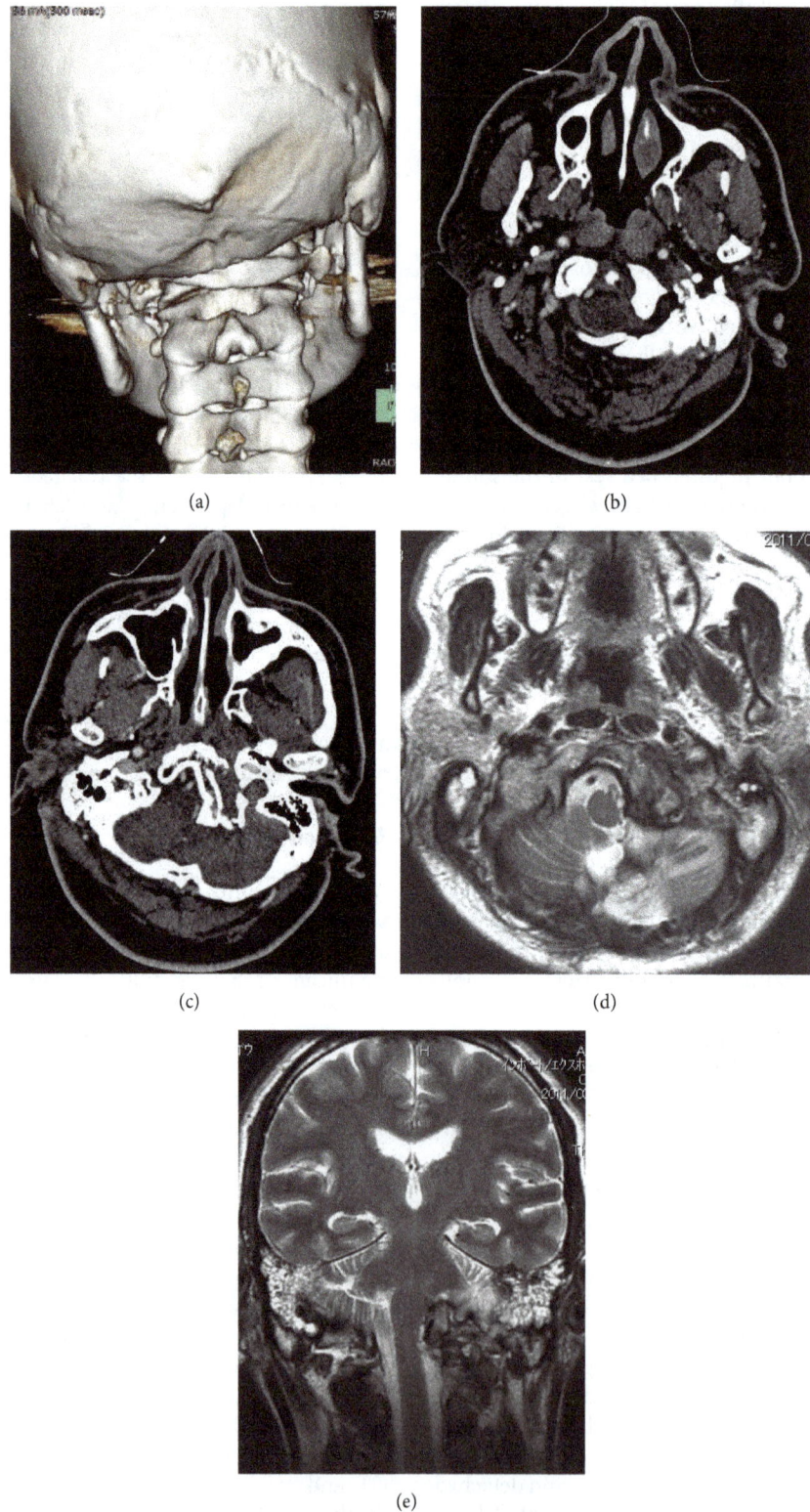

(a)

(b)

(c)

(d)

(e)

FIGURE 1: Images from a three-dimensional computed tomography (a), enhanced computed tomography (b and c), and magnetic resonance imaging (d and e) when the patient was first examined. The dislocated C1 that accompanied the occipital condyle fractures was intracranially impacted (a, b, and c). The left vertebral artery was not revealed by CT angiography (b and c). Cerebellar edema occurred due to traumatic hemorrhagic cerebellar contusions, which compresses the brainstem (d and e).

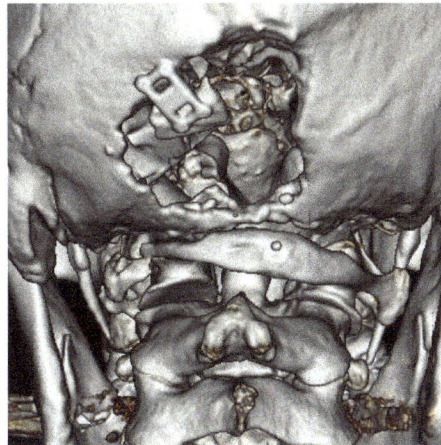

FIGURE 2: Computed tomography of the head and neck when the patient was referred to our hospital. Defects are observed in the left side and midline of the occipital bone.

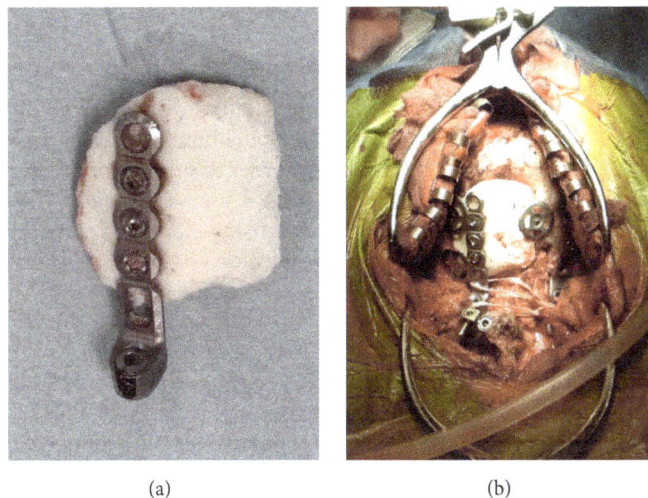

| (a) | (b) |

FIGURE 3: Intraoperative findings. A resin-made occipital bone was anchored with a titanium plate and titanium screws (a). Simultaneous cranioplasty and posterior fusion of the craniovertebral junction were performed. The iliac crest bone was grafted onto the occipital bone-C1-C2 alignment, and this grafted bone was fixed by a cable.

explained that type 2B also includes potentially unstable fractures; therefore, we diagnosed our case as type 2B because it included C1 dislocation and indicated instability.

Because OCFs do not occur frequently, there has been no reported high-level evidence of a therapeutic strategy for OCFs [12]. Some reports have indicated that immobilization of the neck using a cervical collar and halo vest showed good outcomes when compared to those for patients without a medical device [3], but the sample sizes in these studies were small. Many healthcare institutions recommend using a cervical collar or a halo vest for about 6 to 12 weeks [9]. According to Tuli et al. [11], immobilization of the neck is unnecessary for type 1 fractures, but the use of a cervical collar is recommended for type 2A fractures, and the use of a halo vest or posterior fusion of the craniovertebral junction is recommended for type 2B fractures. Since our case was classified as type 2B, we needed to decide between HVI

and posterior fusion of the craniovertebral junction. Surgical treatment was chosen because we estimated that the OCFs could be treated with external fixation using a halo vest, but the stability between two joints (O-C1 and C1-C2) was unlikely to be achieved due to the presence of C1 dislocation. In performing surgery, we considered decompression of the brainstem, jugular foramen, and hypoglossal canal, which is achieved by the removal of the dislocated fragments associated with C1 dislocation and OCFs. Likewise, there are also other reports indicating that the lower cranial nerve symptoms in patients experiencing OCFs complicated by lower cranial nerve palsy resolve after surgical removal of dislocated fragments [13, 14]; however there have only been three such cases, which is insufficient to show the superiority of surgical treatment [3]. On the other hand, removal of dislocated fragments from OCFs is associated with the risk of fatal complications, such as bleeding, caused by stroke and venous

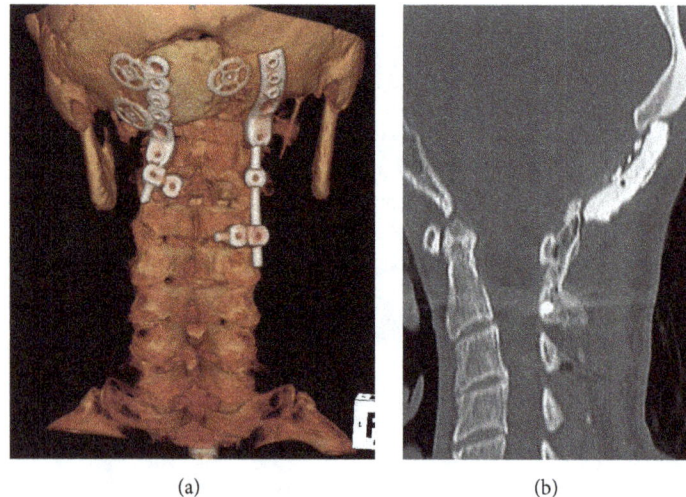

(a)   (b)

FIGURE 4: Clinical findings 50 months after surgery. Obvious implant breakage was not observed during a 5-year postoperative follow-up (a). The grafted bone was fused from the occipital bone through the C1 vertebra to the spinous process and the vertebral arch of the C2 vertebra (b).

sinus injury induced by sigmoid sinus occlusion because of anatomical location close to the sigmoid sinuses, and so forth, and therefore requires careful consideration. There is also another report indicating that conservative management is effective in patients with brainstem compression caused by dislocated fragments [15].

In this case, removal of dislocated fragments, together with the reduction of C1 dislocation, was not performed because the patient had a history of traumatic cerebellar hemorrhage which indicated the risk of complications. Furthermore, although decompression was not performed, swallowing disturbance and dysarthria associated with lower cranial nerve palsy resolved during a follow-up period after posterior fusion. This clinical course also indicates that the removal of dislocated fragments may not always be essential for this type of injury. Additionally, a surgical approach for obtaining stability of the craniovertebral junction reportedly alleviates not only neurological fallout but also pain and actually provided effective pain relief in our patient.

A large number of surgical procedures for craniovertebral junction instability have been reported [16–18]. Many types of occipitocervical fusion systems are currently available, but most of them involve using an occipital bone plate placed in the thickest part of the midline of the occipital bone, which is an anatomically favorable way [19]. When this patient was transferred to our hospital, he had undergone suboccipital craniotomy, and a large skull defect was observed in the left side and midline of the occipital bone. We concluded that, in such a situation, it would be difficult to perform occipitocervical fusion, which requires sufficient occipital bone area and strength. Furthermore, it was difficult to establish the continuity of bone in left side of the occipital bone-C1-C2 because we dropped the plan to reduce C1 dislocation. We also thought that it would be difficult to provide enough stability of the craniovertebral junction by fixing only the right side of the occipital bone. We were further concerned about damaging the hardware after surgery because posterior fusion of the craniovertebral junction on only one side of the occipital bone would increase strain on the screws and rods. In order to solve all of the above issues, we performed cranioplasty by securing a resin-made occipital bone to the defective part using a titanium plate. We also performed occipital cervical fusion on the left side by connecting vertebral arch pedicle screws of the cervical spine with an occipital bone plate that had been secured to the resin-made occipital bone. These enabled us to establish strong stability of the craniovertebral junction on the left side of occipital bone. Therefore, to our knowledge, this is the first case report of the simultaneous performance of cranioplasty and posterior fusion of the craniovertebral junction. Postoperative CT showed good bone graft incorporation at the 5-year follow-up. Although our primary concern was the displacement of the resin-made occipital bone used for cranioplasty, it did not occur.

Competing Interests

The authors declare that there are no competing interests regarding the publication of this paper.

References

[1] T. M. Link, G. Schuierer, A. Hufendiek, C. Horch, and P. E. Peters, "Substantial head trauma: value of routine CT examination of the cervicocranium," *Radiology*, vol. 196, no. 3, pp. 741–745, 1995.

[2] M. F. Blacksin and Huey Jen Lee, "Frequency and significance of fractures of the upper cervical spine detected by CT in patients with severe neck trauma," *American Journal of Roentgenology*, vol. 165, no. 5, pp. 1201–1204, 1995.

[3] I. Alcelik, K. S. Manik, P. S. Sian, and S. E. Khoshneviszadeh, "Occipital condylar fractures. Review of the literature and case report," *The Journal of Bone & Joint Surgery—British Volume*, vol. 88, no. 5, pp. 665–669, 2006.

[4] S. Demisch, A. Lindner, R. Beck, and S. Zierz, "The forgotten condyle: delayed hypoglossal nerve palsy caused by fracture of

the occipital condyle," *Clinical Neurology and Neurosurgery*, vol. 100, no. 1, pp. 44–45, 1998.

[5] F. S. Erol, C. Topsakal, M. Kaplan, H. Yildirim, and M. F. Ozveren, "Collet-sicard syndrome associated with occipital condyle fracture and epidural hematoma," *Yonsei Medical Journal*, vol. 48, no. 1, pp. 120–123, 2007.

[6] M. A. Wani, P. N. Tandon, A. K. Banerji, and R. Bhatia, "Collet-sicard syndrome resulting from closed head injury: case report," *Journal of Trauma—Injury, Infection and Critical Care*, vol. 31, no. 10, pp. 1437–1439, 1991.

[7] A. Leone, A. Cerase, C. Colosimo, L. Lauro, A. Puca, and P. Marano, "Occipital condylar fractures: a review," *Radiology*, vol. 216, no. 3, pp. 635–644, 2000.

[8] A. Krüger, L. Oberkircher, T. Frangen, S. Ruchholtz, C. Kühne, and A. Junge, "Fractures of the occipital condyle clinical spectrum and course in eight patients," *Journal of Craniovertebral Junction and Spine*, vol. 4, no. 2, pp. 49–55, 2013.

[9] N. C. Utheim, R. Josefsen, P. H. Nakstad, T. Solgaard, and O. Roise, "Occipital condyle fracture and lower cranial nerve palsy after blunt head trauma—a literature review and case report," *Journal of Trauma Management and Outcomes*, vol. 9, article 2, 2015.

[10] P. A. Anderson and P. X. Montesano, "Morphology and treatment of occipital condyle fractures," *Spine*, vol. 13, no. 7, pp. 731–736, 1988.

[11] S. Tuli, C. H. Tator, M. G. Fehlings, and M. Mackay, "Occipital condyle fractures," *Neurosurgery*, vol. 41, no. 2, pp. 368–377, 1997.

[12] P. Suchomel and L. Jurák, "Occipital condyle fractures," in *Reconstruction of Upper Cervical Spine and Craniovertebral Junction*, pp. 145–149, Springer, Berlin, Germany, 2011.

[13] M. Bozboga, F. Unal, K. Hepgul, N. Izgi, M. I. Turantan, and K. Turker, "Fracture of the occipital condyle: case report," *Spine*, vol. 17, no. 9, pp. 1119–1121, 1992.

[14] D. N. Jones, A. M. Knox, and M. R. Sage, "Traumatic avulsion fracture of the occipital condyles and clivus with associated unilateral atlantooccipital distraction," *American Journal of Neuroradiology*, vol. 11, no. 6, pp. 1181–1183, 1990.

[15] W. F. Young, R. H. Rosenwasser, C. Getch, and J. Jallo, "Diagnosis and management of occipital condyle fractures," *Neurosurgery*, vol. 34, no. 2, pp. 257–261, 1994.

[16] M. G. Fehlings, T. Errico, P. Cooper et al., "Occipitocervical fusion with a five-millimeter malleable rod and segmental fixation," *Neurosurgery*, vol. 32, no. 2, pp. 198–208, 1993.

[17] G. A. Flint, A. D. Hockley, J. J. McMillan, and A. G. Thompson, "A new method of occipitocervical fusion using internal fixation," *Neurosurgery*, vol. 21, no. 6, pp. 947–950, 1987.

[18] S. K. Singh, L. Rickards, R. I. Apfelbaum, R. J. Hurlbert, D. Maiman, and M. G. Fehlings, "Occipitocervical reconstruction with the Ohio Medical Instruments Loop: results of a multicenter evaluation in 30 cases," *Journal of Neurosurgery*, vol. 98, supplement 3, pp. 239–246, 2003.

[19] A. W. B. Heywood, I. D. Learmonth, and M. Thomas, "Internal fixation for occipito-cervical fusion," *Journal of Bone and Joint Surgery—Series B*, vol. 70, no. 5, pp. 708–711, 1988.

36

A Rare Case of Pheohyphomycotic Lumbar Spondylodiscitis Mistreated as Koch's Spine

Shakti A. Goel,[1] Hitesh N. Modi,[1] Yatin J. Desai,[1] and Harshal P. Thaker[2]

[1]Department of Orthopaedics and Spine Surgery, Zydus Hospitals and Healthcare Research Pvt. Ltd., Thaltej, Ahmedabad, Gujarat, India
[2]Dr. Harshal Thaker's Clinic, Ambawadi, Ahmedabad, Gujarat, India

Correspondence should be addressed to Hitesh N. Modi; modispine@yahoo.co.in

Academic Editor: Mark K. Lyons

Pheohyphomycosis is an uncommon infection and its association in spondylodiscitis has not yet been reported. The purpose of this case report is to describe a rare case of Pheohyphomycotic spondylodiscitis and methods to diagnose and manage the patient with less invasive techniques. A 29-year-old male patient presented to the outpatient department with complaints of gradually increasing low back pain with bilateral lower limbs radicular pain since one and a half years. He had associated fever, weight loss, voice changes, and dry, scaly, erythematous skin with elevated ESR. The patient had been taking anti-Koch's therapy since 1 year with little relief in pain and no radiological improvement. Percutaneous pedicle biopsy of L4 vertebra was taken under local anaesthesia and confirmed Pheohyphomycosis which was treated with antifungal medications. The patient showed sequential improvement with long term antifungal treatment. He was eventually able to walk independently without support.

1. Introduction

Pheohyphomycosis represents infections caused by pigmented filamentous fungi which contain melanin in their cell walls [1]. Their morphologic characteristics include hyphae, yeast-like cells, or combination [2]. They are either associated with *Alternaria or Exophiala jeanselmei* [3, 4].

Pheohyphomycosis is an uncommon infection and almost all reported cases have occurred in immunosuppressed patients with 80 percent mortality rate [5]. The disease is transmissible through air, wind, and water. The contacted individuals and population can be easily affected by it and usually it is too late to be successfully treated by the time the disease is recognized. Whenever seen, these organisms affect the skin and subcutaneous tissue with nodules or cyst [6]. Eye infections and plaques and granulomatous damage on the body have also been reported [7]. However, effect on spine by this organism in Southern Asia has not yet been seen.

Here we report a unique case of Pheohyphomycosis of lumbosacral spine, previously mistaken for Koch's spine (TB) and treated accordingly. The patient did not report any improvement for a long time until the pedicle biopsy was taken and antifungal treatment started.

Tuberculosis (TB) has been described as an ancient infectious disease with evidence being discovered in centuries-old skeletal remains [8]. Moreover, it is the most common cause of spinal infection in south Asian population [9]. In recent decades, there has been a significant resurgence of TB (Tuberculosis), causing 2-3 million deaths annually worldwide [10, 11].

Due to the frequent prevalence of TB in spine, it is a common practice to consider Koch's spine (TB) as the first differential in all spinal infections in developing nations. Many of these patients get better with anti-Koch's therapy without the surgery [12]. Hence it is a common practice to start anti-Koch's therapy in patients while the biopsy report is awaited [12]. However, rarely, other organisms besides TB could be a reason for such an infection [13]. This is the first case report of Pheohyphomycosis causing spinal infection in an immunocompetent host.

2. Case Report

A 29-year-old immunocompetent male patient presented to the outpatient department with complaints of gradually increasing low back pain since one and a half years. The pain

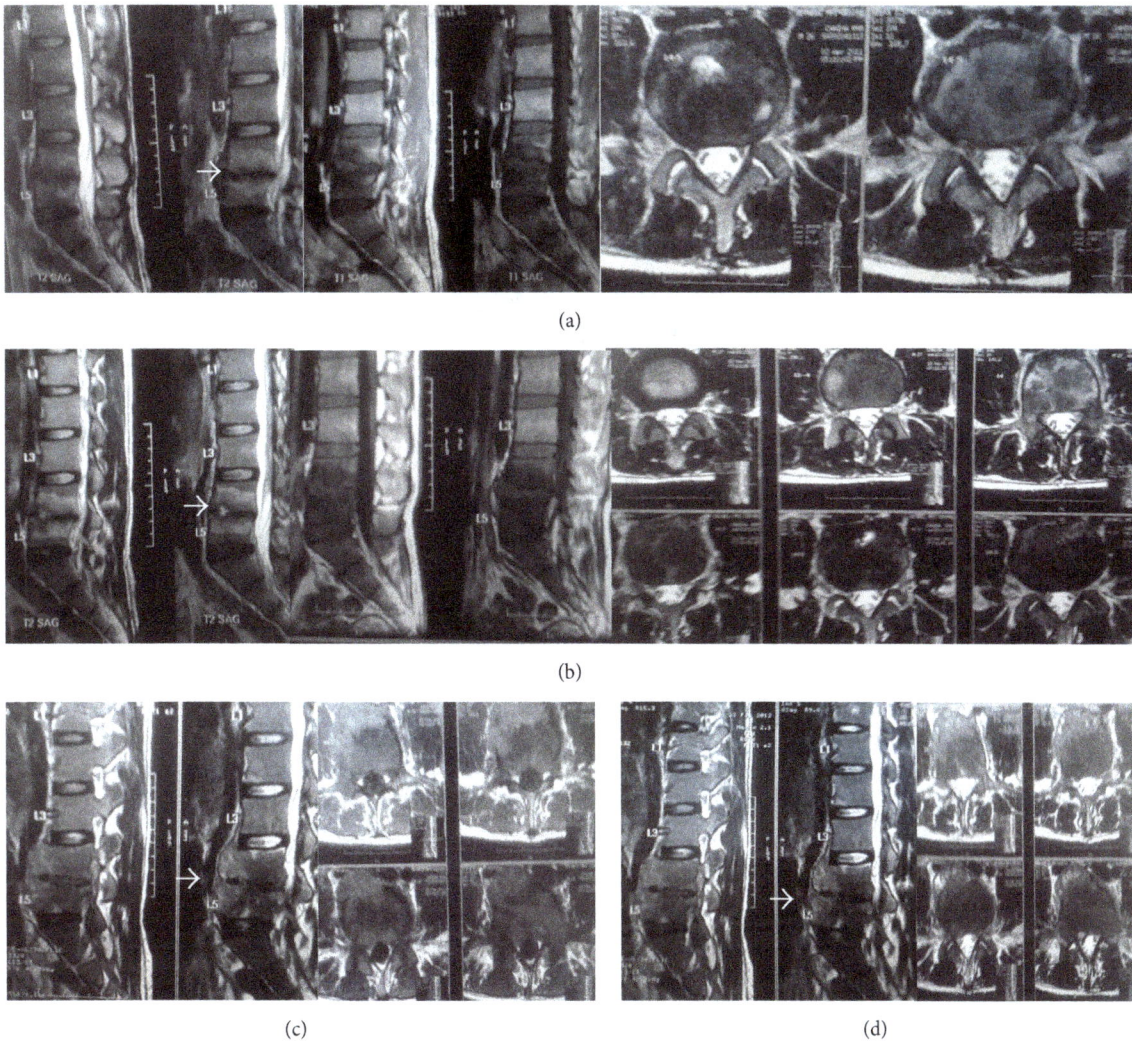

FIGURE 1: Sequential MRI images of the patient. (a) MRI before the initiation of anti-Koch's therapy. (b) MRI image after 4 months of anti-Koch's therapy. (c) MRI image after 9 months of anti-Koch's therapy. (d) MRI image after 12 months of anti-Koch's therapy.

increased on changing position and relieved with rest. There was associated bilateral lower limb radiculopathy which was more on right side as compared to left. Manual muscle testing of upper and lower limbs did not show any reduction in the grade of power but right lower limb straight leg raising was restricted to 50 degrees. Radical involvement of L4, L5, and S1 nerve root was seen. However, there was no motor weakness present. The patient had radicular pain to right lower limb in posterior gluteal region, lateral and anterior shin. The sensations were intact in all four limbs and reflexes were of two plus grade with a flexor Babinski and negative Hoffman's test. He had associated fever and weight loss of seven kilograms in one year. There were associated voice changes and dry, scaly, erythematous skin, the biopsy of which was previously reported to be inconclusive of any infection. He had lumbar kyphosis and elevated ESR (Erythrocyte Sedimentation Rate) of 94 mm per hour. The patient had been taking anti-Koch's therapy since 1 year with little relief in pain.

The patient had a series of MRI (Magnetic Resonance Imaging) images starting with the first one taken 14 months ago (Figure 1(a)). It showed spondylodiscitis at lumbar 4 and lumbar 5 region and patient was started on anti-Koch's therapy. The second MRI taken after 4 months of anti-Koch's therapy did not show any improvement in the disc lesion or symptoms. The lesion rather progressed in the second MRI (Figure 1(b)). The third MRI taken 9 months after anti-Koch's therapy treatment did not even show any improvement (Figure 1(c)). The fourth MRI was taken after the patient completed 1 year of anti-Koch's therapy (Figure 1(d)). It showed further destruction of lumbar 4-lumbar 5 disc areas and bodies. The lesion had further progressed and patient reported no improvement in symptoms.

Considering other differentials like plasmacytoma, lymphocytoma, fungal infection, or metastasis in mind, CT (Computerised Tomography) scan was advised. It showed lesions in the lung and liver (Figure 2). CT guided biopsy of the lung was done which was inconclusive. No specific

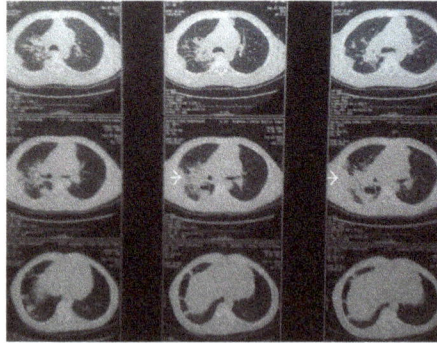

FIGURE 2: CT scan of the chest showing lesion in the lungs. Biopsy of these lesions was inconclusive.

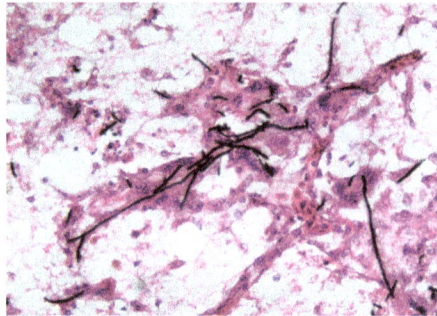

FIGURE 3: Microscopic image (Silver Methenamine, Haemotoxylin and Eosin Staining) of the 4th pedicle biopsy showing hyphae and yeast-like cells suggesting Pheohyphomycosis. The biopsy material was stained with Silver Methenamine with H&E counterstaining. Gram-positive hyphae/pseudohyphae can be appreciated.

pathology in the CT scan of the abdomen and pelvis was found.

Following CT scan, it was decided to take 4th lumbar vertebra's pedicle biopsy under local anaesthesia and look for culture sensitivity and fungal growth. The microscopy showed hyphae and yeast-like cells representing Pheohyphomycosis (Figure 3). The patient was started on intravenous antifungal medications for 2 weeks (Amphotericin B 3–5 mg/Kg body weight). This was followed by 12 months of oral antifungal medications (tablet Voriconazole twice a day). The leg pain of the patient disappeared in one week. The back pain relieved by 90 percent in one month and he started to walk independently without support. The improvements in the radiographs of chest and spine were also evident (Figure 4). At present the patient has no mechanical pain symptoms and is walking independently without support.

3. Discussion

Tuberculosis has been reported to be the commonest cause of spondylodiscitis. Other causes of spinal infection have also been reported [13]. This is the first case report which shows Pheohyphomycosis as a cause of spondylodiscitis in an immunocompetent host which was diagnosed with percutaneous pedicle biopsy.

Pheohyphomycosis is an amalgam of clinical diseases caused by a variety of fungi which often lead to subcutaneous cyst formation at the site of traumatic implantation [1, 3]. It is more commonly found in immunocompromised host; however skin lesion in immunocompetent adults has also been reported. Primary pulmonary infection is usually associated with an endemic area and with the inhalation of a large number of infecting spores. Normal patients exposed to such fungi generally fight off infection easily with no sign of illness. However, if exposed to a large enough inoculum of virulent fungus, a person with an intact immune system may develop a chronic infection. The chronic infection may require treatment such as antifungal drugs and surgery and require the patient to abstain from smoking. A compromised patient may easily develop systemic and progressive illness depending on the specifics surrounding the infection [6, 7]. In this case, the patient was an immunocompetent adult, in contrast to the usual findings of Pheohyphomycotic fungal infection. Moreover, though he did not have any respiratory complaints, the lungs did confirm the fungal lesion on CT scan. This further lays emphasis on the usual findings of the fungal spore entry via pulmonary route.

There is little information on spinal Pheohyphomycosis management. However, based on available data and experience, therapy with Amphotericin B alone may not be adequate. Some successfully treated cases of cerebral Pheohyphomycosis used itraconazole or flucytosine in combination with Amphotericin B, although few have been documented. The newer azole antifungal drugs such as Voriconazole and posaconazole may also play a role in therapy [14, 15]. Prolonged follow-up is essential because relapses are not uncommon [15]. In this case study, the patient was started on intravenous antifungal medications for

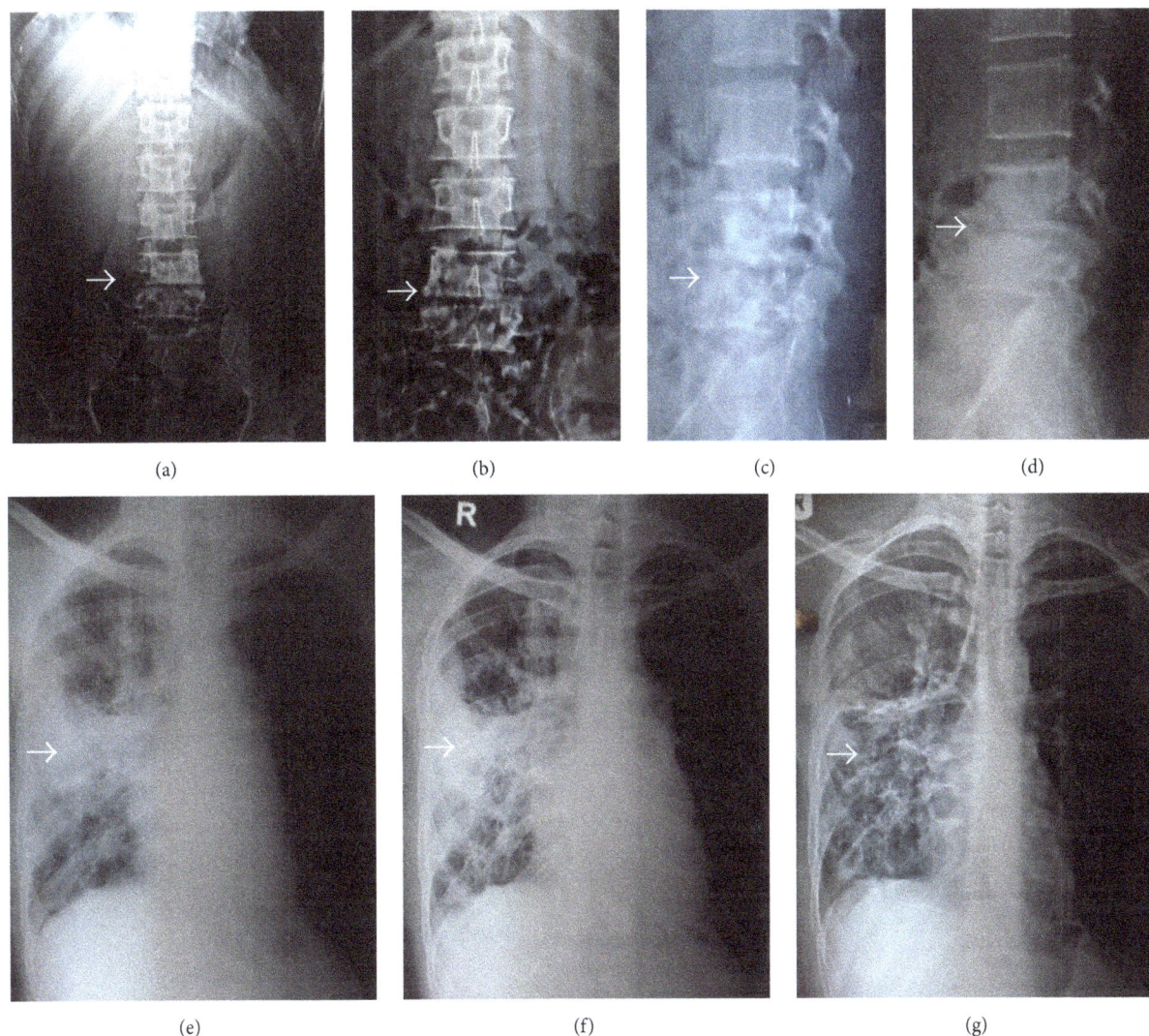

FIGURE 4: Radiographic evidence of improvement in spine and chest after antifungal treatment. (a) and (b) represent anteroposterior X-rays of lumbar spine, before and after treatment, respectively. (c) and (d) represent lateral X-rays of lumbar spine, before and after treatment, respectively. (e), (f), and (g) represent the sequential improvement in chest radiographs after the initiation of antifungal treatment.

2 weeks (Amphotericin B 3–5 mg/Kg body weight). This was followed by 12 months of oral antifungal medications (tablet Voriconazole twice a day). This long term therapy made the patient symptom-free and he started to walk independently without support.

Two important questions have been raised by this case study. First one is if biopsy confirmation is a must after radiological signs of infection in spine before starting the treatment. The pedicle biopsy can be taken by an open technique under general anaesthesia or percutaneous method under local anaesthesia. The percutaneous pedicle biopsy under local anaesthesia is a promising alternative as described fby Dave et al. [16]. In this case study, the biopsy taken was by percutaneous method under local anaesthesia. The importance of this technique lies in the fact that there is a definitive evidence of the microorganism and the patient is not mistreated with inappropriate antimicrobials. The patient in this case study was mistreated as Koch's spine until pedicle biopsy confirmed Pheohyphomycosis as the cause of the disease.

The second question that arises is if anti-Koch's therapy should be started in all patients with spinal infections in Asian nations. It is a common practice to start anti-Koch's therapy in all spondylodiscitis patients and wait for the response in Southern Asia while results of biopsy are awaited or negative [12]. A delay in diagnosing such an infection and mistreating it as Koch's spine will not only keep the patient in pain for a long time but also make him suffer the toxic side effects of anti-Koch's therapy [17, 18].

Here we report a unique case of Pheohyphomycotic spondylodiscitis which was diagnosed and treated by a nonsurgical method. The pedicle biopsy of the 4th lumbar vertebra was taken under local anaesthesia [16]. The patient showed complete recovery after the diagnosis and medical treatment of the fungal infection.

4. Conclusion

A number of differentials can be kept in mind while encountering a case of spondylodiscitis. Besides tuberculosis, plasmacytoma, lymphocytoma, metastasis, chronic nonspecific inflammations, and fungal infections should be considered. It is at the physician's discretion to decide about the next modality of treatment. Should the patient be started on anti-Koch's therapy in south Asian region as it is routinely done or should results of open biopsy/surgery/radiochemotherapy be awaited? Percutaneous pedicle biopsy under local anaesthesia is an efficient alternative.

Here we present a unique case of Pheohyphomycotic spondylodiscitis of lumbar 4-lumbar 5 region which was misdiagnosed and treated as Koch's spine until percutaneous lumbar 4 pedicle biopsy confirmed the diagnosis and patient was treated with antifungal medications.

Competing Interests

The authors declare that they have no competing interests.

References

[1] L. Ajello, L. K. Georg, R. T. Steigbigel, and C. J. Wang, "A case of phaeohyphomycosis caused by a new species of Phialophora," *Mycologia*, vol. 66, no. 3, pp. 490–498, 1974.

[2] W. D. James, "Rosacea: wonderings of a clinician," *Cutis*, vol. 78, no. 2, pp. 91–92, 2006.

[3] R. Boyce, P. Deziel, C. Otley et al., "Phaeohyphomycosis due to Alternaria species in transplant recipients," *Transplant Infectious Disease*, vol. 12, no. 3, pp. 242–250, 2010.

[4] N. Umemoto, T. Demitsu, M. Kakurai et al., "Two cases of cutaneous phaeohyphomycosis due to exophiala jeanselmei: diagnostic significance of direct microscopical examination of the purulent discharge," *Clinical and Experimental Dermatology*, vol. 34, no. 7, pp. e351–e353, 2009.

[5] S. G. Revankar, J. E. Patterson, D. A. Sutton, R. Pullen, and M. G. Rinaldi, "Disseminated phaeohyphomycosis: review of an emerging mycosis," *Clinical Infectious Diseases*, vol. 34, no. 4, pp. 467–476, 2002.

[6] M. Hasei, K. Takeda, K. Anzawa, A. Nishibu, H. Tanabe, and T. Mochizuki, "Case of phaeohyphomycosis producing sporotrichoid lesions," *Journal of Dermatology*, vol. 40, no. 8, pp. 638–640, 2013.

[7] Q. Cai, G.-X. Lv, Y.-Q. Jiang et al., "The first case of phaeohyphomycosis caused by *Rhinocladiella basitona* in an immunocompetent child in China," *Mycopathologia*, vol. 176, no. 1-2, pp. 101–105, 2013.

[8] N. A. S. Kiran, S. Vaishya, S. S. Kale, B. S. Sharma, and A. K. Mahapatra, "Surgical results in patients with tuberculosis of the spine and severe lower-extremity motor deficits: a retrospective study of 48 patients," *Journal of Neurosurgery: Spine*, vol. 6, no. 4, pp. 320–326, 2007.

[9] M. R. Rasouli, M. Mirkoohi, A. R. Vaccaro, K. K. Yarandi, and V. Rahimi-Movaghar, "Spinal tuberculosis: diagnosis and management," *Asian Spine Journal*, vol. 6, no. 4, pp. 294–308, 2012.

[10] M. Kang, S. Gupta, N. Khandelwal, S. Shankar, M. Gulati, and S. Suri, "CT-guided fine-needle aspiration biopsy of spinal lesions," *Acta Radiologica*, vol. 40, no. 5, pp. 474–478, 1999.

[11] N. Al-Khudairi and A. Meir, "Isolated tuberculosis of the posterior spinal elements: case report and discussion of management," *JRSM Open*, vol. 5, no. 9, 2014.

[12] S. M. Tuli, "Results of treatment of spinal tuberculosis by 'middle-path' regime," *Journal of Bone and Joint Surgery—Series B*, vol. 57, no. 1, pp. 13–23, 1975.

[13] V. R. Patil, A. R. Joshi, S. S. Joshi, and D. Patel, "Lumbosacral actinomycosis in an immunocompetent individual: an extremely rare case," *Journal of Craniovertebral Junction and Spine*, vol. 5, no. 4, pp. 173–175, 2014.

[14] H. Badali, G. S. de Hoog, I. Curfs-Breuker, C. H. W. Klaassen, and J. F. Meis, "Use of amplified fragment length polymorphism to identify 42 *Cladophialophora* strains related to cerebral phaeohyphomycosis with in vitro antifungal susceptibility," *Journal of Clinical Microbiology*, vol. 48, no. 7, pp. 2350–2356, 2010.

[15] M. K. Lyons, J. E. Blair, and K. O. Leslie, "Successful treatment with voriconazole of fungal cerebral abscess due to *Cladophialophora bantiana*," *Clinical Neurology and Neurosurgery*, vol. 107, no. 6, pp. 532–534, 2005.

[16] B. R. Dave, A. Nanda, and J. V. Anandjiwala, "Transpedicular percutaneous biopsy of vertebral body lesions: a series of 71 cases," *Spinal Cord*, vol. 47, no. 5, pp. 384–389, 2009.

[17] R. Aggarwal, S. Dwivedi, and M. Aggarwal, "Unfamiliar manifestations of anti-tubercular therapy," *Journal of Family Medicine and Primary Care*, vol. 3, no. 1, pp. 72–73, 2014.

[18] G. Riedel M, "Contaminación ambiental por Clostridium difficile," *Revista chilena de infectología*, vol. 27, no. 4, 2010.

37

Low-Energy Traumatic Obturator Hip Dislocation with Ipsilateral Femoral Shaft Fracture in a Patient with Omolateral Knee Arthroplasty

G. Gazzotti,[1] **L. Patrizio,**[2] **S. Dall'Aglio,**[1] **and E. Sabetta**[1]

[1]*Unit of Orthopedic Surgery, IRCCS-Arcispedale Santa Maria Nuova, Reggio Emilia, Italy*
[2]*Unit of Orthopedic Surgery, Ospedale Santa Maria dello Splendore, Giulianova, Teramo, Italy*

Correspondence should be addressed to G. Gazzotti; gazzotti.g82@gmail.com

Academic Editor: Paul E. Di Cesare

Ipsilateral obturator hip dislocation and femoral shaft fracture are rare. We report such a case in an older woman after a low-energy injury. She had a knee prostheses in the same limb. The patient was treated by open manipulative reduction of the luxation without opening joint and open reduction and internal fixation of the femur with angular stability plate and screws. We could not find a similar case in the literature. An early diagnosis of the dislocation is crucial in order to obtain good results. Great awareness and radiologic examination are fundamental to achieve precocious diagnosis of both these rare combined injuries, as treatment in these cases is considered an emergency. The first step was an attempt to reduce the dislocation by closed means but it failed. Then we performed a short approach at the trochanteric region and used Lambotte forceps to manoeuvre the proximal femur without opening the joint achieving reduction. Thereafter the femoral shaft fracture underwent open reduction and internal fixation with an angular stable plate. After a 2-year follow-up the outcome was very good.

1. Introduction

Anterior hip dislocation with associated ipsilateral femoral shaft fracture is a very rare injury, with few cases reported in the literature. They are generally related to high-energy trauma (sport or traffic accidents) in young people. We report a rare low-energy injury in an elderly woman: obturator hip dislocation associated with ipsilateral femur shaft fracture in a patient with knee arthroplasty. She was treated by open manipulative reduction of the dislocation reduction without opening joint using Lambotte forceps and open reduction and internal fixation of femur with angular stability plate and screws.

2. Case Report

A 78-year-old woman, while on holiday at the seaside, stumbled as she was pushing her son's wheelchair and fell down a flight of stairs in a hotel. She was transferred to the Emergency Room of the local Hospital. Radiologic assessment revealed an obturator hip dislocation with ipsilateral femur shaft fracture in this patient with knee arthroplasty (Figures 1(a)-1(b)). The patient refused treatment in this facility and was transferred to our Hospital (Hospital Arcispedale Santa Maria Nuova) in Reggio Emilia after a three-hour trip. We evaluated the patient 6 hours after trauma. During clinical examination, we noted an anterior hematoma in the proximal thigh, the hip in adduction and external rotation, and the knee and leg in complete external rotation. Neurological and vascular examinations were normal. A CT scan was performed in order to provide further assessment of injuries in order to help the surgical planning (Figures 2(a)-2(b)). No femoral head fracture was present (Figures 2(c)-2(d)), and in the posterior-inferior rim of the acetabular cavity small calcified images compatible with millimetric free fragments were detected (Figure 2(e)). A surgical repair of every lesion was proposed. First, a closed reduction of hip dislocation under general anaesthetic was attempted but the femoral

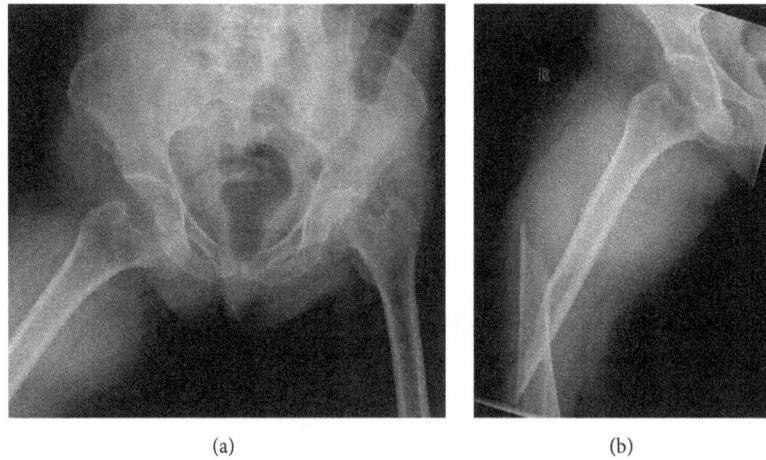

(a)   (b)

FIGURE 1: Preoperative X-ray examination.

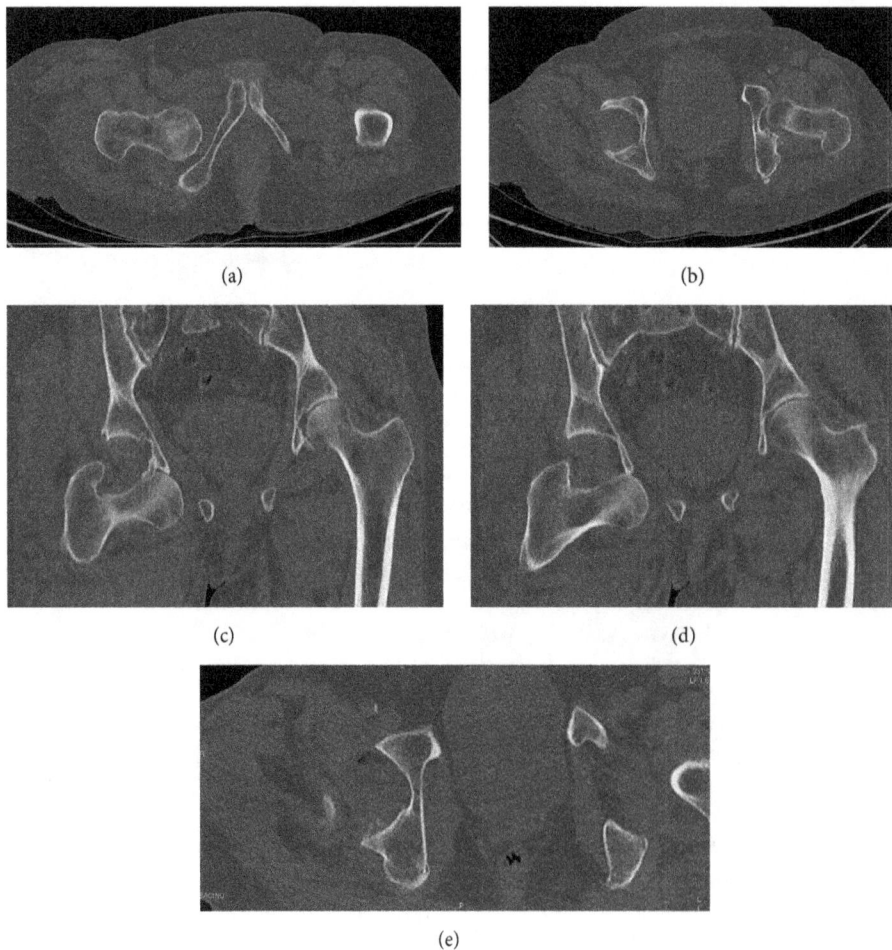

(a)   (b)

(c)   (d)

(e)

FIGURE 2: Preoperative CT scan.

shaft fracture made reduction impossible. A small incision was made under the base of the greater trochanter and manipulation of the proximal femur with a Lambotte forceps without opening the hip joint was successful in reducing the dislocation. A second larger, distal, and lateral incision was made to reduce and fix the femoral shaft fracture with interfragmentary screws and an angular stable plate under fluoroscopic guide (Figures 3(a)-3(b)). During the postoperative period, the patient carried out active and passive mobilization of the hip and knee without bearing

(a)   (b)

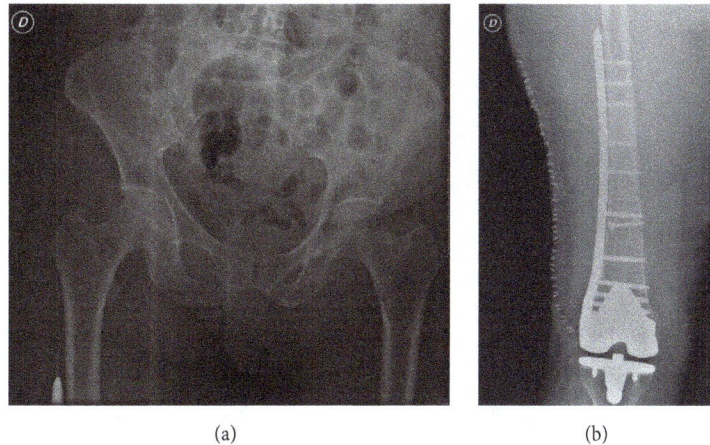

FIGURE 3: Postoperative X-ray examination.

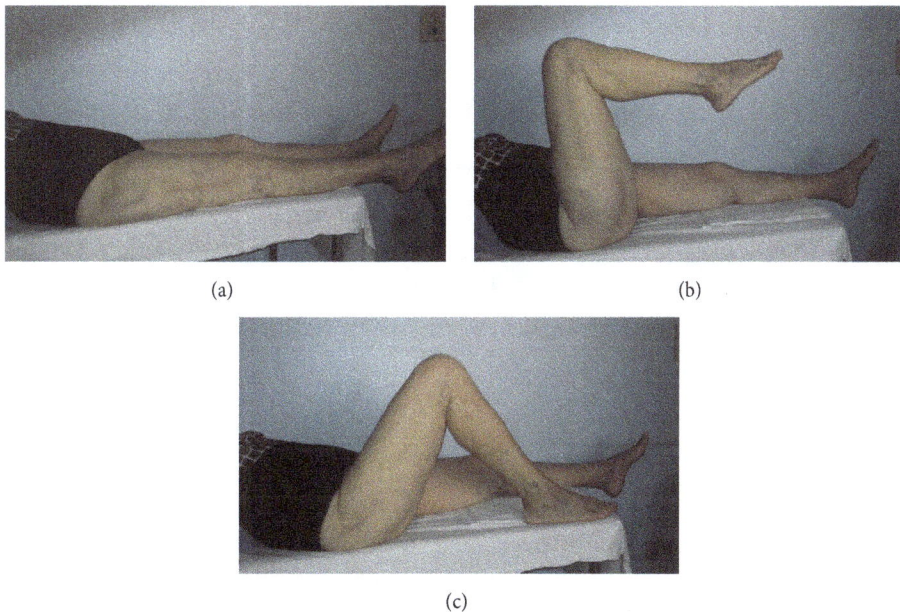

(a)   (b)

(c)

FIGURE 4: Clinical evaluation at 2-year follow-up.

weight for 4 weeks. Then she started walking with crutches, bearing partial weight (20 kg) on the injured limb for 2 weeks, increasing 15 kg per week. After 45 days, she was able to walk with full weight-bearing. Five months after the injury the hip had full range of pain-free motion, there was no limb shortening, and radiographs confirmed shaft fracture healing. At 12 months, she returned on holiday at the seaside with her son. At the 2-year follow-up, there was complete painless hip function (Figures 4(a)–4(c)) and radiographs did not show any evidence of avascular necrosis (Figures 5(a)–5(d)).

3. Discussion

Hip dislocation associated with femoral shaft fracture is a rare condition [1]. Wiltenberger et al. estimated hip dislocation

incidence at 1 in 100000 femur shaft fractures [2]. A literature review of these combined injuries indicates that the hip dislocation is primarily missed in nearly half of the cases, and this is for different reasons [3–5]. First, it is an uncommon combined injury. Second, it is generally associated with severe shock and in the first aid, more attention is paid to resuscitation. Third, shaft fractures often obscure clinical signs of the dislocated hip. A sign that should be searched and might be for diagnosis in an anterior hip dislocation is the palpation of the femoral head in the midinguinal region as well as a less prominent greater trochanter [6]. Generally, these combined injuries occur in young and middle age adults and are caused by high-energy trauma due to sport, pedestrian, or traffic accidents [1]. We could not find low-energy traumas causing this type of injury in the world literature. Helal and Skevis [7] postulated that the trauma mechanism

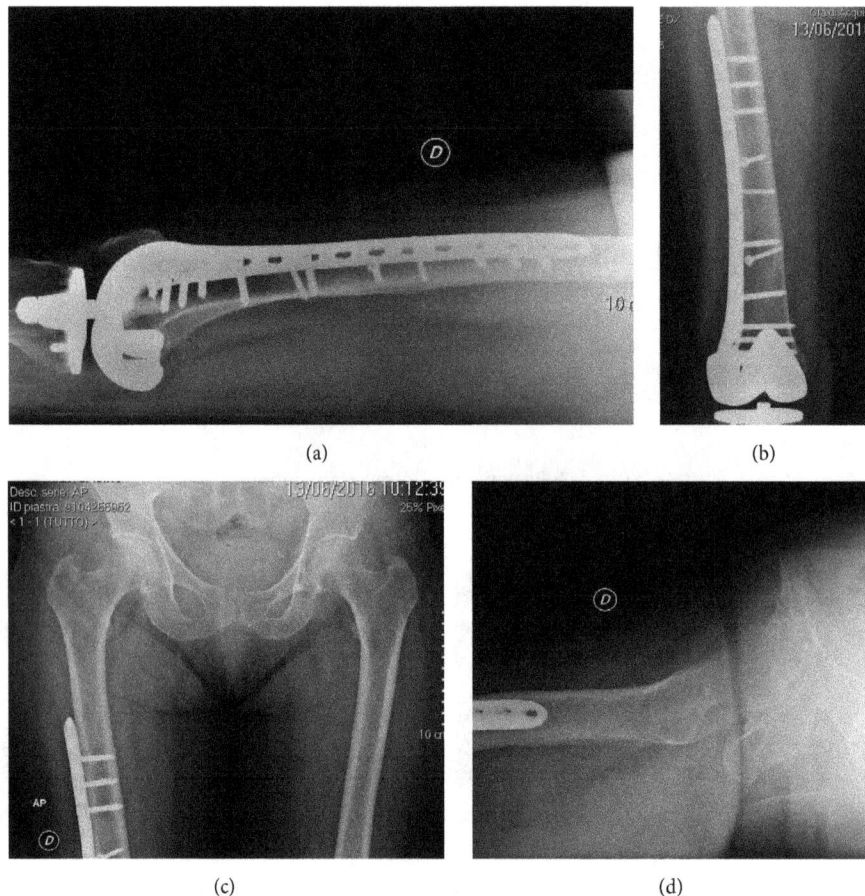

(a)

(b)

(c)

(d)

FIGURE 5: X-ray examination at 2-year follow-up.

in a similar case was related to two separate forces: an axial force on the flexed femur which causes the dislocation and a direct trauma, subsequent to the fall, which causes the shaft fracture. The degree of abduction or adduction of the thigh determines whether the dislocation is anterior or posterior. Most hip dislocations are posterior [8]; anterior hip dislocation is less common and is of two main types: superior (in the iliac or pubic region) or inferior (obturator region). Delayed reduction of hip dislocation is more difficult to obtain and it is related to several complications such as avascular necrosis of femoral head [9]. Reduction, even in acutely diagnosed cases, is extremely difficult because the femur, that is, the lever, is not intact and therefore it does not provide for control on the proximal femur [10, 11]. Therefore, closed manipulation may be attempted but it is effective in less than 50% of the cases [3, 6, 12, 13]. Lyddon and Hartman [14] described a method of closed reduction using a device on the trochanter to facilitate manipulation. Ingram and Turner [15] used a Steinman pin drilled through the greater trochanter. Helal and Skevis [7] suggested using a traction screw into the femoral neck or an intramedullary Denness' device in the proximal shaft of the femur to obtain a better leverage and make reduction easier. Also Dehne and Immermann [3] suggested an operative exposure of the fracture site and direct manipulation of the proximal

fragment. Open reduction of the hip is recommended if previously described closed methods would fail, although this is associated with an increased risk of avascular necrosis of the femoral head [16]. Watson-Jones recommended ORIF of the femoral shaft fracture followed by closed manipulative reduction of hip [17]. Also Sambandan [18] preferred to treat the fracture first. He reported a case report of a twenty-year-old male who sustained a motor vehicle accident with associated injuries and cerebral concussion. He described an obturator dislocation associated with a femur shaft fracture managed by internal fixation of the femur with a Kuntscher nail followed by closed manipulative reduction of hip.

In the case reported here, at the latest follow-up examination (2 years), the patient had full range of passive motion with no pain or disability. Schoenecker et al. [12] reported three cases; one of them was an 18-year-old man involved in a motor vehicle accident with an anterior hip dislocation with ipsilateral femoral shaft fracture. The dislocation was reduced by closed means using a large bone clamp and the fracture was reduced and fixed with an intramedullary rod. At one-year postinjury, the patient had excellent results with no discomfort and radiologic assessment revealed that the fracture had healed and the hip joint appeared normal. We used a similar technique to reduce the hip dislocation without opening the joint even if we agree that closed manipulations might be attempted first. In our case, the shaft fracture was spiroid and we preferred to use interfragmentary screws and an angular stable plate in order to fix the shaft fracture.

Competing Interests

The authors declare that they have no competing interests.

References

[1] M. T. Taylor, B. Banerjee, and E. K. Alpar, "Injuries associated with a fractured shaft of the femur," *Injury*, vol. 25, no. 3, pp. 185–187, 1994.

[2] B. R. Wiltenberger, C. L. Mitchell, and D. W. Hedrick, "Fracture of the femoral shaft complicated by hip dislocation," *The Journal of Bone and Joint Surgery. American*, vol. 30, no. 1, pp. 225–228, 1948.

[3] E. Dehne and E. W. Immermann, "Dislocation of the hip combined with fracture of the shaft of the femur on the same side," *The Journal of Bone & Joint Surgery—American Volume*, vol. 33, no. 3, pp. 731–745, 1951.

[4] P. S. Saxena, "Fracture shaft femur combined with ipsilateral posterior dislocation of hip: report of a case," *Indian Journal of Medical Sciences*, vol. 28, no. 6, pp. 266–268, 1974.

[5] A. P. Singh, A. P. Singh, and V. Mittal, "Traumatic inferior hip dislocation with ipsilateral open subtrochanteric fracture: a rare case," *Injury Extra*, vol. 39, no. 12, pp. 384–385, 2008.

[6] S. M. A. Ehtisham, "Traumatic dislocation of hip joint with fracture of shaft of femur on the same side," *The Journal of Trauma*, vol. 16, no. 3, 1976.

[7] B. Helal and X. Skevis, "Unrecognised dislocation of the hip in fractures of the femoral shaft," *The Journal of Bone & Joint Surgery—British Volume*, vol. 49, no. 2, pp. 293–300, 1967.

[8] B.-C. Qi, Y. Zhao, C.-X. Wang et al., "Posterior dislocation of the hip with bilateral femoral fractures: an unusual combination," *Technology and Health Care*, vol. 24, no. 2, pp. 281–286, 2016.

[9] R. Merle d'Aubigne and G. Lord, "Lésions traumatiques combinées de la diaphyse fémorale et de la hance homologud (onze observations)," *Mémoires. Académie de Chirurgie*, vol. 83, p. 646, 1957.

[10] G. Sharma, M. Chadha, and A. Pankaj, "Hip dislocation associated with ipsilateral femoral neck and shaft fractures: an unusual combination and dilemma regarding head preservation," *Acta Orthopaedica et Traumatologica Turcica*, vol. 48, no. 6, pp. 698–702, 2014.

[11] N. C. Tiedcken, V. Saldanha, J. Handal, and J. Raphael, "The irreducible floating hip: a unique presentation of a rare injury," *Journal of Surgical Case Reports*, vol. 2013, no. 10, Article ID rjt075, 2013.

[12] P. L. Schoenecker, P. R. Manske, and G. O. Sertl, "Traumatic hip dislocation with ipsilateral femoral shaft fractures," *Clinical Orthopaedics and Related Research*, no. 130, pp. 233–238, 1978.

[13] L. Tomcovcík and M. Kitka, "Hip dislocation with ipsilateral femoral shaft fracture," *Acta Chirurgiae Orthopaedicae et Traumatologiae Cechoslovaca*, vol. 67, no. 3, pp. 203–209, 2000.

[14] D. W. Lyddon and J. T. Hartman, "Traumatic dislocation of the hip with ipsilateral femoral fractures. A case report," *The Journal of Bone & Joint Surgery—American Volume*, vol. 53, no. 5, pp. 1012–1016, 1971.

[15] A. J. Ingram and T. C. Turner, "Bilateral traumatic posterior dislocation of the hip complicated by bilateral fracture of the femoral shaft," *The Journal of Bone and Joint Surgery*, vol. 36-A, no. 6, pp. 1249–1255, 1954.

[16] A. K. Henry and M. Bayumi, "Fracture of the femur with luxation of the ipsilateral hip," *British Journal of Surgery*, vol. 22, no. 86, pp. 204–230, 1934.

[17] Watson-Jones, "Injuries of the hip," in *Fractures and Joint Injuries*, J. N. Wilson, Ed., p. 908, Churchill Livingstone, New York, NY, USA, 5th edition, 1976.

[18] S. Sambandan, "Obturator dislocation of the hip associated with fracture shaft of femur: a case report," *Singapore Medical Journal*, vol. 27, no. 5, pp. 442–445, 1986.

38

Simultaneous Bilateral Transient Osteoporosis of the Hip without Pregnancy

Yasuaki Okada, Sachiyuki Tsukada, Masayoshi Saito, and Atsushi Tasaki

Department of Orthopaedic Surgery, St. Luke's International Hospital, 9-1 Akashi-cho, Chuo-ku, Tokyo 104-8560, Japan

Correspondence should be addressed to Sachiyuki Tsukada; s8058@nms.ac.jp

Academic Editor: Koichi Sairyo

Transient osteoporosis of the hip (TOH) is a rare disorder characterized by acute severe coxalgia and temporary osteopenia in the proximal femur. Although most cases were unilateral or staged bilateral TOH, some authors reported that the pregnant patients simultaneously had TOH in their bilateral hips. However, there has been no report of simultaneous bilateral TOH in the patient without pregnancy. A 25-year-old Japanese woman without pregnancy had acute simultaneous bilateral hip pain. Plain X-ray of the bilateral hips did not show a periarticular osteopenia. However, magnetic resonance image obtained one week after the onset demonstrated increased T2-weighted signal intensity and decreased T1-weighted signal intensity in the bilateral femoral heads. She was treated conservatively, and follow-up magnetic resonance image at seven weeks after the onset returned to normal bone marrow signal intensity. Her bilateral coxalgia subsided gradually. At one year after the onset, she had no sign of symptomatic flair. Our experience with this case indicates that recognizing the possibility of simultaneous bilateral TOH is important unless the patient is pregnant, and magnetic resonance image is predictable test to make a diagnosis of TOH, even in the absence of abnormal finding on plain X-ray.

1. Introduction

Transient osteoporosis of the hip (TOH) is a rare condition that causes temporary bone loss in the proximal femur and sudden-onset severe hip pain [1, 2]. Most previously reported cases of TOH affected a unilateral hip joint or staged bilateral hip joints; however, some authors reported cases in which pregnant female patients simultaneously had TOH in bilateral hips [3–6]. To our knowledge, there have been no reports on patients without pregnancy but with simultaneous bilateral TOH. Although the pathophysiology of TOH has not been clarified, the cause of simultaneous bilateral TOH has been believed to be associated with pregnancy based on previous case reports [3–6].

We report a 25-year-old woman without pregnancy who had bilateral simultaneous hip TOH. The patient was informed that data concerning the case would be submitted for publication and provided consent for study.

2. Case Report

A 25-year-old Japanese nonpregnant woman without a significant medical history developed acute bilateral hip pain that progressively increased over the span of a few days. Her occupation was radiology technologist, and she has not been physically active on a regular basis. The onset of hip pain was not associated with trauma, and the patient had no other predisposing factors for osteonecrosis. She was unable to bear weight and walked with a limp. When walking, her right and left hip pain score evaluated via numeric rating scale were eight and six, respectively.

On physical examination, she was 160 cm tall and weighed 53.6 kg with a body mass index of 20.9 kg/m^2. Bilateral hips were positive on the Patrick test. Both anterior and posterior impingement tests were negative for bilateral hips. The following ranges of motion were obtained: flexion, right 90 degrees/left 110 degrees; extension, right 10 degrees/left

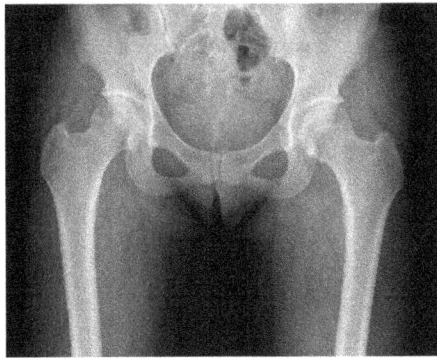

FIGURE 1: Anteroposterior X-ray of pelvis one week after symptom onset. No osteopenia.

20 degrees; abduction, right 20 degrees/left 30 degrees; adduction, right 30 degrees/left 40 degrees; internal rotation, right 20 degrees/left 30 degrees; and external rotation, right 30 degrees/left 40 degrees.

She was afebrile. Her blood tests for hematology, biochemistry, coagulation, erythrocyte sedimentation rate, endocrine, rheumatoid arthritis, and bone metabolism were unremarkable. Calcium was 9.4 mEq/L (normal, 8.4 to 10.2 mEq/L), intact parathyroid hormone was 32 pg/mL (normal, 10.0 to 65.0 pg/mL), and 25-hydroxyvitamin D measured with a DiaSorin radioimmunoassay was 16.4 ng/mL (normal, 9.0 to 37.6 ng/mL).

Plain anteroposterior view X-ray of the pelvis and hips one week after symptom onset did not show an obvious appearance of osteopenia or diffuse thinning of the cortex of the bilateral femoral head and neck (Figure 1). There was no evidence of dysplasia of the bilateral hips (Figure 1). The right hip had a center-edge angle of 27.9 degrees (normal in Japanese women, 27.0 to 34.0 degrees), the sharp angle was 45.3 degrees (normal in Japanese women, 34.0 to 42.0 degrees), and the acetabular head index was 79% (normal in Japanese women, 80 to 89%). The left hip had a center-edge angle of 27.3 degrees and sharp angle of 49.7 degrees. The acetabular head index was 83.7%. A magnetic resonance image obtained on the same day, however, demonstrated increased T2-weighted signal intensity and decreased T1-weighted signal intensity in the bilateral femoral heads consistent with bone marrow edema, and there were no findings to suggest osteonecrosis (Figure 2). Bone mineral density was measured with dual energy X-ray absorptiometry at nine days after onset: the Z-sore of the left femoral neck was −0.5 and that of lumbar spine was 0.3. A 740 MBq Tc 99-labeled methyl diphosphonate bone scintigraphy to distinguish neoplasm showed increased uptake only in bilateral femoral heads (Figure 3).

We recommended conservative treatment with analgesics and protected weight bearing. At first, she remained non-weight-bearing with bed rest and a wheel chair and took an oral nonsteroidal anti-inflammatory drug (25 mg of diclofenac [Voltaren]; Novartis Pharmaceuticals Japan, Tokyo, Japan) three times per day. Despite continued symptoms, magnetic resonance image seven weeks after onset

demonstrated a return of normal bone marrow signal intensity in the bilateral femoral heads (Figure 4). Her symptoms gradually resolved eight weeks after onset. The results of these tests and clinical course led us to make a tentative diagnosis of TOH.

Pain and range of motion in the left hip improved earlier than those in the right hip. Partial weight bearing with crutches was allowed eight weeks after onset. She was discharged from the hospital with crutches and took no analgesics two months after onset. The left hip was fully improved with a normal range of motion three months after onset, and full weight bearing without pain was possible. By four months, the range of motion in bilateral hips had completely recovered. At this point, she was permitted to gradually return to her job. The intensity was gradually increased, and her return to full activity was permitted at nine months after onset.

She was subsequently followed up over a period of 12 months. Follow-up X-ray and magnetic resonance image were normal. She was able to return to her normal level of activity.

3. Discussion

This case suggested two clinical issues. First, a patient without pregnancy may have simultaneous bilateral TOH. Second, magnetic resonance image is useful in detecting this disorder even in the absence of abnormal X-ray and laboratory test findings.

Our case report revealed that a patient without pregnancy could have simultaneous bilateral TOH. TOH usually affects pregnant women in the third trimester or middle-aged men [2, 7]. All patients of previous reports involving simultaneous bilateral TOH were pregnant women [3–6]. Although the cause of TOH of young woman remains unclear, Rajak and Camilleri noted a clear association between pregnancy and TOH [8]. Investigators advocated that the etiology of the TOH involved obturator nerve compressions or local vascular blocks by the fetus, defects in fibrinolysis due to pregnancy causing ischemia in the bone, and deficiencies in bone metabolism such as vitamin D deficiency [7]. In previous simultaneous bilateral TOH cases, Axt-Fliedner et al. reported a pregnant woman with functional recovery after the termination of pregnancy via cesarean section due to limited motion in both hips [4]. Willis-Owen et al. reported a pregnant woman with simultaneous bilateral TOH following a femoral neck fracture [5]. Emami et al. also reported a pregnant woman who had simultaneous bilateral TOH following femoral neck fracture and noted that the mechanism of TOH was considered to be a microvascular disorder leading to tissue ischemia [6]. We believe that our patient (without pregnancy) could provide the new clue in determining the cause of bilateral simultaneous TOH.

Magnetic resonance imaging was useful in detecting TOH when plain X-ray showed no abnormalities. Although plain X-ray is believed to typically show pronounced demineralization and the loss of a trabecular pattern in the femoral head and neck [1, 9], no radiographic evidence

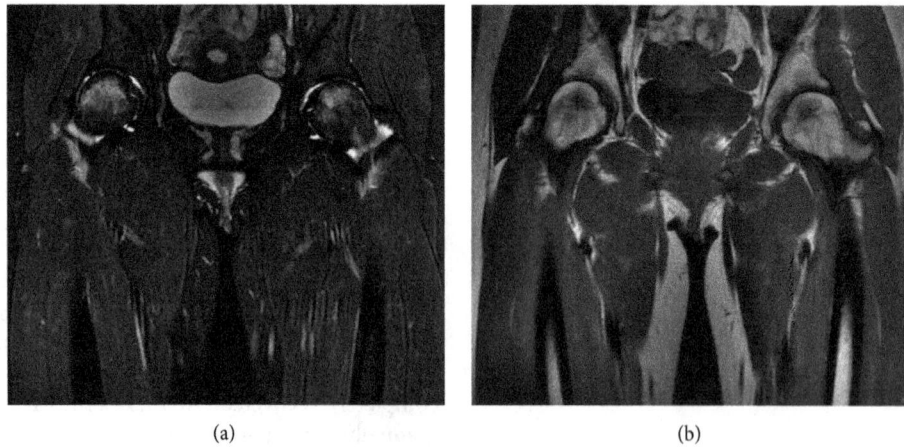

FIGURE 2: Magnetic resonance images of pelvis one week after symptom onset. (a) Coronal T2-weighted magnetic resonance image. Increased signal uptake within the femoral heads and necks bilaterally. There were no signs of osteonecrosis. (b) Coronal T1-weighted magnetic resonance image. Decreased signal uptake within the femoral heads and necks bilaterally.

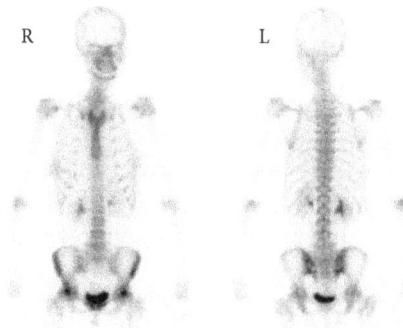

FIGURE 3: Bone scintigraphy of pelvis one month after symptom onset. Increased signal uptake within the femoral heads and necks bilaterally.

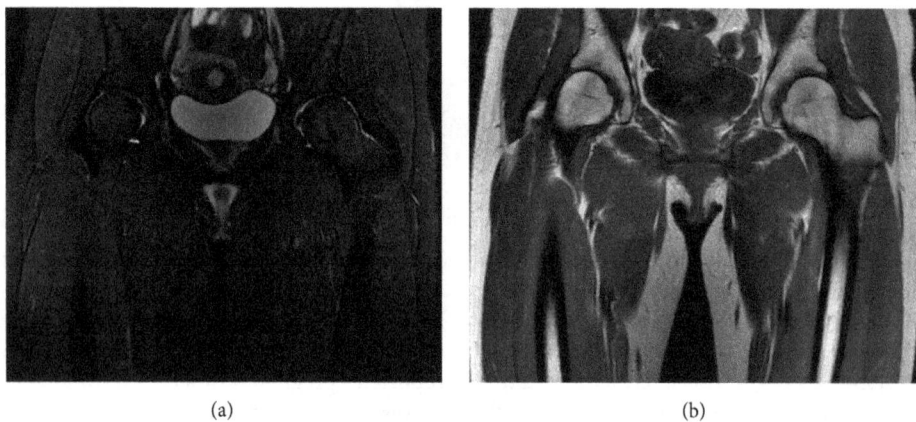

FIGURE 4: Magnetic resonance images of pelvis seven weeks after symptom onset. (a) Coronal T2-weighted magnetic resonance image. Normal signal uptake within the femoral heads and necks bilaterally. (b) Coronal T1-weighted magnetic resonance image. Normal signal uptake within the femoral heads and necks bilaterally.

of demineralization may exist during early symptom onset [10]. Our case had no remarkable plain X-ray findings at one week after symptom onset, and some investigators reported normal plain X-ray findings in the early stage of TOH [11, 12]. Magnetic resonance imaging shows diffuse bone marrow edema with increased signal on T2-weighted images and decreased signal on T1-weighted images in TOH [13]. Characteristic findings of TOH in magnetic resonance imaging include the complete resolution of abnormal signal intensity over several weeks [14]. Our report supported the utility of repeated magnetic resonance imaging in a patient suspected to be affected by TOH.

Several investigators recommend distinguishing TOH from transient bone marrow edema syndrome [14–16]. Hayes et al. advocated that the term "transient bone marrow edema syndrome" should be used for patients in whom the bone marrow edema pattern was not accompanied by radiographic evidence of osteopenia [14]. Our case fulfilled the criteria of Hayes et al. for transient bone marrow edema syndrome. However, we believe that distinguishing between the two terms is rarely useful in clinical practice because it may not impact the therapeutic strategy.

Bone mineral density measured at nine days after onset remained within the normal range in this case. Several reports suggested the relationship between TOH and low bone mineral density [17, 18]. Because bone mineral density changes with time in TOH [18], single-point measurement may cause the normal finding of bone mineral density in this case.

TOH is a rare disorder that cannot be easily diagnosed. Clinicians should be aware of the possibility of simultaneous bilateral hip pain caused by TOH unless the patient is pregnant. We recommend advanced imaging, especially magnetic resonance imaging, if the patient is suspected to be affected by TOH without abnormal findings on plain X-ray.

4. Conclusions

To the best of our knowledge, this is the first case report of simultaneous bilateral TOH in a patient without pregnancy. Notably, unless the patient is pregnant, the patient could be affected by simultaneous bilateral TOH. If the patient is suspected to be affected by TOH without clear abnormal findings via plain X-ray, magnetic resonance imaging is recommended for diagnosis and in monitoring disease progression.

Competing Interests

The authors have no competing interests.

Acknowledgments

The authors thank Yuji Iwata, M.D., Yu Sato, M.D., Kentaro Amaha, M.D., Mikihito Ito, M.D., Souichi Tsuji, M.D., Eishi Kuroda, M.D., and Hajime Inoue, M.D., for their help in this study.

References

[1] P. H. Curtiss Jr. and W. E. Kincaid, "Transitory demineralization of the hip in pregnancy. A report of three cases," *The Journal of Bone & Joint Surgery—American Volume*, vol. 41, pp. 1327–1333, 1959.

[2] S. Lakhanpal, W. W. Ginsburg, H. S. Luthra, and G. G. Hunder, "Transient regional osteoporosis. A study of 56 cases and review of the literature," *Annals of Internal Medicine*, vol. 106, no. 3, pp. 444–450, 1987.

[3] G. W. Keys and J. Walters, "Idiopathic transient osteoporosis of the hip: brief report," *The Journal of Bone & Joint Surgery—British Volume*, vol. 69, no. 5, pp. 773–774, 1987.

[4] R. Axt-Fliedner, G. Schneider, R. Seil, M. Friedrich, D. Mink, and W. Schmidt, "Transient bilateral osteoporosis of the hip in pregnancy: a case report and review of the literature," *Gynecologic and Obstetric Investigation*, vol. 51, no. 2, pp. 138–140, 2001.

[5] C. A. Willis-Owen, J. S. Daurka, A. Chen, and A. Lewis, "Bilateral femoral neck fractures due to transient osteoporosis of pregnancy: a case report," *Cases Journal*, vol. 1, article 120, 2008.

[6] M. J. Emami, H. R. Abdollahpour, A. R. Kazemi, and A. R. Vosoughi, "Bilateral subcapital femoral neck fractures secondary to transient osteoporosis during pregnancy: a case report," *Journal of Orthopaedic Surgery*, vol. 20, no. 2, pp. 260–262, 2012.

[7] G. Maliha, J. Morgan, and M. Vrahas, "Transient osteoporosis of pregnancy," *Injury*, vol. 43, no. 8, pp. 1237–1241, 2012.

[8] R. Rajak and J. Camilleri, "An unusual cause of hip pain," *BMJ Case Reports*, vol. 2011, 2011.

[9] J. D. Brodell, J. E. Burns Jr., and K. G. Heiple, "Transient osteoporosis of the hip of pregnancy. Two cases complicated by pathological fracture," *The Journal of Bone & Joint Surgery—American Volume*, vol. 71, no. 8, pp. 1252–1257, 1989.

[10] D. Szwedowski, Z. Nitek, and J. Walecki, "Evaluation of transient osteoporosis of the hip in magnetic resonance imaging," *Polish Journal of Radiology*, vol. 79, pp. 36–38, 2014.

[11] M. J. Bolland, "Bilateral transient osteoporosis of the hip in a young man," *Journal of Clinical Densitometry*, vol. 11, no. 2, pp. 339–341, 2008.

[12] J. Vogler, J. Caracciolo, and D. Cheong, "Bilateral transient osteoporosis of the hip," *JBJS Case Connector*, vol. 4, no. 3, article e56, 2014.

[13] J. Dhaliwal, J. S. McConnell, and T. Greer, "Bilateral transient osteoporosis of the hip in a 20-year-old man," *BMJ Case Reports*, 2014.

[14] C. W. Hayes, W. F. Conway, and W. W. Daniel, "MR imaging of bone marrow edema pattern: transient osteoporosis, transient bone marrow edema syndrome, or osteonecrosis," *Radiographics*, vol. 13, no. 5, pp. 1001–1012, 1993.

[15] A. V. Korompilias, A. H. Karantanas, M. G. Lykissas, and A. E. Beris, "Bone marrow edema syndrome," *Skeletal Radiology*, vol. 38, no. 5, pp. 425–436, 2009.

[16] A. H. Karantanas, "Acute bone marrow edema of the hip: role of MR imaging," *European Radiology*, vol. 17, no. 9, pp. 2225–2236, 2007.

[17] M. Varenna, L. Sinigaglia, L. Binelli, P. Beltrametti, and M. Gallazzi, "Transient osteoporosis of the hip: a densitometric study," *Clinical Rheumatology*, vol. 15, no. 2, pp. 169–173, 1996.

[18] R. Niimi, A. Sudo, M. Hasegawa, A. Fukuda, and A. Uchida, "Changes in bone mineral density in transient osteoporosis of the hip," *The Journal of Bone & Joint Surgery—British Volume*, vol. 88, no. 11, pp. 1438–1440, 2006.

39

Traumatic Testicular Dislocation Associated with Lateral Compression Pelvic Ring Injury and T-Shaped Acetabulum Fracture

Daniel Howard Wiznia, Mike Wang, Chang Yeon-Kim, Paul Tomaszewski, and Michael P. Leslie

Department of Orthopaedics and Rehabilitation, Yale University School of Medicine, 800 Howard Avenue, New Haven, CT 06510, USA

Correspondence should be addressed to Daniel Howard Wiznia; daniel.wiznia@yale.edu

Academic Editor: Byron Chalidis

We report a case of a unilateral testicular dislocation to the superficial inguinal region associated with a lateral compression type pelvic ring injury (OTA classification 61-C3.3a2, b2, c3) and left T-shaped acetabulum fracture (OTA classification 62-B2) in a 44-year-old male who was in a motorcycle accident. The testicular dislocation was noted during the emergency department primary survey, and its location and viability were verified with ultrasound. The testicle was isolated during surgical stabilization of the left acetabulum through a Pfannenstiel incision and modified-Stoppa approach and returned through the inguinal canal to the scrotum. In follow-up, the patient did not suffer urologic or sexual dysfunction. All motorcycle collision patients presenting with pelvic ring injuries or acetabulum fractures should be worked up for possible testicular dislocation with a scrotal exam. Advanced imaging and a urologic consult may be necessary to detect and treat these injuries.

1. Introduction

Traumatic testicular dislocation is a rare finding most frequently found as part of a spectrum of anterior posterior compression type pelvic ring fractures associated with motorcycle collisions [1–5]. The following report describes a testicular dislocation with a lateral compression type pelvic ring injury and a T-type acetabulum fracture, which is unique to the literature. The purpose of this report is to raise awareness of the potential association of lateral compression type pelvic ring injuries and testicular dislocations in the context of motorcycle-related trauma, as well as describe comanagement of this presentation. Knowledge of this presentation will likely prevent iatrogenic injury and the associated comorbidities of an unrecognized testicular dislocation. We have obtained the patient's written informed consent for print and electronic publication of this report.

2. Case Report

A 44-year-old nonhelmeted motorcycle rider presented to the emergency department after suffering a front end collision. Clinical exam demonstrated a Glasgow Coma Scale of 14. His right arm was positioned overhead with the shoulder in full abduction and elbow in flexion, his left leg was shortened with a foot drop, and only one testicle was palpable in the scrotum. Imaging demonstrated a lateral compression pelvic ring injury which included a type II dens left-sided sacral fracture with dissociation and bilateral superior and inferior pubic rami fractures (OTA classification 61-C3.3a2, b2, c3) [6]. In addition, there was a left-sided T-shaped acetabulum fracture (OTA classification 62-B2) [6] with protrusio and right shoulder luxatio erecta (Figures 1 and 2). Ultrasound demonstrated that the left testicle was in the inguinal canal with normal Doppler wave forms (Figure 3). Urology was unable to relocate the testicle with external pressure.

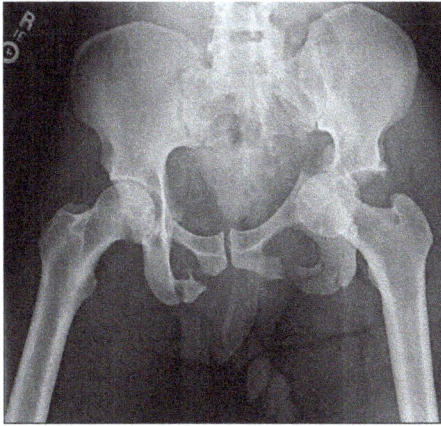

FIGURE 1: Trauma series AP pelvis radiograph.

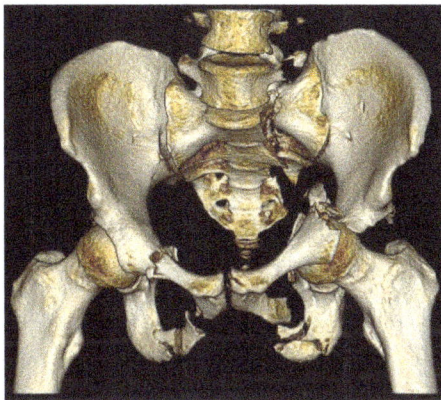

FIGURE 2: 3D pelvis preoperative CT reconstruction.

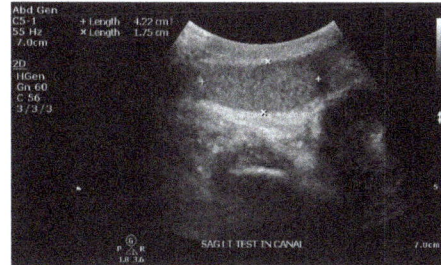

FIGURE 3: Ultrasound of left testicle in the inguinal canal.

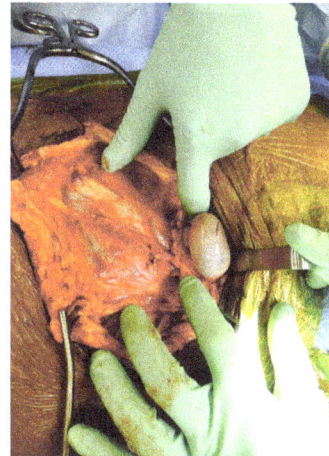

FIGURE 4: Intraoperative photograph of left testicle within the wound superior to the fascia overlying the inguinal canal.

On hospital day three, the patient went to the operating room for an open reduction and internal fixation of the left acetabular fracture. The posterior column of the acetabulum was addressed via a Kocher Langenbeck approach [7] and the anterior column was addressed with a Pfannenstiel incision and a modified-Stoppa approach [8]. As dissection was carried down to the level of the rectus fascia, the inguinal canal was noted to be completely disrupted and the left testicle was noted to be within the wound superior to the fascia overlying the inguinal canal (Figure 4). Soft tissue trauma suggested that the testicle was ejected through the superficial ring. Urology assisted in returning the testicle to the scrotum and confirmed blood flow with ultrasound.

Subsequently, the patient returned to the operating room on hospital day six for further stabilization of the pelvis (Figure 5). The patient underwent open reduction of the left sacral fracture, percutaneous screw fixation of the posterior pelvic ring (right sacroiliac joint and left zone 2 sacral fracture), and stabilization of the anterior pelvic ring with anterior external fixation.

At the twelfth week of follow-up, the patient had no urologic or sexual dysfunction. His left-sided foot drop improved. At one year of follow-up, the patient is ambulating with a cane.

3. Discussion

As noted above, testicular dislocation often presents with a wide variety of traumatic injuries, most frequently due to a motorcycle collision, and it can easily be overlooked due to the severity of other injuries [2]. Testicular dislocation occurs when an upward force is applied directly to the scrotum, forcing either one or both testicles into the surrounding tissues [2, 3]. The most common region to be dislocated to is the superficial inguinal area [2, 9], and dislocations to the deep inguinal canal and the abdominal cavity have been reported as well [2, 10]. In cases associated with motorcycle collisions, the force to the scrotum is likely caused by the gasoline tank striking the rider's perineum and scrotal region due to rapid deceleration of the vehicle [3]. In the above case, the testicular dislocation in the presence of a lateral compression pelvic ring injury is suggestive of two separate traumas, as a testicular dislocation requires an upward force, and the lateral compression of the pelvic ring is the result of a laterally directed force. This insight can be useful in reconstructing the sequence of events of the motorcycle accident.

There are case reports describing testicular dislocation associated with anterior-posterior pelvic ring injuries and various types of non-pelvic ring-associated lesions, such as femoral, tibial, and foot fractures, as well as soft tissue injuries [1–5, 9–13]. Specifically, Boudissa et al. described

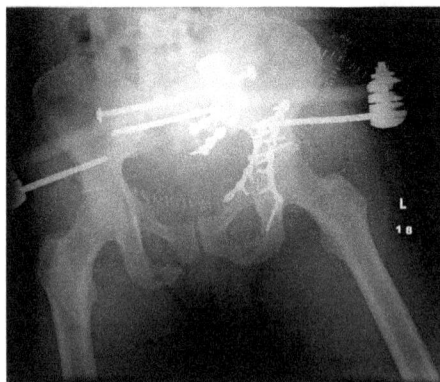

FIGURE 5: AP pelvis radiograph status after stabilization of the pelvis.

a bilateral testicular dislocation presenting with a Tile B1 pelvic ring fracture [1] and Smith et al. reported a bilateral testicular dislocation presenting with a type II anterior-posterior compression pelvic ring injury [2]. Our case is particularly interesting as no other reports to our knowledge have presented a testicular dislocation with an associated lateral compression type injury of the pelvic ring or with an associated acetabulum fracture.

All motorcycle collision patients presenting with pelvic ring injuries or acetabulum fractures should be worked up for possible testicular dislocation with a scrotal exam. Pelvic ring injuries presenting with testicular dislocation should be managed with a urologic consultation, as the location of the dislocated testicle is intimately tied with the pelvic ring fixation surgical approach [1]. The initial diagnosis of testicular dislocation should be made during the patient's workup by physical exam. Direct palpation of the scrotum for the presence of two testicles will suffice [1, 2]. Any concern for a missing testicle should be confirmed with either ultrasound or CT [3–5].

Once the diagnosis is confirmed, surgical reduction and orchidopexy are required to prevent urologic and sexual sequelae, which include spermatogenesis, fertility, and endocrine issues [1, 2]. Open reduction is indicated when the testicle cannot be relocated via external manipulation or if testicular and/or spermatic cord integrity is in doubt [1].

For our patient, the Pfannenstiel approach was used to stabilize the anterior column of the acetabulum fracture [8]. As the most common location of the dislocated testicle is the superficial inguinal region [8], which is directly in the path of the Pfannenstiel approach, the unaware surgeon performing this procedure may risk causing iatrogenic injuries to the dislocated testicle [1].

Patients with pelvic ring injuries or testicular dislocations should be examined for signs of additional urological injuries, such as bleeding at the urethral meatus, a high riding prostate, or hematuria [14]. Studies have demonstrated that urogenital injuries may be present in 12–20% of patients with pelvic ring fractures and that there is a higher incidence in males [14, 15]. Posterior urethral tears and bladder rupture are the most common urogenital injuries associated with pelvic

ring fractures [15]. Diagnosis is made with a retrograde urethrocystogram. Patients may require a temporary suprapubic catheter. Urological repairs should be done concomitantly with anterior ring stabilization to reduce the risk of infection [14]. Complications include urethral stricture, impotence, infection, anterior pelvic ring nonunion, and urinary incontinence [15].

Consent

For this case report, the authors have obtained the patient's written informed consent for print and electronic publication of the report and for reprinting in foreign editions of the journal.

Competing Interests

None of the authors have any competing interests with respect to the authorship and/or publication of this article.

Authors' Contributions

All authors have read the manuscript, agreed the work is ready for submission, and accepted responsibility for the manuscript's contents. Each author is a major contributor to the design of the study, analyzed the data and interpreted the results, prepared and edited the manuscript, and approved the final version of the paper. In addition, each author agrees to be accountable for all aspects of the work in ensuring that questions related to the accuracy or integrity of any part of the work are appropriately investigated and resolved.

References

[1] M. Boudissa, S. Ruatti, N. Maisse et al., "Bilateral testicular dislocation with pelvic ring fracture: a case report and literature review," *Orthopaedics and Traumatology: Surgery and Research*, vol. 99, no. 4, pp. 485–487, 2013.

[2] C. S. Smith, C. S. Rosenbaum, and A. M. Harris, "Traumatic bilateral testicular dislocation associated with an anterior posterior compression fracture of the pelvis: a case report," *Journal of Surgical Orthopaedic Advances*, vol. 21, no. 3, pp. 162–164, 2012.

[3] E. Perera, S. Bhatt, and V. S. Dogra, "Traumatic ectopic dislocation of testis," *Journal of Clinical Imaging Science*, vol. 1, article 17, 2011.

[4] N. Ezra, A. Afari, and J. Wong, "Pelvic and scrotal trauma: CT and triage of patients," *Abdominal Imaging*, vol. 34, no. 4, pp. 541–544, 2009.

[5] R. G. Gómez, O. Storme, G. Catalán, P. Marchetti, and M. Djordjevic, "Traumatic testicular dislocation," *International Urology and Nephrology*, vol. 46, no. 10, pp. 1883–1887, 2014.

[6] J. L. Marsh, T. F. Slongo, J. Agel et al., "Fracture and dislocation classification compendium—2007: Orthopaedic Trauma Association Classification, Database and Outcomes Committee," *Journal of Orthopaedic Trauma*, vol. 21, no. 10, supplement, pp. S1–S133, 2007.

[7] Y. Zhuang, J.-L. Lei, X. Wei, D.-G. Lu, and K. Zhang, "Surgical treatment of acetabulum top compression fracture with sea gull sign," *Orthopaedic Surgery*, vol. 7, no. 2, pp. 146–154, 2015.

[8] A. Khoury, Y. Weill, and R. Mosheiff, "The Stoppa approach for acetabular fracture," *Operative Orthopadie und Traumatologie*, vol. 24, no. 4-5, pp. 439–448, 2012.

[9] W. Bromberg, C. Wong, S. Kurek, and A. Salim, "Traumatic bilateral testicular dislocation," *The Journal of Trauma*, vol. 54, no. 5, pp. 1009–1011, 2003.

[10] S. Toranji and Z. Barbaric, "Testicular dislocation," *Abdominal Imaging*, vol. 19, no. 4, pp. 379–380, 1994.

[11] W. Kochakarn, V. Choonhaklai, P. Hotrapawanond, and V. Muangman, "Traumatic testicular dislocation a review of 36 cases," *Journal of the Medical Association of Thailand*, vol. 83, no. 2, pp. 208–212, 2000.

[12] S. Meena, N. Barwar, and B. Chowdhury, "Double trouble: testicular dislocation associated with hip dislocation," *Journal of Emergencies, Trauma and Shock*, vol. 7, no. 1, pp. 58–59, 2014.

[13] M. Tauber, H. Joos, S. Karpik, S. Lederer, and H. Resch, "Urogenital injuries accompanying pelvic ring fractures," *Unfallchirurg*, vol. 110, no. 2, pp. 116–123, 2007.

[14] N. F. Watnik, M. Coburn, and M. Goldberger, "Urologic injuries in pelvic ring disruptions," *Clinical Orthopaedics and Related Research*, no. 329, pp. 37–45, 1996.

[15] M. L. Routt, P. T. Simonian, A. J. Defalco, J. Miller, and T. Clarke, "Internal fixation in pelvic fractures and primary repairs of associated genitourinary disruptions: a team approach," *The Journal of Trauma*, vol. 40, no. 5, pp. 784–790, 1996.

40

Morel-Lavallée Lesion of the Knee in a Recreational Frisbee Player

Alison Shmerling,[1] Jonathan T. Bravman,[2] and Morteza Khodaee[3]

[1]*Department of Family Medicine, University of Colorado School of Medicine, Denver, CO 80238, USA*
[2]*CU Sports Medicine, Division of Sports Medicine and Shoulder Surgery, Department of Orthopaedics,*
 University of Colorado School of Medicine, Denver, CO 80238, USA
[3]*Department of Family Medicine, AFW Clinic, University of Colorado School of Medicine, 3055 Roslyn Street, Denver, CO 80238, USA*

Correspondence should be addressed to Morteza Khodaee; morteza.khodaee@ucdenver.edu

Academic Editor: John Nyland

Traumatic swelling/effusion in the knee region is a relatively common presenting complaint among athletes and nonathletes. Due to its broad differential diagnosis, a comprehensive evaluation beginning with history and physical examination are recommended. Knee joint effusion can be differentiated from other types of swelling by careful physical examination. Imaging, including plain radiography, ultrasound, and magnetic resonance imaging (MRI), is preferred modality. Aspiration of a local fluctuating mass may help with the diagnosis and management of some of these conditions. We present a case of a 26-year-old gentleman with superomedial Morel-Lavallée lesion (MLL) of the knee with history of a fall during a Frisbee game. His MLL was successfully treated with therapeutic aspiration and compression wrap without further sequelae. MLL is a rare condition consisting of a closed degloving injury caused by pressure and shear stress between the subcutaneous tissue and the superficial fascia or bone. Most commonly, MLL is found over the greater trochanter and sacrum but in rare cases can occur in other regions of the body. In most cases, concurrent severe injury mechanisms and concomitant fractures are present. MLL due to sports injuries are very rare. Therapeutic strategies may vary from compression wraps and aspiration to surgical evacuation.

1. Introduction

Effusions and swelling in the knee region are common presenting complaints among athletes and nonathletes. With a thorough history and physical examination, particularly with a history of trauma, infectious and inflammatory causes can often be ruled out. The time course of a traumatic knee effusion is also important to incorporate, as an effusion evolving within four hours of injury increases the likelihood of major osseous, ligamentous, or meniscal injury [1]. Morel-Lavallée lesions (MLL) is a rare condition presenting with superficial fluid collection between subcutaneous tissue and the superficial fascia or bone mainly caused by direct trauma. MLLs are a structural cause of knee swelling which are often missed or late diagnosed, in part because their occurrence at the knee is only more recently appreciated [2]. With MLL, the lesion can present anywhere from a few hours after the injury or as late as 13 years later, making the diagnosis more challenging [3]. Fortunately, with imaging techniques such as ultrasound and MRI, and procedures such as aspiration, MLL is increasingly diagnosed as the etiology of traumatic periarticular knee swelling. This case describes an uncharacteristic MLL found in the knee of a recreational Frisbee player. There have been only few case reports of sports related knee MLL.

2. Case Report

A 26-year-old gentleman presented to his primary care physician with right knee swelling after a direct fall on his knee during a Frisbee game 2 days earlier. He denied hearing or feeling a popping sensation. The swelling had developed over a few hours but started diminishing since the day before the visit. His moderate pain has been improving since the incident. He had been able to walk with minimum discomfort. His past medical, social, and family histories were unremarkable. On physical examination, he had a mild ecchymosis

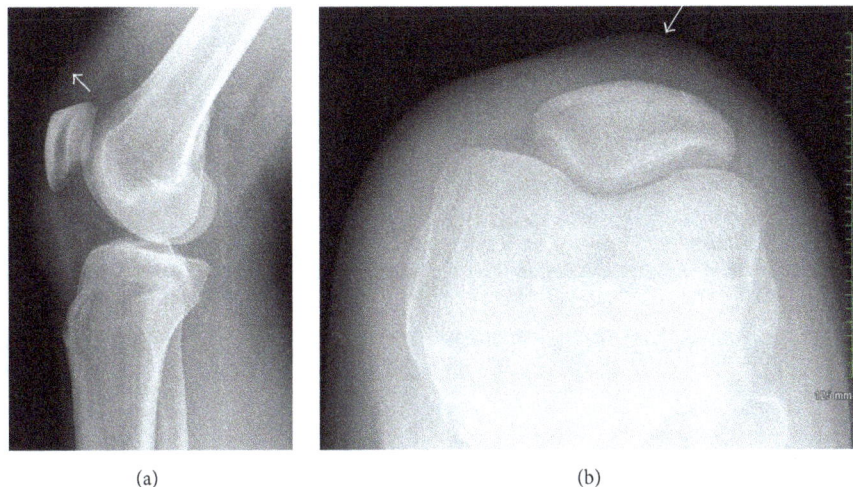

FIGURE 1: Plain radiography of the right knee. Lateral (a) and sunrise (b) views revealed anterior soft tissue swelling particularly in the superomedial patellar region (arrows).

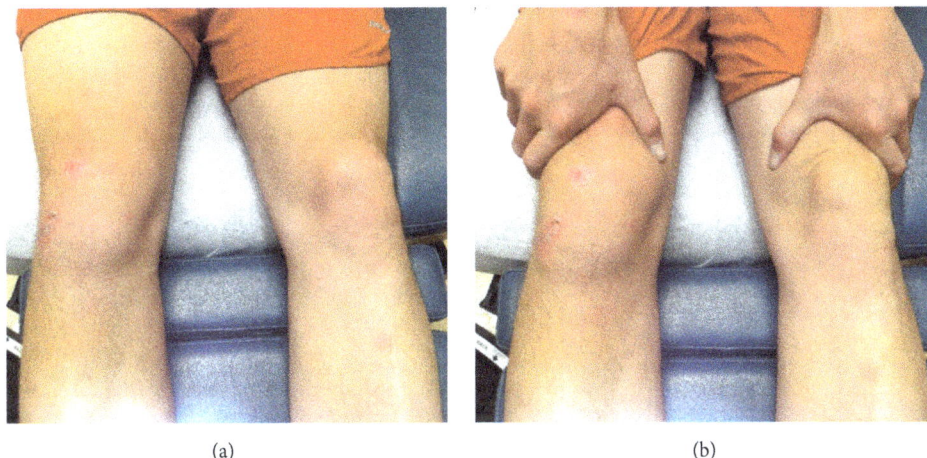

FIGURE 2: Moderate swelling/effusion in the superomedial aspect of right knee (a) which is accentuated by milking the suprapatellar tissue inferiorly (b).

and abrasion in the superior aspect of his knee with mild swelling. Plain radiography demonstrated soft tissue swelling anteriorly without osseous abnormality (Figure 1). He was advised to rest and use ibuprofen as needed for pain. He presented to our sports medicine clinic with continuous, painless swelling in the same region 19 days after injury. He denied mechanical symptoms and his physical examination was significant for a nontender, moderate sized swelling in the superomedial aspect of his right knee (Figure 2). There was no palpable joint effusion. In-office ultrasound revealed a homogeneous, anechoic fluid collection with scattered hyperechoic substance between the superficial quadriceps fascia and subcutaneous tissue which was compressible (Figure 3). After proper cleansing and local anesthesia with 1% lidocaine, using ultrasound for needle placement and an 18-gauge needle, 38 mL serosanguinous fluid was aspirated (Figure 4). Patient was advised to use a compression wrap following the procedure. He presented for recurrence of his knee swelling on day 25 after injury. Another aspiration provided 35 mL of serosanguinous fluid. After the second aspiration, his symptoms were completely resolved with no reaccumulation of the fluid. At latest follow-up, 4 weeks from injury, he is asymptomatic and had returned to full, unrestricted activity.

3. Discussion

MLL is a rare condition consisting of a closed degloving injury caused by tangential impact and shear stress between the subcutaneous tissue and the muscle fascia or bone [4]. The potential space between these tissues is subsequently filled with serous, blood, lymphatic fluid, or necrotic fat [5, 6]. Most commonly, this lesion is found over the greater trochanter but can be found in other regions of the body [5–7]. Classic history includes crush injury, with soft fluctuant area appreciable on physical examination [3, 5]. MLL has been rarely reported in the knee region [2, 8–12] and as a result of sports injuries [10, 13–16]. In some chronic cases, the history of a significant trauma may not be present [16].

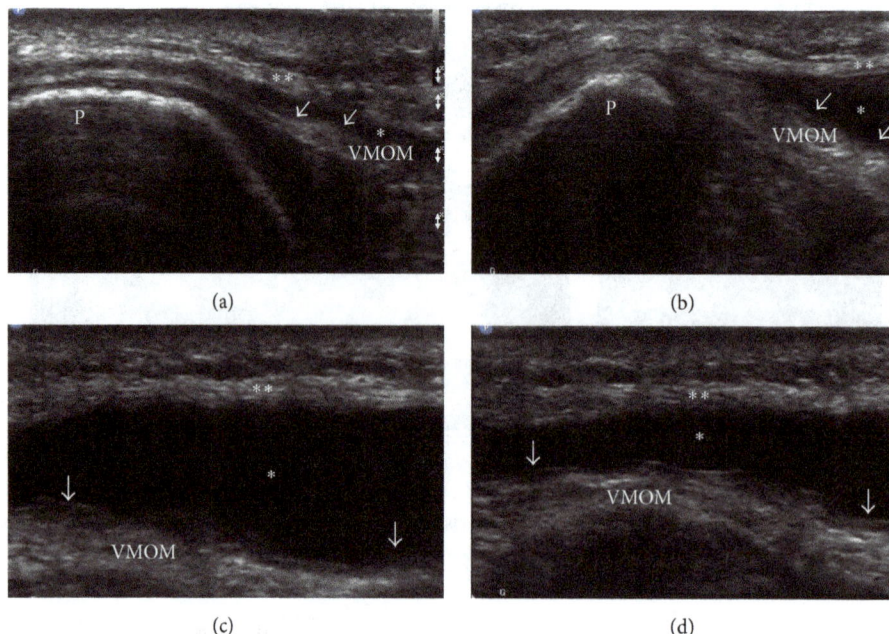

(a)

(b)

(c)

(d)

FIGURE 3: Using a linear transducer (Philips L12–3 MHz) an area of homogenous anechoic fluid collection with scattered hyperechoic substance (∗) between subcutaneous tissue (∗∗) and superficial quadriceps fascia (arrows) was visualized. Long-axis middle suprapatellar view (a), long-axis medial suprapatellar view (b), short-axis medial suprapatellar view (c), and compressible fluid collection in short-axis suprapatellar view (d). Patellae (P) and vastus medialis oblique muscle (VMOM) look unremarkable with no signs of prepatellar bursal enlargement.

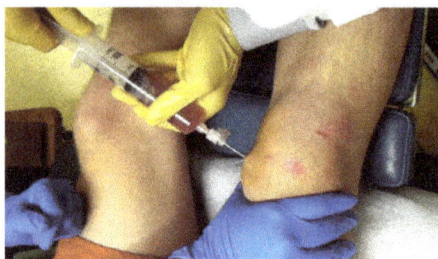

FIGURE 4: Using ultrasound for needle placement, 38 mL serosanguinous fluid was aspirated.

For these reasons, MLLs are often misdiagnosed. The natural course is not well understood, with the lesion potentially enlarging in size, remaining stable, or self-resolving. This depends on the content of the fluid and stages of hematoma formation [5, 17, 18]. In some cases, it may recur [5, 18].

Diagnosis can be made clinically. Ultrasound may reveal hypoechoic or anechoic collection which is typically compressible and usually located between deep fat and overlying fascia, regardless of age of the lesion [4]. Lesions <1 month old appear heterogeneous with irregular margins and lobular shape, while lesions >18 months old tend to appear more homogenous and have a flat or fusiform shape with smooth margins [4, 17]. MRI can also be used to diagnose MLL [4, 5, 11, 12, 17] and can help classify MLL into different types based on T1 and T2 characteristics of the lesions [5]. Mellado and Bencardino classified the MLL into six types [18]. Type I is a serohematic effusion, type II is a subacute hematoma, type III is a chronic organizing hematoma, type IV is perifascial dissection with closed fatty laceration, type V is a

perifascial pseudonodular lesion, and type VI characterizes as an infected lesion with multiple sinus tract formation, internal septations, and thick capsule [5, 18]. With MRI, the age of the lesion is more easily appreciated [5].

Treatment varies from watchful waiting to drainage and compression/pressure, with surgical intervention as a last resort [3, 5, 19]. Percutaneous aspiration with a large-bore needle (14–22 gauges) is recommended, particularly being performed with ultrasound guidance, both to aid with diagnosis and to treat the lesion. Depending on the stage of hematoma formation, aspiration may not provide any fluid. Immediate compression after aspiration may help prevent reaccumulation [10, 11]. Sclerosing agents such as doxycycline, erythromycin, alcohol, bleomycin, or talc can be used on chronic lesions [5] and surgery may be performed for refractory cases, which may involve excision of the pseudocapsule and necrotic tissue debridement [3, 5, 19]. The wound is then either left open, placed to vacuum seal, or closed with or without a drain [11].

Based on few case reports including this case, it seems that MLLs as a result of low energy and sports injuries typically have a favorable outcome with full return to physical activities and no further sequelae.

Consent

The patient gave the informed consent to the publication of the case study.

Competing Interests

The authors declare no competing interests and do not have any financial disclosures.

References

[1] M. W. Johnson, "Acute knee effusions: a systematic approach to diagnosis," *American Family Physician*, vol. 61, no. 8, pp. 2391–2400, 2000.

[2] S. van Gennip, S. C. van Bokhoven, and E. van den Eede, "Pain at the knee: the Morel-Lavallée lesion, a case series," *Clinical Journal of Sport Medicine*, vol. 22, no. 2, pp. 163–166, 2012.

[3] T. P. Nickerson, M. D. Zielinski, D. H. Jenkins, and H. J. Schiller, "The Mayo clinic experience with morel-lavallée lesions: establishment of a practice management guideline," *Journal of Trauma and Acute Care Surgery*, vol. 76, no. 2, pp. 493–497, 2014.

[4] C. Neal, J. A. Jacobson, C. Brandon, M. Kalume-Brigido, Y. Morag, and G. Girish, "Sonography of Morel-Lavallée lesions," *Journal of Ultrasound in Medicine*, vol. 27, no. 7, pp. 1077–1081, 2008.

[5] I. Bonilla-Yoon, S. Masih, D. B. Patel et al., "The Morel-Lavallée lesion: pathophysiology, clinical presentation, imaging features, and treatment options," *Emergency Radiology*, vol. 21, no. 1, pp. 35–43, 2014.

[6] F. H. Chokshi, J. Jose, and P. D. Clifford, "Morel-Lavallée lesion," *American Journal of Orthopedics*, vol. 39, no. 5, pp. 252–253, 2010.

[7] A. Harma, M. Inan, and K. Ertem, "The Morel-Lavallée lesion: a conservative approach to closed degloving injuries," *Acta Orthopaedica et Traumatologica Turcica*, vol. 38, no. 4, pp. 270–273, 2004.

[8] M. Ciaschini and M. Sundaram, "Prepatellar Morel-Lavallée Lesion," *Orthopedics*, vol. 31, no. 7, pp. 626–721, 2008.

[9] S. Kumar and S. Kumar, "Morel-Lavallee lesion in distal thigh: a case report," *Journal of Clinical Orthopaedics and Trauma*, vol. 5, no. 3, pp. 161–166, 2014.

[10] S. G. Tejwani, S. B. Cohen, and J. P. Bradley, "Management of Morel-Lavallee lesion of the knee: twenty-seven cases in the national football league," *The American Journal of Sports Medicine*, vol. 35, no. 7, pp. 1162–1167, 2007.

[11] I. S. Vanhegan, B. Dala-Ali, L. Verhelst, P. Mallucci, and F. S. Haddad, "The Morel-Lavallée Lesion as a rare differential diagnosis for recalcitrant bursitis of the knee: case report and literature review," *Case Reports in Orthopedics*, vol. 2012, Article ID 593193, 5 pages, 2012.

[12] N. A. Weiss, J. J. Johnson, and S. B. Anderson, "Morel-lavallee lesion initially diagnosed as quadriceps contusion: ultrasound, MRI, and importance of early intervention," *Western Journal of Emergency Medicine*, vol. 16, no. 3, pp. 438–441, 2015.

[13] R. Depaoli, E. Canepari, C. Bortolotto, and G. Ferrozzi, "Morel-Lavallée lesion of the knee in a soccer player," *Journal of Ultrasound*, vol. 18, no. 1, pp. 87–89, 2015.

[14] RJ. Fawcett, "Morel-Lavallee lesion in a male cyclist," *BMJ Case Reports*, 2013.

[15] M. J. Matava, E. Ellis, N. R. Shah, D. Pogue, and T. Williams, "Morel-lavallée lesion in a professional american football player," *The American Journal of Orthopedics*, vol. 39, no. 3, pp. 144–147, 2010.

[16] M. Khodaee and R. S. Deu, "Ankle Morel-Lavallée lesion in a recreational racquetball player," *The Journal of Sports Medicine and Physical Fitness*, In press.

[17] B. S. Goodman, M. T. Smith, S. Mallempati, and P. Nuthakki, "A comparison of ultrasound and magnetic resonance imaging findings of a morel-lavallée lesion of the knee," *PM & R*, vol. 5, no. 1, pp. 70–73, 2013.

[18] J. M. Mellado and J. T. Bencardino, "Morel-Lavallée lesion: review with emphasis on MR imaging," *Magnetic Resonance Imaging Clinics of North America*, vol. 13, no. 4, pp. 775–782, 2005.

[19] S. Tseng and P. Tornetta III, "Percutaneous management of Morel-Lavallee lesions," *Journal of Bone and Joint Surgery—Series A*, vol. 88, no. 1, pp. 92–96, 2006.

41

Interdigital Neuroma in the Second Intermetatarsal Space Associated with Metatarsophalangeal Joint Instability

Takumi Matsumoto, Song Ho Chang, Naohiro Izawa, Yohei Ohshiro, and Sakae Tanaka

Department of Orthopaedic Surgery, Faculty of Medicine, The University of Tokyo, 7-3-1 Hongo, Bunkyo-ku, Tokyo 113-8655, Japan

Correspondence should be addressed to Takumi Matsumoto; matumot-tky@umin.ac.jp

Academic Editor: Koichi Sairyo

The entrapment theory is the most commonly accepted theory concerning the development of interdigital neuroma; it incriminates the deep transverse metatarsal ligament as the major causative factor of the condition. This report presents a patient with interdigital neuroma in the second intermetatarsal space, which was strongly suspected to be caused by the metatarsophalangeal joint instability due to plantar plate injury. Surgical intervention revealed that the neuroma was located more distally and dorsally than the deep transverse metatarsal ligament and was pinched between the adjacent metatarsal heads, suggesting the involvement of the metatarsophalangeal joint instability and chronic trauma as etiologies in this case.

1. Introduction

Interdigital neuroma in the foot, generally known as Morton's neuroma, is a painful condition that produces neuropathic pain in the distribution of the affected interdigital nerve [1]. Other conditions that cause forefoot pain can be differential diagnoses of Morton's neuroma and include stress fracture, metatarsalgia, degenerative and inflammatory arthritis, Freiberg disease, tarsal tunnel syndrome, tumors, and metatarsophalangeal (MTP) joint instability [1, 2]. Caution must also be exercised in case of the concomitant existence of these pathologies with interdigital neuroma. In particular, a high prevalence of coexisting second intermetatarsal space neuroma and second MTP joint instability has been reported [3]; however, there has been little discussion about the possible etiologic relationship between these two pathologies [3]. Because overlooking MTP joint instability can lead to residual pain after neurectomy for interdigital neuroma [4], it is important to understand the relationship between these two pathologies.

Here, we report a case of interdigital neuroma in the second intermetatarsal space accompanied with MTP joint instability of the second and third toes due to plantar plate rupture. The interdigital nerve was deflected dorsally and a spatulate-shaped neuroma was formed between the second and third metatarsal heads. The neuroma had a dent in the center, which was assumed to have been made by the impression between the metatarsal heads. The symptoms were completely resolved after neurectomy and plantar plate reconstruction of the second and third MTP joints. This case strongly supports the chronic trauma theory as one of the etiologies of interdigital neuroma and indicates a possible causal relationship between interdigital neuroma and MTP joint instability.

2. Case Report

The patient was a 62-year-old male with an 11-year history of dialysis due to chronic renal failure. He had complained of pain around the second and third metatarsal heads and numbness in the second and third lesser toes five to six years ago, which was accentuated by ambulation and shoes with a tight toe box. He had received conservative treatment including intermittent local analgesic injection a few years ago from other physicians and was referred to our hospital due to the gradual worsening of symptoms, which were unresponsive to conservative treatment.

When he presented at our hospital, he could not walk for more than 10 minutes at a time because of pain accentuated

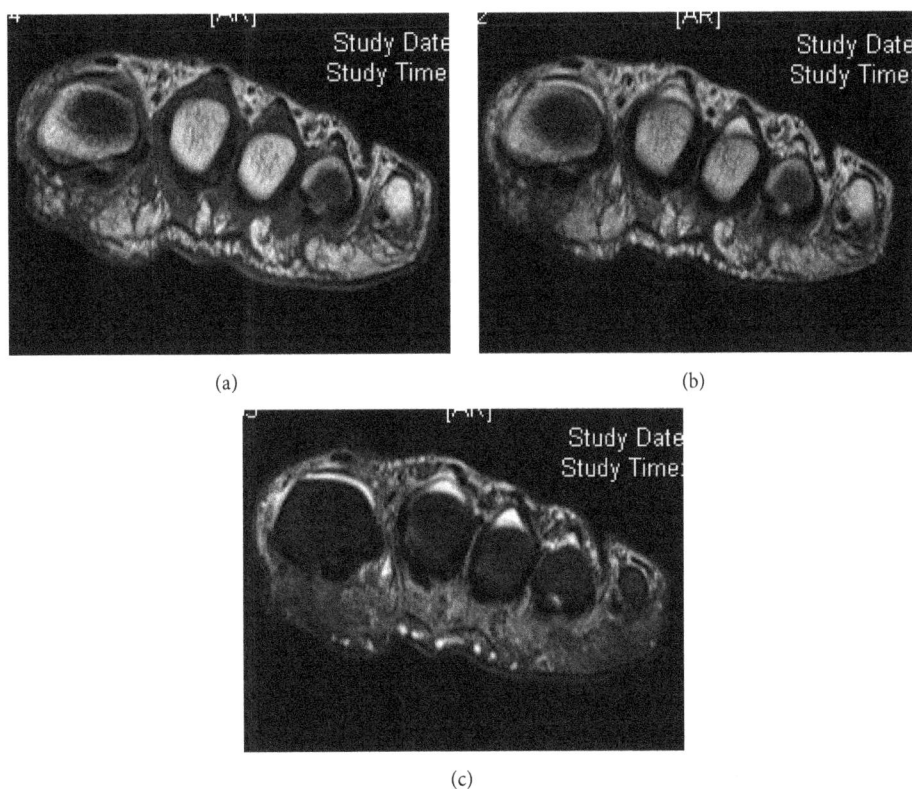

(a)

(b)

(c)

FIGURE 1: Magnetic resonance images of the distal metatarsals showing an upside-down bulbous-shaped mass with low-signal intensity in T1-weighted (a), T2-weighted (b), and short-tau inversion recovery image (c) extending dorsally between the second and third metatarsal heads.

by ambulation. The static observation of the feet in the standing position showed hammertoe deformities of the second and third toes, which did not touch the ground. Clinical examination revealed tenderness to palpation in the second and third MTP joints and the second intermetatarsal space. The foot squeeze test examining Mulder's sign elicited a severe radiating pain but not the click [5]. The drawer test was positive in both the second and third MTP joints showing more than 50% subluxation and producing intolerable radiating pain in the second and third toes. Radiographs of the feet showed no apparent deviation of the toes but demonstrated a slight opening of the joint space at the second MTP joint. T1-weighted magnetic resonance imaging scans in the coronal plane showed an upside-down bulbous-shaped neuroma with low-signal intensity between the second and third metatarsal heads (Figure 1). Although taping in order to stabilize the toe in the neutral position was effective in reducing the pain accentuated by ambulation, it did not change the numbness in the toes. The taping was not continued for over a month by the patient because of discomfort; therefore, surgical treatment with excision of the interdigital neuroma and plantar plate repair was offered to the patient.

The operation was performed under tourniquet control through a 3 cm dorsal incision over the second intermetatarsal space. Before dividing the deep transverse metatarsal ligament (DTML), the visibly enlarged interdigital nerve was observed which was deflected dorsally and was located between the second and third metatarsal heads (Figure 2(a)).

The neuroma had a spatulate shape and had a dent in the center, which was plausibly due to the impression by the metatarsal heads (Figures 2(b) and 3). After the transection of the DTML, the second common digital nerve was dissected as proximally as practical before cutting it and any adjacent capsular nerve branches were served in order to allow the proximal nerve stump to retract into the intrinsic muscles of the foot. The nerve including the neuroma was resected with a length of 3 cm. Subsequently, the second and third MTP joints were exposed through the interval between the extensor digitorum longus and brevis tendons. The metatarsal head transected using Weil osteotomy was shifted proximally about 10 mm and temporarily fixed with a K-wire. An incomplete tear of the plantar plate was noted at the insertion of the plantar plate into the base of the proximal phalanx, which was a grade II tear in the second MTP joint with greater than 50% tear laterally and a grade I tear in the third MTP joint with less than 50% tear medially according to the grading by Nery et al. [6]. The plantar plates of the second and third MTP joints were repaired by sewing them back on the plantar base of the proximal phalanx following the method described by Watson et al. [7]. Shortly, a partially attached plantar plate was detached completely from the base of the proximal phalanx. A mattress suture was created in the plantar plate using the Mini Scorpion DX loaded with 0-Fiberwire (Arthrex, Naples, FL). Then, the sutures were retrieved into the two oblique holes which were made at the base of the proximal phalanx using a 0.062-inch K-wire.

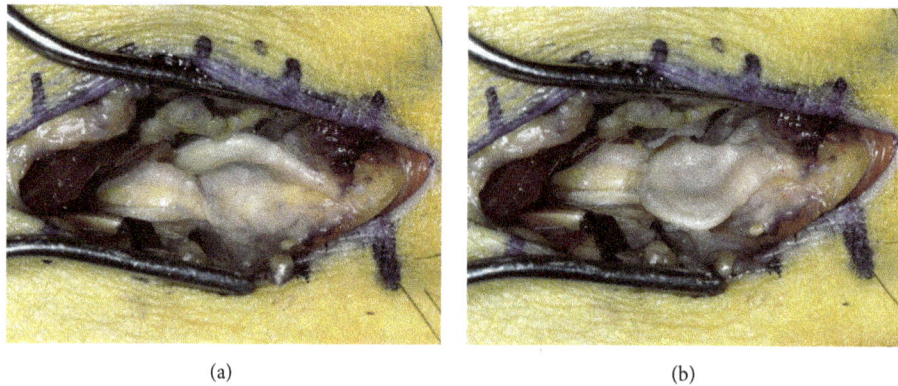

(a)   (b)

FIGURE 2: Intraoperative photograph. (a) Dorsally deviated course of the interdigital nerve and neuroma; (b) transversely reclined neuroma showing the impression in its center assumedly made by the adjacent metatarsal heads.

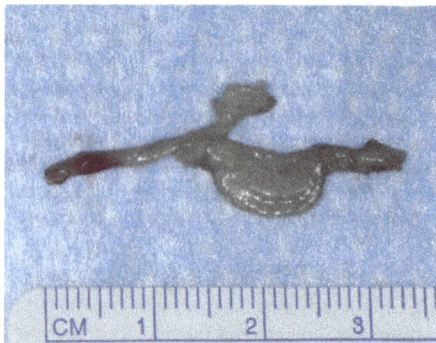

FIGURE 3: Excised interdigital nerve including a neuroma located distal to the bifurcation point.

The K-wire in the Weil osteotomy was removed, and the metatarsal head was relocated in the position with 3 mm of shortening and fixed with an Asnis micro 2.0 mm cannulated titanium screw (Stryker Japan, Tokyo, Japan). Then, the sutures were tied over the dorsal aspect of the proximal phalanx with the toe plantar-flexed in 15 degrees at the MTP joint. Postoperatively, the patient was allowed to walk in a postoperative shoe with no weight on the forefoot for 3 weeks and with weight through the entire foot for another 3 weeks. Comfortable shoes and normal gait were permitted 6 weeks after the surgery. The histopathology result reported neural fibrosis, which was consistent with an interdigital neuroma.

The postoperative course was uneventful. At one year postoperatively, the patient could walk unrestricted in normal shoes. He had no pain but had a reduction of sensation in the supplying area of the resected nerve, which did not affect the patient's satisfaction. The Japanese Society for Surgery of the Foot (JSSF) ankle/hindfoot scale improved from 64 preoperatively to 85 one year postoperatively. The Self-Administered Foot Evaluation Questionnaire [8], which was developed and validated by JSSF as a patient-based outcome measure, improved or remained unchanged from the preoperative period to one year postoperatively in each subscale as follows: 71 to 81 in pain and pain-related, 75 to 89 in physical functioning and daily living, 83 to 88 in social functioning, 33 to 75 in shoe-related, and 100 to 100 in general health and well-being.

3. Discussion

Open neurectomy for interdigital neuroma is the most common procedure in patients with persistent symptoms unresponsive to the conservative treatment; however, some patients complain of continued forefoot pain even after the procedure. The rate of residual pain after neurectomy for interdigital neuroma has been reported to be from 4 to 35% [9–14]. While some of the continued pain after neurectomy might be attributed to inadequate resection or secondary conditions such as stump neuroma, some might be attributed to misdiagnosis or an overlooking of other concomitant pathologies. Haddad et al. reported that some cases with residual pain after neuroma resection in the second inter-metatarsal space were successfully treated by flexor tendon transfer for correction of the crossover second toe deformity [4]. This study promotes awareness about concurrent MTP joint instability when treating interdigital neuroma. The study by Coughlin et al. involving 121 patients with symptomatic interdigital neuroma reported that 24 patients (20%) had a concurrent second MTP joint instability [3]. They also reported that 81% of these cases with two concurrent pathologies had neuromas in the second intermetatarsal space, a proportion markedly higher than in generally reported cases concerning the location of interdigital neuromas. The incidence of interdigital neuroma in the second intermetatarsal space has been reported to be from 5 to 32% [10, 11, 13, 15–18]. A reported higher prevalence of the second intermetatarsal space neuroma in cases with the second MTP joint instability compared to the prevalence of the second intermetatarsal space neuroma in the general population strongly suggests an association between these two pathologies.

Many histological studies have demonstrated that interdigital neuroma is not a true neuroma but a perineural fibrosis [15, 19–21]. Several theories have been advocated as etiologies of interdigital neuroma including the chronic repetitive trauma theory, entrapment theory, ischemic theory, and intermetatarsal bursitis theory [22]. Among these, the entrapment theory is the most common where the neuroma is considered to be formed by the entrapment of the interdigital nerve at the point where the nerve passes underneath the DTML [23, 24]. This theory is supported by the success of Gauthier's surgical technique consisting of the release of

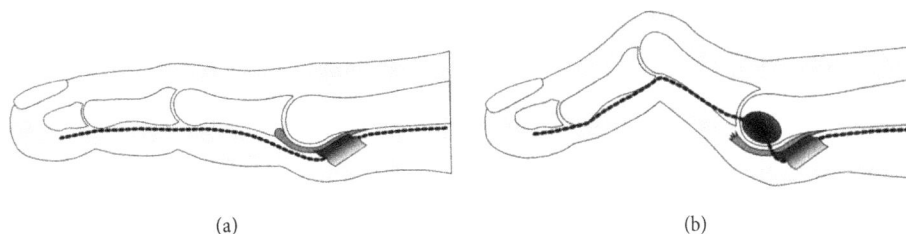

(a)   (b)

FIGURE 4: Diagram showing the etiology of interdigital neuroma associated with metatarsophalangeal joint instability. (a) The interdigital nerve runs consistently along the bottom side of the toe passing under the deep transverse metatarsal ligament at the distal metatarsal. (b) Metatarsophalangeal joint instability can curve the interdigital nerve with the distal end of deep transverse metatarsal ligament as a flexion point predisposing the nerve to impingement by the adjacent metatarsal heads.

the anterior edge of the DTML without resection of the neuroma [23]. In 206 patients treated with this technique, 83% reportedly had rapid and stable improvement [23]. On the other hand, the chronic repetitive trauma theory suggests that repeated trauma to the interdigital nerve by mechanical effects during walking causes neuroma [15, 25]. The frequent involvement of the third common digital nerve has been explained anatomically since the third common digital nerve is generally formed by branches of the medial and lateral plantar nerves, which possibly make the nerve vulnerable to tethering [26]. Electron microscopic evaluation of the resected specimens of interdigital neuroma reported edema of the endoneurium, fibrosis beneath the perineurium, axonal degeneration, and necrosis, which suggested nerve damage secondary to mechanical impingement by adjacent structures [27]. While the DTML is necessarily involved in the pathology of the interdigital neuroma as demonstrated by the success of Gauthier's surgical technique, some authors have advocated the involvement of the metatarsal heads [5, 25, 28]. An anatomical study examining the relationship between the location of interdigital neuromas and the DTML demonstrated that the interdigital neuromas were located more distally than the DTML in both the mid-stance and the heel-off stage during walking, which raised an objection against an entrapment by the DTML and supported chronic repetitive trauma by the metatarsal heads as an etiology [28]. The eliciting procedure known as Mulder's click, which has high sensitivity and specificity in diagnosing interdigital neuroma, is considered to replicate the compression of neuromas by the metatarsal heads [5, 29, 30]. The neuroma in our case was located between the metatarsal heads distally apart from the DTML and showed the peculiar configuration suggesting mechanical compression by the adjacent metatarsal heads.

Like the collateral ligaments, the plantar plate is a major static-stabilizing structure of the lesser MTP joint [6, 31] and its rupture has been well-documented as a primary pathology of MTP joint instability [31–33]. The plantar plate originates from the proximal neck of the metatarsal metaphysis with a thin synovial attachment and inserts distally into the plantar base of the proximal phalanx with a firm fibrocartilaginous attachment. Several structures have an attachment with the plantar plate including the plantar fascia, tendon sheath of the flexor tendons, DTML, collateral ligaments, and the interossei tendons [33, 34]. The insertion area of the DTML into the plantar plate is located at its proximal two-thirds and plantar

one-third [34]. Although a plantar plate tear can be caused by trauma, most of the tears occur as degenerative changes around its distal attachment to the proximal phalanx [6]. A cadaveric study transecting the plantar plate at the distal attachment demonstrated an increase of displacement of the proximal phalanx by over 70% [31]. Clinically, the severest stage of plantar plate tear is even associated with dorsal dislocation of the proximal phalanx [6, 35]. Considering the course of the interdigital nerve under the DTML, MTP joint instability due to the plantar plate insufficiency is expected to cause pulling or dorsal deviation of the interdigital nerve with tethering at the distal end of the DTML (Figure 4). As plantar plate insufficiency occurs most commonly at the second MTP joint, the interdigital nerve most likely affected will be the one running through the second intermetatarsal space [6, 36].

When MTP joint instability and interdigital neuroma coexist, it is not easy to confirm which pathology produces the patient's chief complaint. Patients with interdigital neuroma generally complain of a burning pain localized to the plantar aspect of the forefoot, which may radiate into the toes. Conversely, patients with plantar plate insufficiency demonstrate a hammer toe or crossover toe if the deformity progresses; however, they only complain of a pain localized to the plantar aspect of the forefoot mimicking interdigital neuroma in the early stage with no toe deformity. Sequential xylocaine injections may help to differentiate the two pathologies; however, the possible spreading of injected fluid around adjacent structures makes the interpretation of results ambiguous [3, 37]. Recently, the direct repair of plantar plate rupture through a dorsal approach has been established with good clinical outcome [6, 7, 38]. The present case was successfully treated with neurectomy and direct repair of the plantar plate with no residual pain or toe deformity. We recommend that MTP joint instability accompanied with the interdigital neuroma should be treated with neurectomy in order to exclude the risk of residual pain or toe deformity progression.

4. Conclusion

We reported a case of interdigital neuroma in the second intermetatarsal space which could be attributed to the MTP joint instability. Considering the possible causal relationship between these two pathologies, MTP instability should be examined for carefully in patients diagnosed with interdigital neuromas, especially in neuromas occurring in the second intermetatarsal space.

Competing Interests

The authors declare that there are no competing interests regarding the publication of this paper.

References

[1] S. Jain and K. Mannan, "The diagnosis and management of Morton's neuroma: a literature review," *Foot & Ankle Specialist*, vol. 6, no. 4, pp. 307–317, 2013.

[2] K. K. Wu, "Morton's interdigital neuroma: a clinical review of its etiology, treatment, and results," *Journal of Foot and Ankle Surgery*, vol. 35, no. 2, pp. 112–119, 1996.

[3] M. J. Coughlin, R. C. Schenck Jr., P. S. Shurnas, and D. M. Bloome, "Concurrent interdigital neuroma and MTP joint instability: long-term results of treatment," *Foot & Ankle International*, vol. 23, no. 11, pp. 1018–1025, 2002.

[4] S. L. Haddad, R. C. Sabbagh, S. Resch, B. Myerson, and M. S. Myerson, "Results of flexor-to-extensor and extensor brevis tendon transfer for correction of the crossover second toe deformity," *Foot and Ankle International*, vol. 20, no. 12, pp. 781–788, 1999.

[5] J. D. Mulder, "The causative mechanism in Morton's metatarsalgia," *The Journal of Bone & Joint Surgery—British Volume*, vol. 33, no. 1, pp. 94–95, 1951.

[6] C. Nery, M. J. Coughlin, D. Baumfeld, and T. S. Mann, "Lesser metatarsophalangeal joint instability: prospective evaluation and repair of plantar plate and capsular insufficiency," *Foot and Ankle International*, vol. 33, no. 4, pp. 301–311, 2012.

[7] T. S. Watson, D. Y. Reid, and T. L. Frerichs, "Dorsal approach for plantar plate repair with weil osteotomy: operative technique," *Foot and Ankle International*, vol. 35, no. 7, pp. 730–739, 2014.

[8] H. Niki, S. Tatsunami, N. Haraguchi et al., "Validity and reliability of a self-administered foot evaluation questionnaire (SAFE-Q)," *Journal of Orthopaedic Science*, vol. 18, no. 2, pp. 298–320, 2013.

[9] G. Dereymaeker, I. Schroven, A. Steenwerckx, and P. Stuer, "Results of excision of the interdigital nerve in the treatment of morton's metatarsalgia," *Acta Orthopaedica Belgica*, vol. 62, no. 1, pp. 22–25, 1996.

[10] M. J. Coughlin and T. Pinsonneault, "Operative treatment of interdigital neuroma. A long-term follow-up study," *The Journal of Bone & Joint Surgery—American Volume*, vol. 83, no. 9, pp. 1321–1328, 2001.

[11] A. Pace, B. Scammell, and S. Dhar, "The outcome of Morton's neurectomy in the treatment of metatarsalgia," *International Orthopaedics*, vol. 34, no. 4, pp. 511–515, 2010.

[12] K. T. Lee, J. B. Kim, K. W. Young, Y. U. Park, J. S. Kim, and H. Jegal, "Long-term results of neurectomy in the treatment of Morton's neuroma: more than 10 years' follow-up," *Foot & Ankle Specialist*, vol. 4, no. 6, pp. 349–353, 2011.

[13] M. Kasparek and W. Schneider, "Surgical treatment of Morton's neuroma: clinical results after open excision," *International Orthopaedics*, vol. 37, no. 9, pp. 1857–1861, 2013.

[14] T. Bauer, E. Gaumetou, S. Klouche, P. Hardy, and N. Maffulli, "Metatarsalgia and Morton's disease: comparison of outcomes between open procedure and neurectomy versus percutaneous

[15] N. Hingertz and L. Unander-Scharin, "Morton's disease: a clinical and patho-anatomical study," *Acta Orthopaedica*, vol. 19, no. 3, pp. 327–348, 1950.

[16] C. J. Gudas and G. M. Mattana, "Retrospective analysis of intermetatarsal neuroma excision with preservation of the transverse metatarsal ligament," *Journal of Foot Surgery*, vol. 25, no. 6, pp. 459–463, 1986.

[17] D. A. Friscia, D. E. Strom, J. W. Parr, C. L. Saltzman, and K. A. Johnson, "Surgical treatment for primary interdigital neuroma," *Orthopedics*, vol. 14, no. 6, pp. 669–672, 1991.

[18] J. Valero, J. Gallart, D. González, J. Deus, and M. Lahoz, "Multiple interdigital neuromas: a retrospective study of 279 feet with 462 neuromas," *Journal of Foot and Ankle Surgery*, vol. 54, no. 3, pp. 320–322, 2015.

[19] G. B. Ha'Eri, V. L. Fornasier, and J. Schatzker, "Morton's neuroma—pathogenesis and ultrastructure," *Clinical Orthopaedics and Related Research*, no. 141, pp. 256–259, 1979.

[20] R. J. Guiloff, J. W. Scadding, and L. Klenerman, "Morton's metatarsalgia. Clinical electrophysiological and histological observations," *Journal of Bone and Joint Surgery—Series B*, vol. 66, no. 4, pp. 586–591, 1984.

[21] E. W. Morscher, J. Ulrich, and W. Dick, "Morton's intermetatarsal neuroma: morphology and histological substrate," *Foot and Ankle International*, vol. 21, no. 7, pp. 558–562, 2000.

[22] H. Hassouna and D. Singh, "Morton's metatarsalgia: pathogenesis, aetiology and current management," *Acta Orthopaedica Belgica*, vol. 71, no. 6, pp. 646–655, 2005.

[23] G. Gauthier, "Thomas Morton's disease: a nerve entrapment syndrome. A new surgical technique," *Clinical Orthopaedics and Related Research*, no. 142, pp. 90–92, 1979.

[24] S. L. Shapiro, "Endoscopic decompression of the intermetatarsal nerve for Morton's neuroma," *Foot and Ankle Clinics*, vol. 9, no. 2, pp. 297–304, 2004.

[25] T. G. Morton, "A peculiar and painful affliction of the fourth metatarsophalangeal joint articulation," *The American Journal of the Medical Sciences*, vol. 71, pp. 37–45, 1876.

[26] J. R. Jones and L. Klenerman, "A study of the communicating branch between the medial and lateral plantar nerves," *Foot and Ankle*, vol. 4, no. 6, pp. 313–315, 1984.

[27] M. J. Shereff and D. A. Grande, "Electron microscopic analysis of the interdigital neuroma," *Clinical Orthopaedics and Related Research*, no. 271, pp. 296–299, 1991.

[28] J.-Y. Kim, H. C. Jae, J. Park, J. Wang, and I. Lee, "An anatomical study of Morton's interdigital neuroma: the relationship between the occurring site and the deep transverse metatarsal ligament (DTML)," *Foot and Ankle International*, vol. 28, no. 9, pp. 1007–1010, 2007.

[29] D. J. Cloke and M. E. Greiss, "The digital nerve stretch test: a sensitive indicator of Morton's neuroma and neuritis," *Foot and Ankle Surgery*, vol. 12, no. 4, pp. 201–203, 2006.

[30] R. Owens, N. Gougoulias, H. Guthrie, and A. Sakellariou, "Morton's neuroma: clinical testing and imaging in 76 feet, compared to a control group," *Foot and Ankle Surgery*, vol. 17, no. 3, pp. 197–200, 2011.

[31] L. A. Ford, K. B. Collins, and J. C. Christensen, "Stabilization of the subluxed second metatarsophalangeal joint: flexor tendon transfer versus primary repair of the plantar plate," *Journal of Foot and Ankle Surgery*, vol. 37, no. 3, pp. 217–222, 1998.

metatarsal osteotomies and ligament release with a minimum of 2 years of follow-up," *Journal of Foot and Ankle Surgery*, vol. 54, no. 3, pp. 373–377, 2015.

[32] J. T. Deland, M. Sobel, S. P. Arnoczky, and F. M. Thompson, "Collateral ligament reconstruction of the unstable metatarsophalangeal joint: an in vitro study," *Foot and Ankle*, vol. 13, no. 7, pp. 391–395, 1992.

[33] R. B. Johnston III, J. Smith, and T. Daniels, "The plantar plate of the lesser toes: an anatomical study in human cadavers," *Foot and Ankle International*, vol. 15, no. 5, pp. 276–282, 1994.

[34] J. T. Deland, K.-T. Lee, M. Sobel, and E. F. DiCarlo, "Anatomy of the plantar plate and its attachments in the lesser metatarsal phalangeal joint," *Foot and Ankle International*, vol. 16, no. 8, pp. 480–486, 1995.

[35] F. M. Thompson and W. G. Hamilton, "Problems of the second metatarsophalangeal joint," *Orthopedics*, vol. 10, no. 1, pp. 83–89, 1987.

[36] M. J. Coughlin, "Second metatarsophalangeal joint instability in the athlete," *Foot and Ankle*, vol. 14, no. 6, pp. 309–319, 1993.

[37] L. Yao, H. M. Do, A. Cracchiolo, and K. Farahani, "Plantar plate of the foot: findings on conventional arthrography and MR imaging," *American Journal of Roentgenology*, vol. 163, no. 3, pp. 641–644, 1994.

[38] J. A. V. Sanhudo and J. L. Ellera Gomes, "Pull-out technique for plantar plate repair of the metatarsophalangeal joint," *Foot and Ankle Clinics*, vol. 17, no. 3, pp. 417–424, 2012.

42

A Subdermal Osteochondroma in a Young Girl

Heather A. Cole,[1] Hernan Correa,[2] and Jonathan G. Schoenecker[1,2,3,4,5]

[1]Department of Orthopaedics and Rehabilitation, Vanderbilt University Medical Center, 4202 Doctors' Office Tower,
2200 Children's Way, Nashville, TN 37232-9565, USA
[2]Department of Pathology, Vanderbilt University Medical Center, 4202 Doctors' Office Tower, 2200 Children's Way,
Nashville, TN 37232-9565, USA
[3]Department of Pediatrics, Vanderbilt University Medical Center, 4202 Doctors' Office Tower, 2200 Children's Way,
Nashville, TN 37232-9565, USA
[4]Vanderbilt Center for Bone Biology, Vanderbilt University Medical Center, 4202 Doctors' Office Tower, 2200 Children's Way,
Nashville, TN 37232-9565, USA
[5]Department of Pharmacology, Vanderbilt University Medical Center, 4202 Doctors' Office Tower, 2200 Children's Way,
Nashville, TN 37232-9565, USA

Correspondence should be addressed to Jonathan G. Schoenecker; jon.schoenecker@vanderbilt.edu

Academic Editor: Elke R. Ahlmann

Osteochondromas are common benign tumors of cartilage and bone. They are usually found as contiguous bone with a cartilage cap at the end of the growth plate of long bones. Similar to structure are extraskeletal osteochondromas. However, unlike typical osteochondromas, extraskeletal osteochondromas are noncontinuous with bone. To our knowledge, all reported extraskeletal osteochondromas have been contained within fascial compartments. Here we present the case of a 5-year-old female who had a slow growing mass of the anterior distal right thigh. Imaging studies revealed an ossified mass extending from dermal layer of the subcutaneous tissue with no connection to the underlying deep fascia. An excisional biopsy was performed and proved to be a subdermal extraskeletal osteochondroma.

1. Introduction

An osteochondroma by definition is a benign tumor that includes components of both cartilage and bone [1–4]. A conventional osteochondroma occurs in the metaphysis of a long bone, is continuous with the adjacent bone, and extends into the soft tissues led by a proliferative cartilaginous cap. In reality, an osteochondroma can occur anywhere in which a population of undifferentiated chondrocytes exists, and there have been numerous reports of extraskeletal osteochondromas [1–17]. These rare, benign soft-tissue lesions must be differentiated from other mineralizing lesions, such as myositis ossificans, and more aggressive lesions such as synovial chondromas and synovial sarcomas. To our knowledge, all reported extraskeletal osteochondromas have been contained within fascial compartments. Here we present a case of a subcutaneous osteochondroma in a young girl.

2. Case Presentation

A 5-year-old female was seen at clinic, with a chief complaint of a mass in the anterior distal right thigh. The mass was noted to be slow growing but unknown when it first appeared. There were no complaints of pain, no history of trauma in the region, and no other lesions identified. On physical examination, the mass was firm and well adhered to the dermis but freely mobile over the underlying fascia. There were no skin changes or discoloration and the knee exam was otherwise normal.

Plain radiographs showed an oval, calcified mass within the soft tissue of the suprapatellar region (Figures 1(a) and 1(b)). Magnetic resonance imagining revealed a mass confined to the subcutaneous soft tissues along the anteromedial aspect of the thigh superficial to the vastus medialis causing extrinsic mass-effect without deep invasion (Figures 1(c) and

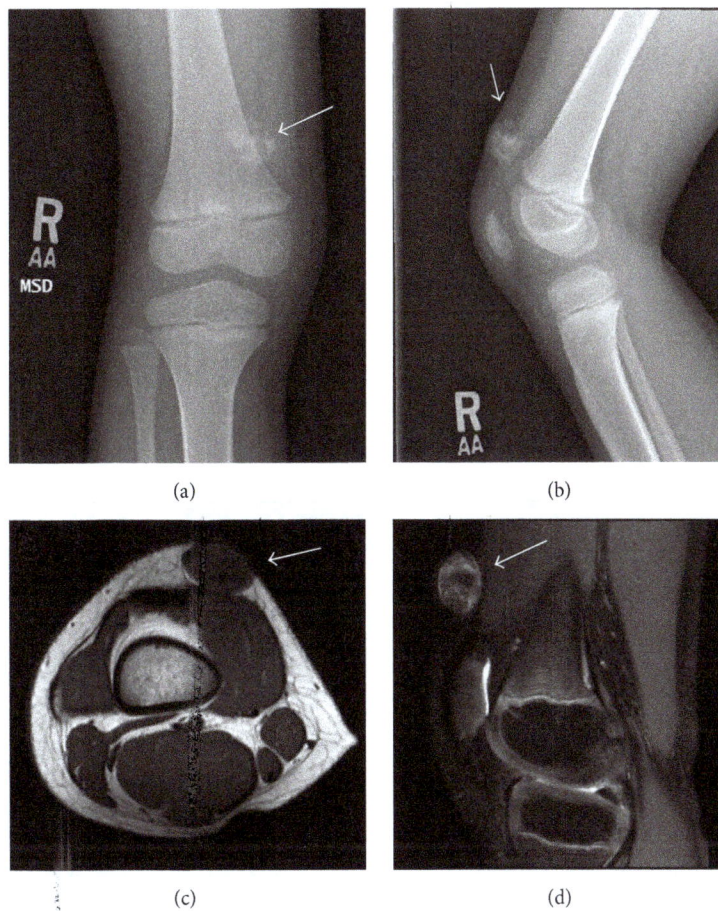

FIGURE 1: AP (a) and lateral (b) radiographic imaging of distal femur demonstrates aberrant calcification of the suprapatellar region within the soft tissue. Transverse (c) and lateral magnetic resonance imaging (d) reveals that the calcified mass is confined to the subcutaneous tissue with no connections to the underlying bone.

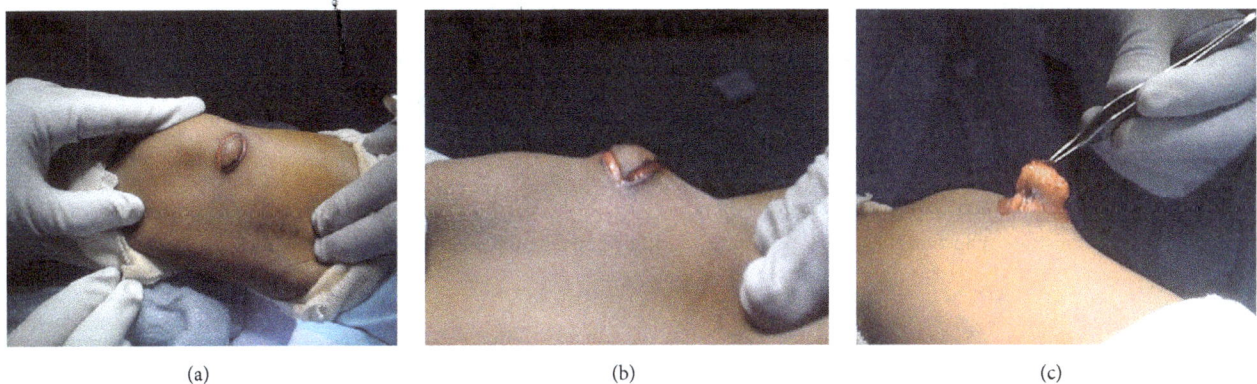

FIGURE 2: Intraoperative imagining demonstrates the mass within the subcutaneous tissue in the anteromedial region of the distal femur (a). An elliptical incision was made (b) and the calcified mass was carefully dissected and removed (c).

1(d)). This mass measured 2.0 cm medial-lateral by 1.4 cm anteroposterior by 1.9 cm cranial caudal with the underlying musculature appearing normal. This mass was predominantly low signal intensity both eccentrically and centrally on all imaging sequences. These findings were considered to show

an extraskeletal osteochondroma and an excisional biopsy was discussed with the family.

For the excision biopsy, an elliptical incision was made surrounding the nonadhesive area of the skin in Langer's lines (Figure 2). The mass was then dissected circumferentially

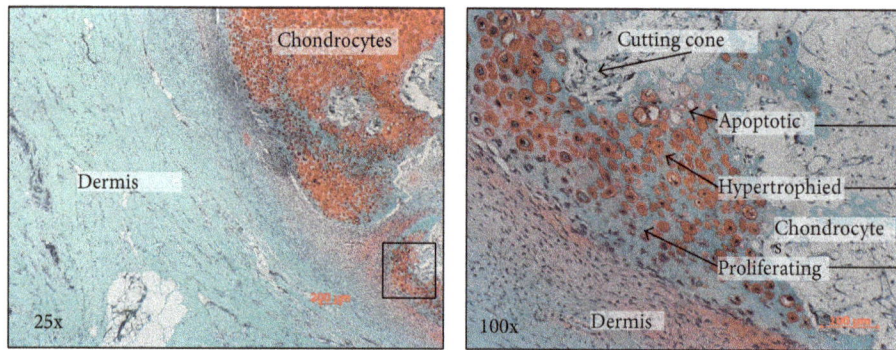

FIGURE 3: Safranin-O (25x) demonstrates cartilage cap with endochondral bone formation underlying the dermis. Zone of proliferation, hypertrophy, and apoptosis with new bone formation are identified at 100x. These findings are consistent with osteochondroma.

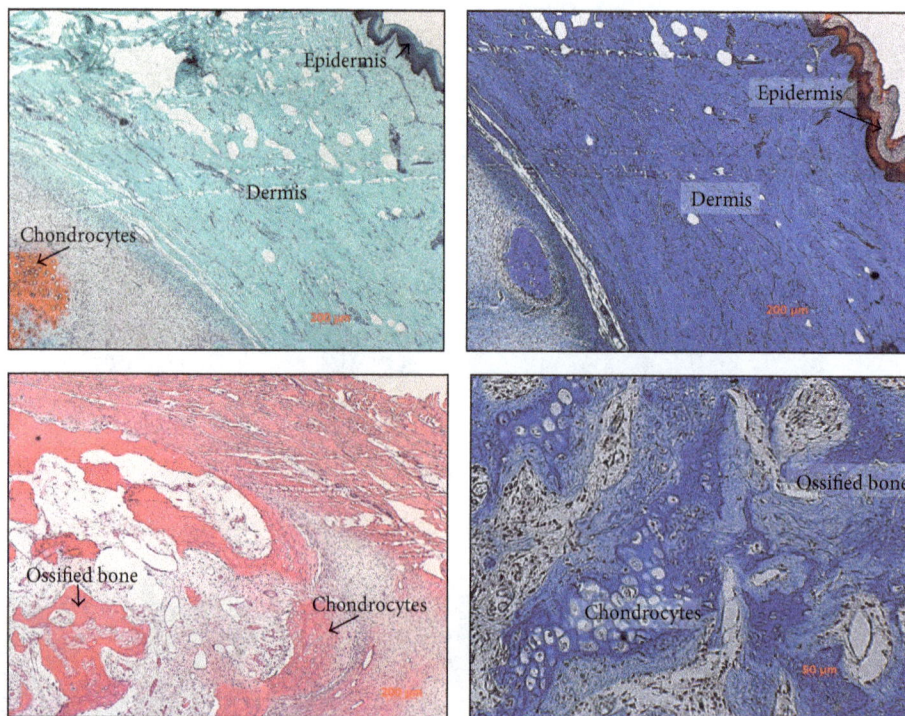

FIGURE 4: Safranin-O staining (25x) demonstrates calcified chondrocytes located just deep to the dermal area of the tissue (red). Masson's Trichrome (25x) demonstrates the epidermal (red) and dermal (blue) layer that is directly adjacent to the chondrocytic area. H&E and Masson's Trichrome (25x) demonstrate endochondral bone formation adjacent to a cartilaginous cap indicating the formation of an osteochondroma.

and easily removed as there were no attachments to the deep fascia. Grossly, the specimen was hard, tan-pale pink, bony cut surface with multifocal areas of firm, white, glistening, cartilaginous tissue. No discrete areas of hemorrhage or necrosis were grossly identified. A representative portion of tissue was submitted for histopathology. The sections demonstrated a nodular, slightly disorganized cartilaginous cap surrounding the lesion that progressed to endochondral-like bone formation (Figures 3 and 4). No evidence of malignancy was identified. No reoccurrence had developed at last follow-up clinic visit at age 9. No photographs or radiographs were available.

3. Discussion

Osteochondromas are the most common benign tumors occurring in the metaphysis of long bones [1, 2, 5]. Most commonly they present as an extension of the metaphysis consisting of trabecular bone with a cartilaginous cap. Germline mutation and functional loss of EXT1 or EXT2 are commonly found in multiple osteochondromas [6]. These proteins are expressed in the growth plate and it is known that mutations of these proteins can lead to heparin sulfate deficiency [6]. Heparin sulfate is an essential component of cell surface and matrix-associated proteoglycans and significant in regulating distribution and activity of signaling proteins [6]. Therefore, aberrant signaling factors are thought to lead to exostosis formation [6].

Rarely are these lesions extraskeletal or independent of the bone, but they have been reported in the hand, feet [3, 7, 8, 10–12], knee [13–15], and hip [16, 17], most commonly near tendon sheaths, joint capsule, or periosteum and most commonly found within the deep fascia. It has been suggested that the pathogenesis of such tumors occurs through either cellular migration, precartilaginous tissue persisting in the tendon, or metaplasia of mesenchymal cells or fibroblasts. Here we show for the first time to our knowledge as searched from English literature that osteochondroma extended from the dermal layer of the skin with complete containment within the subcutaneous tissue.

When presented with a well-circumscribed calcified lesion various possible differential diagnoses should be considered. These include myositis ossificans, lipomatous lesion, tumoral calcinosis, synovial sarcoma, and extraskeletal osteosarcoma, the most common being myositis ossificans. This diagnosis was considered initially with radiographic and magnetic resonance imaging. However, this lesion was confirmed by histopathology with the presence of trabecular bone surrounded by a cartilaginous cap and fibrous capsule (Figure 3). This is distinctly different than myositis ossificans, which is characterized by a zonal phenomenon of peripheral calcification and able to change size within a few weeks. While we acknowledge that extraskeletal osteochondromas are rare, the purpose of this paper is to present awareness to alternative diagnoses to circumscribed, calcified lesions.

Competing Interests

The authors declare that they have no competing interests.

Acknowledgments

The authors would like to thank the Caitlin Lovejoy Fund. Furthermore, the authors would like to recognize Dr. Bill Sales, Mrs. Sally A. Schoenecker, and Dr. Perry L. Schoenecker for their generous contributions to the laboratory.

References

[1] R. A. Marcial-Seoane, M. A. Marcial-Seoane, E. Ramos, and R. A. Marcial-Rojas, "Extraskeletal chondromas," *Boletin de la Asociacion Medica de Puerto Rico*, vol. 82, no. 9, pp. 394–402, 1990.

[2] D. W. Purser, "Extraskeletal osteochondromata," *The Journal of Bone and Joint Surgery*, vol. 38-B, no. 4, pp. 871–873, 1956.

[3] J. S. Sheff and S. Wang, "Extraskeletal osteochondroma of the foot," *Journal of Foot and Ankle Surgery*, vol. 44, no. 1, pp. 57–59, 2005.

[4] M. J. Kransdorf and J. M. Meis, "From the archives of the AFIP. Extraskeletal osseous and cartilaginous tumors of the extremities," *Radiographics*, vol. 13, no. 4, pp. 853–884, 1993.

[5] R. Singh, A. K. Sharma, N. K. Magu, K. P. Kaur, R. Sen, and S. Magu, "Extraskeletal osteochondroma in the nape of the neck:

a case report," *Journal of Orthopaedic Surgery*, vol. 14, no. 2, pp. 192–195, 2006.

[6] J. Huegel, F. Sgariglia, M. Enomoto-Iwamoto, E. Koyama, J. P. Dormans, and M. Pacifici, "Heparan sulfate in skeletal development, growth, and pathology: the case of hereditary multiple exostoses," *Developmental Dynamics*, vol. 242, no. 9, pp. 1021–1032, 2013.

[7] E. L. Gayle, W. B. Morrison, J. A. Carrino, T. W. Parsons, C. Y. Liang, and A. Stevenson, "Extraskeletal osteochondroma of the foot," *Skeletal Radiology*, vol. 28, no. 10, pp. 594–598, 1999.

[8] R. J. Spencer and N. M. Blitz, "Giant extraskeletal osteochondroma of the plantar midfoot arch," *Journal of Foot and Ankle Surgery*, vol. 47, no. 4, pp. 362–367, 2008.

[9] T. Ueno, S.-I. Ansai, T. Omi, and S. Kawana, "Extraskeletal osteochondroma arising on the plantar region," *Case Reports in Dermatology*, vol. 3, no. 2, pp. 147–150, 2011.

[10] V. K.-S. Kho and W.-C. Chen, "Extraskeletal osteochondroma of the foot," *Journal of the Chinese Medical Association*, vol. 73, no. 1, pp. 52–55, 2010.

[11] D. S. Williams and S. Zichichi, "Extraskeletal chondroma of the foot," *Journal of the American Podiatric Medical Association*, vol. 88, no. 10, pp. 506–509, 1998.

[12] P. J. Papagelopoulos, O. D. Savvidou, A. F. Mavrogenis, G. D. Chloros, K. T. Papaparaskeva, and P. N. Soucacos, "Extraskeletal chondroma of the foot," *Joint Bone Spine*, vol. 74, no. 3, pp. 285–288, 2007.

[13] A. V. Maheshwari, A. K. Jain, and I. K. Dhammi, "Extraskeletal paraarticular osteochondroma of the knee—a case report and tumor overview," *Knee*, vol. 13, no. 5, pp. 411–414, 2006.

[14] F. Oliva, A. Marconi, S. Fratoni, and N. Maffulli, "Extra-osseous osteochondroma-like soft tissue mass of the patello-femoral space," *BMC Musculoskeletal Disorders*, vol. 7, article no. 57, 2006.

[15] K. E. Ozturan, I. Yucel, H. Cakici, M. Guven, K. Gurel, and S. Dervisoglu, "Patellar tendinopathy caused by a para-articular/extraskeletal osteochondroma in the lateral infrapatellar region of the knee: a case report," *Cases Journal*, vol. 2, no. 12, article no. 9341, 2009.

[16] Z. J. Liu, Q. Zhao, and L. J. Zhang, "Extraskeletal osteochondroma near the hip: a pediatric case," *Journal of Pediatric Orthopaedics Part B*, vol. 19, no. 6, pp. 524–528, 2010.

[17] S.-C. Lim, Y.-S. Kim, Y.-S. Kim, and Y.-R. Moon, "Extraskeletal osteochondroma of the buttock," *Journal of Korean Medical Science*, vol. 18, no. 1, pp. 127–130, 2003.

Permissions

All chapters in this book were first published in CRIO, by Hindawi Publishing Corporation; hereby published with permission under the Creative Commons Attribution License or equivalent. Every chapter published in this book has been scrutinized by our experts. Their significance has been extensively debated. The topics covered herein carry significant findings which will fuel the growth of the discipline. They may even be implemented as practical applications or may be referred to as a beginning point for another development.

The contributors of this book come from diverse backgrounds, making this book a truly international effort. This book will bring forth new frontiers with its revolutionizing research information and detailed analysis of the nascent developments around the world.

We would like to thank all the contributing authors for lending their expertise to make the book truly unique. They have played a crucial role in the development of this book. Without their invaluable contributions this book wouldn't have been possible. They have made vital efforts to compile up to date information on the varied aspects of this subject to make this book a valuable addition to the collection of many professionals and students.

This book was conceptualized with the vision of imparting up-to-date information and advanced data in this field. To ensure the same, a matchless editorial board was set up. Every individual on the board went through rigorous rounds of assessment to prove their worth. After which they invested a large part of their time researching and compiling the most relevant data for our readers.

The editorial board has been involved in producing this book since its inception. They have spent rigorous hours researching and exploring the diverse topics which have resulted in the successful publishing of this book. They have passed on their knowledge of decades through this book. To expedite this challenging task, the publisher supported the team at every step. A small team of assistant editors was also appointed to further simplify the editing procedure and attain best results for the readers.

Apart from the editorial board, the designing team has also invested a significant amount of their time in understanding the subject and creating the most relevant covers. They scrutinized every image to scout for the most suitable representation of the subject and create an appropriate cover for the book.

The publishing team has been an ardent support to the editorial, designing and production team. Their endless efforts to recruit the best for this project, has resulted in the accomplishment of this book. They are a veteran in the field of academics and their pool of knowledge is as vast as their experience in printing. Their expertise and guidance has proved useful at every step. Their uncompromising quality standards have made this book an exceptional effort. Their encouragement from time to time has been an inspiration for everyone.

The publisher and the editorial board hope that this book will prove to be a valuable piece of knowledge for researchers, students, practitioners and scholars across the globe.

List of Contributors

Yoshifumi Kudo, Tomoaki Toyone, Toshiyuki Shirahata, Tomoyuki Ozawa, AkiraMatsuoka and Katsunori Inagaki
Department of Orthopaedic Surgery, Showa University School of Medicine, 1-5-8 Hatanodai, Shinagawa-ku, Tokyo 142-8666, Japan

Yoichi Jin
Department of Orthopaedic Surgery, Ebara Hospital, 4-5-10 Higashiyukigaya, Ota-ku, Tokyo 145-0065, Japan

Andreas Panagopoulos, Konstantinos Pantazis, Ilias Iliopoulos, Ioannis Seferlis and Zinon Kokkalis
Department of Shoulder & Elbow Surgery, Patras University Hospital, Papanikolaou 1, 26504 Patras, Greece

Song Ho Chang, Takumi Matsumoto, Masashi Naito and Sakae Tanaka
Department of Orthopaedic Surgery, Faculty of Medicine,The University of Tokyo, 7-3-1 Hongo, Bunkyo-ku, Tokyo 113-8655, Japan

Bárbara Rosa, Pedro Campos, André Barros, Samir Karmali, Carlos Durão, João Alves da Silva and Nuno Coutinho
Trauma and Orthopaedics Department, Hospital Vila Franca de Xira, 2600 009 Lisbon, Portugal

Esperança Ussene
Department of Pathology, Hospital Vila Franca de Xira, 2600 009 Lisbon, Portugal

George I. Mataliotakis, Nikolaos Bounakis and Enrique Garrido-Stratenwerth
Royal Hospital for Sick Children, Scottish National Spine Deformity Centre, Sciennes Road, Edinburgh EH9 1LF, UK

Tayfun Hakan
The Vocational School of Health Services, Okan University, 34959 Tuzla, Turkey
Neurosurgery Clinic, International Kolan Hospital, Şişli, Istanbul, Turkey

Serkan Gürcan
İstanbul Gelişim University, Avcılar, 34315 İstanbul, Turkey

Bridget Ellsworth
Perelman School of Medicine, University of Pennsylvania, Philadelphia, PA, USA

Atul F. Kamath
Department of Orthopaedic Surgery, Perelman School of Medicine, University of Pennsylvania, Philadelphia, PA, USA

Fernando Diaz Dilernia, Ezequiel E. Zaidenberg, Sebastian Gamsie, Danilo E. R. Taype Zamboni, Guido S. Carabelli, Jorge D. Barla and Carlos F. Sancineto
Institute of Orthopaedics "Carlos E. Ottolenghi" Italian Hospital of Buenos Aires, C1199ACK Buenos Aires, Argentina

Luca Daniele, Michael Le, Adam Franklin Parr and Lochlin Mark Brown
Department of Orthopaedics, Gold Coast Health Service, Gold Coast University Hospital, 1 Hospital Blvd., Southport, QLD 4215, Australia

Shuhei Ito, Nobuyuki Fujita, Narihito Nagoshi, Mitsuru Yagi, Akio Iwanami, Kota Watanabe, Masaya Nakamura, Morio Matsumoto and Ken Ishii
Department of Orthopaedic Surgery, Keio University School of Medicine, Tokyo, Japan

Naobumi Hosogane
Department of Orthopaedic Surgery, National Defence Medical College, Saitama, Japan

Takashi Tsuji
Department of Orthopaedic Surgery, Fujita Health University School of Medicine, Aichi, Japan

F. Manfreda
1Department of Orthopedics and Traumatology, University of Perugia, Perugia, Italy

G. Rinonapoli and A. Caraffa
Department of Orthopedics and Traumatology, University of Perugia, Perugia, Italy
Division of Orthopedics and Trauma Surgery, Santa Maria della Misericordia Hospital, Perugia, Italy

A. Nardi and P. Antinolfi
Division of Orthopedics and Trauma Surgery, Santa Maria della Misericordia Hospital, Perugia, Italy

Jan Svacina
Department of Orthopaedic Surgery, Bodden-Kliniken Ribnitz-Damgarten GmbH, 18311 Ribnitz Damgarten, Germany

Alejandro Ordas Bayon and Enrique Sandoval
Department of Orthopedic Surgery, Hospital Universitario Severo Ochoa, Avenida de Orellana SN, 28914 Leganés, Spain

María Valencia Mora
Department of Orthopedic Surgery,Hospital Universitario Fundación Jiménez Díaz, Avenida Reyes Católicos 2, 28040 Madrid, Spain

Benjamin K. Buchanan, Jesse P. DeLuca and Kyle P. Lammlein
Primary Care Sports Medicine Department, Fort Belvoir Community Hospital, Fort Belvoir, VA, USA

Patrick Goetti, Nicolas Gallusser and Olivier Borens
Department of Orthopedics and Traumatology, Lausanne University Hospital, rue du Bugnon 46, 1011 Lausanne, Switzerland

TakeshiMorioka and Kiyohisa Ogawa
Department of Orthopedic Surgery, Eiju General Hospital, 2-23-16 Higashi-Ueno, Taito-ku, Tokyo 110-8645, Japan

Masaaki Takahashi
Department of Orthopedic Surgery, National Hospital Organization Tokyo Medical Center, 2-5-1 Higashigaoka, Meguro-ku, Tokyo 152-8902, Japan

Shaul Beyth and Ori Safran
Orthopedic Surgery Department, Hadassah Medical Center, 91120 Jerusalem, Israel

Binbin Wu, Qingquan Lian and Gonghao Zhan
Department of Anesthesiology and Pain Medicine,The Second Affiliated Hospital and Yuying Children's Hospital of Wenzhou Medical University,Wenzhou 325027, China

Shaobo Zhang
Department of Anesthesiology and Pain Medicine, The Hospital of Integrated Traditional and Western Medicine, Taizhou 317500, China

Haibo Yan
Department of Orthopaedics,The First People's Hospital ofWenling, Taizhou 317500, China

Xianfa Lin
Department of Anesthesiology and Pain Medicine,The First People's Hospital ofWenling, Taizhou 317500, China

Kenya Watanabe, Takuma Fukuzawa and Katsuhiro Mitsui
Department of Orthopedics, Nagano Prefectural Suzaka Hospital, Suzaka, Nagano, Japan

Wakyo Sato
Department of Rehabilitation Medicine, Tokyo Metropolitan Tama Medical Center, 2-8-29 Musashidai, Fuchu-Shi, Tokyo 183-8524, Japan

Hiroshi Okazaki
Department of Orthopedic Surgery, Japan Labour Health andWelfare Organization, Kanto Rosai Hospital, 1-1 Kizukisumiyoshi-cho, Nakahara-ku, Kawasaki City, Kanagawa 211-8510, Japan

Takahiro Goto
Department of Musculoskeletal Oncology, Tokyo Metropolitan Cancer and Infectious Diseases Center Komagome Hospital, 3-18-22 Honkomagome, Bunkyo-ku, Tokyo 113-8677, Japan

Claudia R. Libertin
Division of Infectious Diseases, Mayo Clinic Health System (MCHS-W), Waycross, GA, USA
Departments of Pathology and Laboratory Medicine, Mayo Clinic Health System-Waycross,Waycross, GA, USA
Division of Infectious Diseases, Mayo Clinic, Jacksonville, FL, USA

Joy H. Peterson
Departments of Pathology and Laboratory Medicine, Mayo Clinic Health System-Waycross,Waycross, GA, USA

Mark P. Brodersen and Tamara Huff
Department of Orthopedics, Mayo Clinic Health System-Waycross,Waycross, GA, USA
Department of Orthopedic Surgery, Mayo Clinic, Jacksonville, FL, USA

John Macy
Copley Hospital, Morrisville, VT 05661, USA

Nobuaki Tadokoro, Yusuke Kasai, Katsuhito Kiyasu, Motohiro Kawasaki, Ryuichi Takemasa and Masahiko Ikeuchi
Department of Orthopaedic Surgery, Kochi Medical School, Kochi University, Kochi, Japan

Yu Ozaki, Tomonori Baba, Hironori Ochi, Yasuhiro Homma, Taiji Watari, Mikio Matsumoto and Kazuo Kaneko
Department of Orthopedic Surgery, Juntendo University School of Medicine, 2-1-1 Hongo, Bunkyo-ku, Tokyo, Japan

Baris Beytullah Koc, Martijn Schotanus and Pieter Tilman
Department of Orthopedic Surgery, Zuyderland Medical Centre, Dr. H. van der Hoffplein 1, 6162 BG Sittard-Geleen, Netherlands

Bob Jong
Department of Radiology, Zuyderland Medical Centre, Dr. H. van der Hoffplein 1, 6162 BG Sittard-Geleen, Netherlands

William E. Daner, III and Norman D. Boardman, III
Department of Orthopaedic Surgery, Virginia Commonwealth University Health System, Richmond, VA 23298, USA

Yusuf Erdem
Orthopedics and Traumatology Department, Girne Military Hospital, Kyrenia, Cyprus

Zafer Atbasi
Orthopedics and Traumatology Department, Ankara Military Hospital, Ankara, Turkey

Tuluhan Yunus Emre
Orthopedics and Traumatology Department, Memorial Hizmet Hospital, Istanbul, Turkey

Gülis Kavadar
Physical Medicine and Rehabilitation Department, Medicine Hospital, Istanbul, Turkey

Bahtiyar Demiralp
Orthopedics and Traumatology Department, Medipol University Hospital, Istanbul, Turkey

Ali J. Electricwala and Jaffer T. Electricwala
Electricwala Hospital and Clinics, HimalayanHeights, Pune, Maharashtra 411013, India

Alice Wichelhaus, Judith Emmerich, and Thomas Mittlmeier
Department of Trauma, Hand and Reconstructive Surgery, University Faculty of Medicine Rostock, Schillingallee 35, 18057 Rostock, Germany

Ahmad Jabir Rahyussalim, Yoshi Pratama Djaja and Ifran Saleh
Department of Orthopaedic and Traumatology, Faculty of Medicine, Universitas Indonesia, Dr. Cipto Mangunkusumo General Hospital, Jakarta 10320, Indonesia

Ahmad Yanuar Safri
Neurophysiology Division, Neurology Department, Faculty of Medicine, Universitas Indonesia, Dr. Cipto Mangunkusumo General Hospital, Jakarta 10320, Indonesia

Tri Kurniawati
Stem Cell and Tissue Engineering Cluster, MERC Faculty of Medicine, University of Indonesia, Dr. Cipto Mangunkusumo Hospital, Jakarta, Indonesia

Walid Osman, Thabet Mouelhi and Nader Nawar
Department of Orthopedic Surgery, MES Medical College, Sahloul University Hospital, 4051 Sousse, Tunisia

Meriem Braiki
MES Medical College, Sahloul University Hospital, 4051 Sousse, Tunisia

Zeineb Alaya
Department of Rheumatology, MES Medical College, University Farhat Hached Hospital, 4051 Sousse, Tunisia

Mohamed Ben Ayeche
Department of Orthopedics, MES Medical College, Sahloul University Hospital, 4051 Sousse, Tunisia

Tomoya Takasago, Tomohiro Goto, KeizoWada, Daisuke Hamada, Toshiyuki Iwame, Tetsuya Matsuura, Akihiro Nagamachi and Koichi Sairyo
Department of Orthopedics, Institute of Biomedical Sciences, Tokushima University Graduate School, Tokushima, Japan

Christopher Hein, Barry Watkins and Lee M. Zuckerman
Department of Orthopaedic Surgery, Loma LindaUniversityMedical Center, 11406 Loma LindaDrive,
Suite 218, Loma Linda, CA 92354, USA

Stéphane Pelet
Centre de Recherche FRSQ du CHU de Québec, Hôpital de l'Enfant-Jésus, 1401 18ème rue, Ville de Québec, QC, Canada G1J 1Z4
Department of Orthopedic Surgery, CHU de Québec, Hôpital de l'Enfant-Jésus, 1401 18ème rue, Ville de Québec, QC, Canada G1J 1Z4

Mathieu Hébert, Amerigo Balatri and Pierre-Alexandre LeBlanc
Department of Orthopedic Surgery, CHU de Québec, Hôpital de l'Enfant-Jésus, 1401 18ème rue, Ville de Québec, QC, Canada G1J 1Z4

Shigeo Ueda, Nobuhiro Sasaki, Miyuki Fukuda and Minoru Hoshimaru
Shin-Aikai Spine Center, Katano Hospital, Katano City, Osaka, Japan

Shakti A. Goel, Hitesh N. Modi and Yatin J. Desai
Department of Orthopaedics and Spine Surgery, Zydus Hospitals and Healthcare Research Pvt. Ltd.,Thaltej, Ahmedabad, Gujarat, India

Harshal P. Thaker
Dr. HarshalThaker's Clinic, Ambawadi, Ahmedabad, Gujarat, India

G. Gazzotti, S. Dall'Aglio and E. Sabetta
Unit of Orthopedic Surgery, IRCCS-Arcispedale Santa Maria Nuova, Reggio Emilia, Italy

L. Patrizio
Unit of Orthopedic Surgery, Ospedale Santa Maria dello Splendore, Giulianova, Teramo, Italy

Yasuaki Okada, Sachiyuki Tsukada, Masayoshi Saito and Atsushi Tasaki
Department of Orthopaedic Surgery, St. Luke's International Hospital, 9-1 Akashi-cho, Chuo-ku, Tokyo 104-8560, Japan

Daniel Howard Wiznia,MikeWang, Chang Yeon-Kim, Paul Tomaszewski and Michael P. Leslie
Department of Orthopaedics and Rehabilitation, Yale University School of Medicine, 800 Howard Avenue, New Haven, CT 06510, USA

Heather A. Cole
Department of Orthopaedics and Rehabilitation, Vanderbilt University Medical Center, 4202 Doctors' Office Tower, 2200 Children'sWay, Nashville, TN 37232-9565, USA

Hernan Correa
Department of Pathology, Vanderbilt University Medical Center, 4202 Doctors' Office Tower, 2200 Children'sWay, Nashville, TN 37232-9565, USA

Jonathan G. Schoenecker
Department of Orthopaedics and Rehabilitation, Vanderbilt University Medical Center, 4202 Doctors' Office Tower, 2200 Children'sWay, Nashville, TN 37232-9565, USA Department of Pathology, Vanderbilt University Medical Center, 4202 Doctors' Office Tower, 2200 Children'sWay, Nashville, TN 37232-9565, USA Department of Pediatrics, Vanderbilt University Medical Center, 4202 Doctors' Office Tower, 2200 Children'sWay, Nashville, TN 37232-9565, USA Vanderbilt Center for Bone Biology, Vanderbilt University Medical Center, 4202 Doctors' Office Tower, 2200 Children'sWay, Nashville, TN 37232-9565, USA Department of Pharmacology, Vanderbilt University Medical Center, 4202 Doctors' Office Tower, 2200 Children'sWay, Nashville, TN 37232-9565, USA

Index